Introduction to
Nutrition and
Metabolism

Fifth Edition

David A. Bender

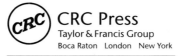

CRC Press
Taylor & Francis Group
Boca Raton   London   New York

CRC Press is an imprint of the
Taylor & Francis Group, an **informa** business

CRC Press
Taylor & Francis Group
6000 Broken Sound Parkway NW, Suite 300
Boca Raton, FL 33487-2742

© 2014 by David A. Bender
CRC Press is an imprint of Taylor & Francis Group, an Informa business

No claim to original U.S. Government works

Printed on acid-free paper
Version Date: 20140124

Printed and bound in India by Replika Press Pvt. Ltd.

International Standard Book Number-13: 978-1-4665-7224-9 (Paperback)

Visit the Taylor & Francis Web site at
http://www.taylorandfrancis.com

and the CRC Press Web site at
http://www.crcpress.com

Contents

v

List of figures

List of tables

Preface

The food we eat has a major effect on our physical health and psychological well-being. An understanding of the way in which nutrients are metabolised, and hence of the principles of biochemistry, is essential for an understanding of the scientific basis of what we would call a prudent or healthy diet.

My aim in the following pages is both to explain the conclusions of the many expert committees that have deliberated on the problems of nutritional requirements, diet, and health over the years and also the scientific basis on which these experts have reached their conclusions. Much of what is now presented as "facts" may well be shown to be incorrect in years to come. This book is intended to provide a foundation of scientific knowledge and understanding from which to interpret and evaluate future advances in nutrition and health sciences.

Nutrition is one of the basic sciences that underlie a proper understanding of health and medical and human sciences and the ways in which human beings and their environment interact. In its turn, the science of nutrition is based on biochemistry and physiology on one hand and the social and behavioural sciences on the other. This book contains such biochemistry as is essential to an understanding of the science of nutrition.

In a book of this kind, which is an introduction to nutrition and metabolism, it is not appropriate to cite the original scientific literature that provides the (sometimes conflicting) evidence for the statements made; in some of the tables of data, I have acknowledged my sources of data as a simple courtesy to my follow scientists and also to guide readers to the original sources of information.

I am grateful to those of my students whose perceptive questions have helped me to formulate and clarify my thoughts and especially those who responded to my enquiry as to what they would like to see (for the benefit of future generations of students) in this new edition. At their request, but somewhat against my better judgement, I have included a list of key points at the end of each chapter—against my better judgement because I think that it is the student's task to summarise the key points from reading.

This book is dedicated to those who will use it as a part of their studies, in the hope that they will be able, in their turn, to advance the frontiers of knowledge, and help their clients, patients, and students to understand the basis of the advice they offer.

David A. Bender

Additional resources on the CD

As a student who has bought a copy of *Introduction to Nutrition and Metabolism, 5th edition*, or borrowed it from a library, you are permitted to make a copy of the CD onto the hard drive of your computer—if you have more than one computer, you may make copies on all of them, but only for your own private study. If you are sharing a copy of the book with a fellow student then you may also allow him/her to make a copy on his/her computer for private study. (You would probably do so anyway, and I could not stop you!)

As a teacher, instructor, or tutor, you are welcome to use part or all of the PowerPoint presentations in your lectures, but I ask that you acknowledge the source and my intellectual property rights. This also applies if you make your PowerPoint presentations available to your students online. You may make all or part of the contents of the CD available *to your students only* on a password-protected network that cannot be accessed by people from outside your institution.

You are welcome to edit the html files as you see fit for your teaching, provided that it is clear where you have done so, and that my copyright is acknowledged and respected. You are welcome to edit the question banks for the *testme* self-assessment program and to add foods to the database for the *food composition* program. There are instructions for this with links from the file licence.htm in the Notes folder.

How to use the CD

The CD contains a number of additional resources to supplement each chapter. All of these can be run directly from the CD, but it is better to copy the files onto a hard disc. You will need to copy all the files in the folder *support*, since these are needed to run the simulation programs in the Virtual Laboratory and the Food Composition program.

To access the resources on the CD you will require an IBM-compatible PC running Windows®, with a minimum screen resolution of 1024×768 pixels for the programs; the PowerPoint presentations, animations, and html files are not dependent on screen resolution. Users of Apple Mac® computers will have to install Windows® emulation software to run the programs but should be able to view the PowerPoint presentations and html files without.

All of the resources on the CD can be accessed with links from the welcome file, although you may wish to set up short cuts to specific sections. If the program on the CD does not autostart when you insert the disc in your CD drive, run the program *welcome. htm*.

What is on the CD

A review of simple chemistry

The file 'Chemistry' on the CD provides a very elementary review of the chemistry you may need to know to understand some aspects of this book. It is an Adobe Acrobat (.pdf) file, and there is a link to download the Acrobat reader in the welcome file.

PowerPoint presentations

There is a PowerPoint® presentation to accompany each chapter as well as one that provides a tour of the cell. In most cases, the slides build with simple animations as you click the mouse or press the spacebar. If you have Microsoft PowerPoint® installed on your computer, then you can view these presentations immediately. If not, the Microsoft PowerPoint viewer is on the CD and can be installed by running the program *ppviewer.exe* from the CD.

Self-assessment quizzes

For each chapter, there is a computer-based self-assessment quiz on the CD. This consists of a series of statements to be marked true or false; you assess your confidence in your answer and gain marks for being correct or lose marks for being incorrect, scaled according to your confidence in your answer. These quizzes are accessed from the welcome screen or from the program *testme.exe* on the CD.

The virtual laboratory

There are a number of simulations of laboratory experiments on the CD; they can be accessed from the welcome file or by going directly to *simulations.htm* in the *simulations* folder. There are html screens to explain the theory for each program:

- Energy balance
- Enzyme assay
- Enzyme purification
- Mutations in a peptide
- Nitrogen balance
- Oxygen electrode studies
- Peptide sequence
- Radioimmunoassay of steroid hormones
- Urea synthesis

Food composition

This program permits you to analyse the nutrients in more than 2700 foods and display the results in the format of a 'food facts' or 'nutrition information' label. You can also add each food you analyse to one of four meals and see the summary of each meal in the same format.

When you start the program, you are offered the choice of using the U.S./Canadian Daily Value (DV) figures or the EU labeling RDA (RDA), and only this value will be used for onscreen display with the nutrient analysis. However, when you print out the results, both %DV and %RDA are shown.

chapter one

Why eat?

An adult eats about a tonne of food a year. This book attempts to answer the question 'why?' by exploring the need for food and the uses to which that food is put in the body. Some discussion of chemistry and biochemistry is obviously essential to understand the fate of food in the body and why there is a continual need for food throughout life. Therefore, in the following chapters, various aspects of biochemistry and metabolism will be discussed. This should provide not only the basis of our present understanding, knowledge, and concepts in nutrition, but also, more importantly, a basis from which to interpret future research findings and evaluate new ideas and hypotheses as they are formulated.

We eat because we are hungry. Why have we evolved complex physiological and psychological mechanisms to control not only hunger and satiety but also our appetite for different types of food? Why do meals form such an important part of our life?

Objectives

After reading this chapter you should be able to

- Describe the need for water and fluid balance
- Describe the need for metabolic fuels and, in outline, the relationship between food intake, energy expenditure, and body weight
- Describe in outline the importance of an appropriate intake of dietary fat
- Describe the mechanisms involved in short- and long-term control of food intake
- Describe the mechanisms involved in the sense of taste
- Explain the various factors that influence peoples' choices of foods
- Describe disorders of appetite: anorexia and bulimia

1.1   The need for water

The body's first need is for water. The human body contains about 60% water—a total of 42 L in a 70-kg person. Water is excreted in the urine as a way of ridding the body of the end products of metabolism, and obviously, there is a need for an intake of water to balance the losses from the body. It is possible to survive for several weeks without any food, using body reserves of fat and protein, but without water, death from dehydration occurs within a few days.

Average daily output of urine is often said to be 1.5 L (although the figures in Table 1.1 show that this is an overestimate), and advertisements for bottled water suggest that we should drink at least this much water per day. At first glance, it might seem obvious that we would need an intake of the same amount of fluid to replace the loss in urine. However, as shown in the table, total daily fluid output from the body is about 3 L for an adult man and about 2.1 L for a woman; urine accounts for less than half of this. Equally, fluid consumption in beverages accounts for only about two thirds of total fluid intake.

Table 1.1 Daily Fluid Balance

		Adult man mL/day	% of total	Adult woman mL/day	% of total
Intake	Fluids	1950	65	1400	67
	Water in food	700	23	450	21
	Metabolic water	350	12	250	12
	Total	3000		2100	
Output	Urine	1400	47	1000	48
	Sweat	650	22	420	20
	Exhaled air	320	11	320	15
	Insensible losses through the skin	530	17	270	13
	Water in faeces	100	3	90	4
	Total	3000		2100	

In addition to the obvious water in beverages, food provides a significant amount of water; around 22% of total intake, and more if you eat the recommended five servings of fruit and vegetables per day (Section 6.3). Most fruits and vegetables contain 60%–90% water.

A further source of water is metabolic water—the water produced when fats, carbohydrates, and proteins are oxidised to yield energy. This accounts for about 12% of total water 'intake', and more on a high fat diet, or when metabolising fat reserves. The camel is able to survive for a considerable time in desert conditions without drinking because it metabolises the fat stored in its hump; the water produced in fat oxidation meets its needs.

Urine accounts for less than half the total fluid output from the body; as shown in Table 1.1, the remainder is made up of sweat, water in exhaled air, so-called insensible losses through the skin (this is distinct from the loss in sweat produced by sweat glands), and a relatively small amount in faeces. The last will also increase on a diet rich in fruit and vegetables because of their content of dietary fibre—part of the beneficial effect of a high-fibre diet (Section 6.3.3.2) is that the fibre retains water in the intestinal tract, thus softening the faeces.

Sweat losses obviously depend on the temperature and physical activity, and we do indeed need to drink more in a hot environment or after strenuous exercise. Losses in exhaled air, faeces, and other insensible losses are relatively constant; urine output varies widely, depending on how much fluid has been consumed. Although average urine volume is between 1 and 1.4 L/day, this reflects average fluid intake; the output of urine required to ensure adequate excretion of waste material and maintain fluid balance without becoming dehydrated is no more than about 500 mL. Put simply, the more you drink, the more urine you will produce.

A final problem is whether water is the most appropriate liquid to drink to balance large losses in sweat after vigorous exercise or in a hot climate. The answer is probably not—sweating involves loss of mineral salts as well as water, and these losses have to be made good. Various sports drinks contain balanced mixtures of mineral salts in the same proportions as they are lost in sweat, together, usually, with glucose or another carbohydrate as a source of metabolic fuel. Milk and fruit juices also provide mineral salts.

1.2   The need for energy

There is an obvious need for energy to perform physical work. Work has to be done to lift a load against the force of gravity, and there must be a source of energy to perform that work. The energy used in various activities can be measured (Section 5.1.3.2), as can the metabolic energy yield of the foods that provide the fuel for that work (Section 1.3). This means that it is possible to calculate a balance between the intake of energy, as metabolic fuels, and the body's energy expenditure. Obviously, energy intake has to be appropriate for the level of energy expenditure; as discussed in Chapters 7 and 8, neither excess intake nor a deficiency is desirable.

Figure 1.1 shows the relationship between food intake, physical work, and changes in body reserves of metabolic fuels, as shown by changes in body weight. This was a study in Germany at the end of the second world war, when there was a great deal of rubble from bomb damaged buildings to be cleared, and a large number of people to be fed and found employment. Increasing food intake resulted in an increase in work output—initially with an increase in body weight, indicating that the food supply was greater than was required to meet the (increased) work output. When a financial reward was offered as well, the work output increased to such an extent that people now drew on their (sparse) reserves, and there was a loss of body weight.

Quite apart from obvious work output, the body has a considerable requirement for energy, even at rest. Only about one third of the average person's energy expenditure is for voluntary work (Section 5.1.3). Two thirds is required for maintenance of the body's functions, homeostasis of the internal environment, and metabolic integrity. This energy requirement at rest, the basal metabolic rate (BMR, Section 5.1.3.1) can be measured by the output of heat, or the consumption of oxygen, when the subject is completely at rest. Figure 1.2 shows the proportion of this resting energy expenditure that is accounted for by different organs.

Part of this basal energy requirement is obvious—the heart beats to circulate the blood; breathing continues, and there is considerable electrical activity in nerves and muscles, whether they are 'working' or not. The brain and nervous system comprise only about 2% of body weight, but consume some 20% of resting energy expenditure, because of the

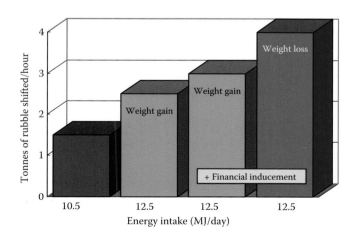

Figure 1.1 The relationship between food intake, work output, and body weight. (From Widdowson, E.M., MRC Special Report Series No. 275, London, HMSO, 1951.)

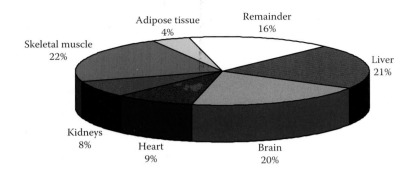

Figure 1.2 Percentage of resting energy expenditure by different organs of the body.

active transport of ions across nerve membranes to maintain electrical activity (Section 3.2.2). This requires a metabolic energy source. Less obviously, there is also a requirement for energy for the wide variety of biochemical reactions occurring all the time in the body: laying down reserves of fat and carbohydrate (Sections 5.6.1 and 5.6.3); turnover of tissue proteins (Section 9.2.3.3); transport of substrates into, and products out of, cells (Section 3.2.2); and the synthesis and secretion of hormones and neurotransmitters.

1.2.1   Units of energy

Energy expenditure is measured by the output of heat from the body (Section 5.1). The unit of heat used in the early studies was the calorie—the amount of heat required to raise the temperature of 1 g of water by 1°C. The calorie is still used to some extent in nutrition; in biological systems, the kilocalorie, kcal (sometimes written as 'Calorie', i.e., with a capital C) is used. One kilocalorie is 1000 calories (10^3 cal), and hence, the amount of heat required to raise the temperature of 1 kg of water by 1°C.

Correctly, the joule is used as the unit of energy. The joule is an SI unit, named after James Prescott Joule (1818–1889), who first showed the equivalence of heat, mechanical work, and other forms of energy. In biological systems, the kilojoule (kJ, = 10^3 J) and megajoule (MJ, = 10^6 J) are used.

To convert between calories and joules:

$$1 \text{ kcal} = 4.186 \text{ kJ (normally rounded off to 4.2 kJ)}$$

$$1 \text{ kJ} = 0.239 \text{ kcal (normally rounded off to 0.24 kcal)}$$

The average total daily energy expenditure of adults is between 7.5 and 10 MJ for women and between 8 and 12 MJ for men.

1.3   Metabolic fuels

The dietary sources of metabolic energy (the metabolic fuels) are carbohydrates, fats, protein, and alcohol. The metabolism of these fuels results in the production of carbon dioxide and water (and also urea in the case of proteins, Section 9.3.1.4). They can be converted to the same end products chemically by burning in air. Although the process of metabolism in the body is more complex, it is a fundamental law of chemistry that if the starting

Table 1.2 The Energy Yield of Metabolic Fuels

	kcal/g	kJ/g
Carbohydrate	4	17
Protein	4	16
Fat	9	37
Alcohol	7	29

Note: 1 kcal = 4.186 kJ or 1 kJ = 0.239 kcal.

material and end products are the same, the energy yield is the same, regardless of the route taken. Therefore, the energy yield of foodstuffs can be determined by measuring the heat produced when they are burnt in air, making allowance for the extent to which they are digested and absorbed from foods. The physiological energy yields of the metabolic fuels in the body, allowing for digestion and absorption, are shown in Table 1.2.

1.3.1 *The need for carbohydrate and fat*

Although there is a requirement for energy sources in the diet, it does not matter unduly how that requirement is met. There is no requirement for a dietary source of carbohydrate; the body can synthesise carbohydrates from amino acids derived from proteins (the pathways of gluconeogenesis, Section 9.3.2). However, there is an average requirement of about 100 g of carbohydrate per day to maintain a normal blood glucose concentration to provide for brain and red blood cell metabolism without the need for gluconeogenesis from amino acids. This is less than 2% of total energy intake; as discussed in Section 6.3.3, a desirable level of carbohydrate intake is 50%–55% of energy. An intake of 50 g of carbohydrate per day is adequate to prevent the development of ketosis (Section 5.5.3), whilst very low carbohydrate diets for weight reduction (Section 7.3.4.4) that provide less than 20 g of carbohydrate per day are associated with significant ketosis.

Similarly, there is no requirement for a dietary source of fat, apart from the essential fatty acids (Sections 4.3.1.1 and 5.6.1.1), and there is certainly no requirement for a dietary source of alcohol. Diets that provide more than about 35%–40% of energy from fat are associated with increased risk of heart disease and some cancers (Section 6.3.2), and there is some evidence that diets that provide more than about 20% of energy from protein are also associated with chronic diseases. Therefore, the general consensus is that diets should provide about 55% of energy from carbohydrates, 30% from fat, and 15% from protein (Section 6.3).

Although there is no requirement for fat in the diet, fats are nutritionally important, and there is a specific mechanism for detecting the taste of fats in foods (Section 1.4.3.1).

- It is difficult to eat enough of a very low-fat diet to meet energy requirements. As shown in Table 1.2, the energy yield per gram of fat is more than twice that of carbohydrate or protein. The problem in many less developed countries, where undernutrition is a problem (Chapter 8), is that diets provide only 10%–15% of energy from fat, and it is difficult to consume a sufficient bulk of food to meet energy requirements. By contrast, the problem in Western countries is an undesirably high intake of fat, contributing to the development of obesity (Chapter 7) and chronic diseases (Section 6.3.2).
- Four of the vitamins, A, D, E, and K (Chapter 11) are fat-soluble, and are found in fatty and oily foods. They are absorbed dissolved in fat; thus, with a very low-fat diet, the absorption of these vitamins may be inadequate to meet requirements, even if the diet provides an adequate amount.

- There is a requirement for small amounts of two essential fatty acids (Sections 4.3.1.1 and 5.6.1.1) that cannot be synthesised in the body but must be provided in the diet.
- In many foods, a great deal of the flavour (and hence the pleasure of eating) is carried in the fat.
- Fat lubricates food and makes it easier to chew and swallow.

1.3.2   The need for protein

Unlike fats and carbohydrates, there is a requirement for protein in the diet. In a growing child, this need is obvious. As the child grows, the size of its body increases; thus, there is an increase in the total amount of protein in the body.

Adults also require protein in the diet (Section 9.1.2). There is a continual loss of protein from the body, for example, in hair, shed skin cells, enzymes and other proteins secreted into the gut and not completely digested. More importantly, there is turnover of tissue proteins, which are continually being broken down and replaced. Although there is no change in the total amount of protein in the body, an adult with an inadequate intake of protein will be unable to replace this loss, and will lose tissue protein.

1.3.3   The need for micronutrients—minerals and vitamins

In addition to metabolic fuels and protein, the body has a requirement for a variety of mineral salts. If a metal or ion has a function in the body, it must be provided by the diet, since the different chemical elements cannot be interconverted. Again, the need is obvious for a growing child; as the body grows, the total amounts of minerals in the body will likewise increase. In adults, there is a turnover of minerals in the body, and losses must be replaced from the diet (Section 11.15).

There is a requirement for a different group of nutrients, in small amounts—the vitamins. These are organic compounds that have a variety of functions. They cannot be synthesised in the body, and so must be provided by the diet. There is metabolic turnover of the vitamins; thus, there must be replacement of losses (Chapter 11).

Other compounds in the diet (especially from fruit and vegetables) are not considered to be nutrients, since they are not dietary essentials, but they may have beneficial effects in reducing the risk of developing a variety of chronic diseases (Section 6.7).

1.4   Hunger and appetite

Human beings have evolved an elaborate system of complex, overlapping, and sometimes apparently redundant, physiological mechanisms to ensure that the body's needs for metabolic fuels and nutrients are met and to balance energy expenditure with food intake. The physiological systems for the control of appetite interact with psychological, social, environmental, and genetic factors, all of which have to be understood to gain a full explanation of eating behaviour.

1.4.1   Hunger and satiety—short-term control of feeding

Early studies showed that there are hunger centres in the brain that stimulate us to begin eating and satiety centres that signal us to stop eating when hunger has been satisfied. The hunger centres are in the lateral hypothalamus, and the satiety centres in the ventromedial

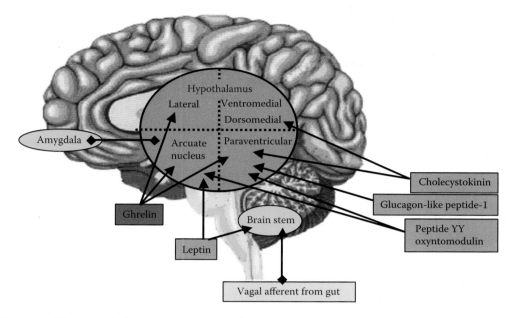

Figure 1.3 The hypothalamic appetite control centres and sites of action of hormones secreted by the gastrointestinal tract.

hypothalamus (see Figure 1.3). In experimental animals, destruction of the hunger centres leads to anorexia—complete loss of appetite, whilst electrical stimulation leads to feeding even if the animal has eaten enough. Similarly, destruction of the satiety centres leads to more frequent, uncontrolled eating (hyperphagia), and electrical stimulation leads to cessation of feeding, even in a physiologically hungry animal.

Other hypothalamic centres are also involved, and destruction of the paraventricular and arcuate nuclei of the hypothalamus also leads to hyperphagia and obesity. The arcuate nucleus responds to hormones and other signals and integrates signalling to the hunger and satiety centres. The hunger centres act through neurons that use neuropeptide Y and the agouti-related protein as their transmitters; the satiety centres act through neurons that use two other peptides: proopiomelanocortin (POMC) and the so-called cocaine- and amphetamine-regulated transcript (CART). The satiety centres to reduce feeding act primarily by reducing the activity of neurons arising from the hunger centres.

The hunger and satiety centres in the hypothalamus have neuronal connections to the temporal lobe of the amygdala, the nucleus accumbens, the brainstem, and higher brain centres, including the cortex. The amydala controls learned food behaviour—i.e., how you know that something is a food, as opposed to non-food. A young child will put almost anything into its mouth and gradually learns what is, and what is not, food. The nucleus accumbens is part of the reward system of the brain, and is concerned with the hedonistic value of food—the pleasure of eating. The brainstem receives direct input via the vagus nerve from the gastrointestinal tract and the liver, signalling the presence of food in the gut and the arrival of nutrients to the liver. The connections to the cortex and other higher brain centres mean that psychological factors (including individual likes and dislikes, Section 1.4.4) can override physiological control of appetite.

The hypothalamic centres control food intake remarkably precisely. Without conscious effort, most people regulate their food intake to match energy expenditure very closely—they neither waste away from lack of metabolic fuel for physical activity nor lay down excessively large reserves of fat. Even people who have excessive reserves of body fat and can be considered to be so overweight or obese as to be putting their health at risk (Section 7.2.2) balance their energy intake and expenditure relatively well considering that the average intake is a tonne of food a year, whilst very severely obese people weigh about 250–300 kg (compared with average weights between 60 and 100 kg), and it takes many years to achieve such a weight. A gain or loss of 5 kg body weight over 6 months would require only a 1% daily mismatch between food intake and energy expenditure (Section 5.2).

A number of drugs can modify responses to hunger and satiety and can be used to reduce appetite in the treatment of obesity (Section 7.3.4.11) or stimulate it in people with loss of appetite or anorexia. The synthesis and release of neuropeptide Y are dependent on zinc, and the loss of appetite associated with zinc deficiency is a result of impaired secretion of this neurotransmitter.

In addition to direct neuronal input from the gastrointestinal tract and liver, a variety of factors act on the hunger and satiety centres to initiate nerve impulses, including

- The relative concentrations of the hormones insulin (secreted by the pancreas in response to increased blood concentrations of glucose and amino acids, Section 5.3.1) and glucagon (secreted by the pancreas in response to a decreased concentration of blood glucose, Section 5.3.2).
- The relative concentrations of glucose, triacylglycerols, non-esterified fatty acids, and ketone bodies available as metabolic fuels in the fed and fasting states (Section 5.3). The plasma concentrations of metabolic fuels are mainly regulated by three hormones:
  - Insulin stimulates the uptake of glucose into tissues and its intracellular utilisation.
  - Glucagon stimulates the synthesis and release of glucose and non-esterified fatty acids into the circulation, and the synthesis of ketone bodies from non-esterified fatty acids.
  - Amylin, which is secreted by the pancreas together with insulin, regulates the output of metabolic fuels from tissue reserves into the circulation.
- Hormones secreted by the gastrointestinal tract, including ghrelin (secreted mainly by the stomach, Section 1.4.1.2), cholecystokinin, which is secreted by the duodenum and acts mainly to stimulate gall bladder contraction and gastrointestinal tract motility and secretion, glucagon-like peptide, and oxyntomodulin (both derived from the glucagon gene, and secreted by gut endocrine cells) and peptide YY (also secreted by gut endocrine cells, largely in response to the energy yield of a meal). Ghrelin acts to stimulate appetite; the other gut-derived hormones act to suppress it. A peptide derived from the ghrelin gene, obestatin, has anti-ghrelin, appetite-suppressing actions.

1.4.1.1   Nutrient sensing in the hypothalamus

There are neurons in the hypothalamus that respond to glucose; some are excited by it, whilst others are inhibited. In both cases, these neurons contain glucokinase, the high K_m isoenzyme of hexokinase (Section 5.3.1), and in response to a modest increase in the concentration of glucose in the cell, there is a considerable increase in the rate of formation of glucose 6-phosphate and its onward metabolism (Section 5.4), leading to an increase in the ratio of ATP/ADP and the closing of a potassium channel in the cell membrane. POMC neurons, which signal satiety, are excited in response to glucose and increase their rate of firing; neuropeptide Y and agouti-related peptide neurons, which signal hunger, are inhibited in response to glucose, and decrease their rate of firing.

1.4.1.2   *Ghrelin—the appetite-stimulating hormone*

Ghrelin is a small peptide (28 amino acids) that was originally discovered as the hormone that stimulates the secretion of growth hormone, but it also acts to increase the synthesis of both neuropeptide Y (thus increasing hunger—an orexigenic action) and a peptide that antagonises the appetite-suppressing action of POMC. The action of ghrelin in stimulating neuropeptide Y neurons is antagonised by insulin and leptin. The secretion of ghrelin increases before an expected meal, suggesting that as well as responding to emptiness of the stomach, there is also central nervous system regulation of secretion.

In addition to its role in stimulating appetite and suppressing satiety signalling, ghrelin is involved in reinforcing the reward system of the nucleus accumbens in response to food, alcohol, and narcotics, by activating dopaminergic and cholinergic neurons. This means that it has a role in the hedonistic responses to food and motivation to eat as well as stimulating feeding behaviour.

Paradoxically, ghrelin secretion is low in obese people, and increases as weight is lost, suggesting that the state of body reserves of adipose tissue, which is signalled by the hormone leptin (Section 1.4.2), may affect ghrelin secretion. This may explain why it is relatively difficult to lose excess weight and maintain a reduced body weight. A short-term weight loss leads to a long-term increase in ghrelin secretion and decrease in peptide YY secretion; thus, even after the lost weight has been regained, there will be increased hunger signalling and decreased satiety signalling. Ghrelin secretion is paradoxically high in anorexia nervosa (Section 1.4.5), suggesting decreased sensitivity of the ghrelin receptor, and some studies have shown that the administration of ghrelin leads to increased food intake in anorexia. The Prader–Willi syndrome involves a voracious appetite and the development of severe obesity; here the problem is indeed excessive secretion of ghrelin.

The main site of ghrelin secretion is the stomach; it is synthesised in, and secreted by, entero-endocrine cells in the gastric fundus—the upper part of the stomach. This is the region that is removed in the surgical procedure of banded gastroplasty for treatment of severe morbid obesity (Section 7.3.4.12), and part of the success of surgery may be due to reduced secretion of ghrelin as well as the physical effect of reduced stomach capacity. Ghrelin is also secreted by ε-cells of the pancreas and, to some extent, the small intestine.

Ghrelin undergoes postsynthetic modification by acetylation. Unacetylated ghrelin is inactive, and inhibitors of ghrelin *O*-acetyltransferase are potential drugs for control of hunger and treatment of obesity (Section 7.3.4.11).

1.4.2   *Long-term control of food intake and energy expenditure—the hormone leptin*

In addition to the immediate control of feeding by sensations of hunger and satiety, there is long-term regulation of food intake and energy expenditure, in response to the size of the body's fat reserves. This is largely a function of the peptide hormone leptin, which is secreted by adipose tissue. It was discovered as the normal product of the gene that is defective in the homozygous recessive mutant (*ob/ob*) obese mouse; administration of the peptide to the obese mice caused them to lose weight. Further studies showed that the administration of leptin to the genetically obese diabetic (*db/db*) mouse had no effect on body weight, and indeed they secreted a normal or greater than normal amount of leptin. The defect in these animals is in the receptor for leptin in the hypothalamus.

The circulating concentration of leptin is determined largely by the mass of adipose tissue in the body, and leptin signals the size of body fat reserves. Low levels of leptin, reflecting adipose tissue reserves that are inadequate to permit a normal pregnancy, not only increase food intake, but also lead to cessation of ovulation and menstruation (by decreasing the secretion of gonadotrophin-releasing hormone); a loss of weight to below about 45 kg is associated with amenorrhoea. In undernourished children, low levels of leptin, reflecting levels of adipose tissue reserves that are inadequate to permit growth, reduce skeletal growth by inhibiting the secretion of growth hormone.

There is reduced food intake in response to leptin, associated with a decrease in the synthesis of neuropeptide Y (the transmitter for neurons from the hunger centres of the hypothalamus) and increased synthesis of POMC (the transmitter for neurons from the satiety centres). However, the resultant weight loss is greater than can be accounted for by reduced food intake alone, and in response to leptin there is a specific loss of adipose tissue, whilst in response to reduced food intake, there is a loss of both adipose and lean tissue. Leptin receptors are found in a variety of tissues, including muscle and adipose tissue itself. In addition to its role in appetite control, leptin acts to increase energy expenditure and promote the loss of adipose tissue by several mechanisms, including

- Increased expression of uncoupling proteins (Section 3.3.1.5) in adipose tissue and muscle. This results in relatively uncontrolled oxidation of metabolic fuel, unrelated to requirements for physical and chemical work, and increased heat output from the body (thermogenesis).
- Increased activity of lipase in adipose tissue (Section 5.3.2), resulting in the breakdown of triacylglycerol reserves and release of non-esterified fatty acids that may either be oxidised or be re-esterified in the liver and transported back to adipose tissue. This is metabolically inefficient because of the energy cost of synthesising triacylglycerol from fatty acids (Section 5.6.1.2); such cycling of lipids is one of the factors involved in the weight loss associated with advanced cancer (Section 8.4).
- Decreased expression of acetyl CoA carboxylase in adipose tissue (Section 5.6.1)—this results in both decreased synthesis and increased oxidation of fatty acids, as a result of decreased formation of malonyl CoA (Sections 5.6.1 and 10.5.2).
- Increased apoptosis (programmed cell death) in adipose tissue, thus reducing the number of adipocytes available for storage of fat in the body.

The result of these actions of leptin on adipose tissue and muscle is that there is an increase in metabolic rate, and hence energy expenditure, in addition to the reduction in food intake.

Although most leptin is secreted by adipose tissue, it is also secreted by muscle and the gastric mucosa. After a meal, there is an increase in circulating leptin, suggesting that as well as its role in long-term control of food intake and energy expenditure, it may also be important in short-term responses to food intake. Some of this leptin comes from the gastric mucosa, but in response to food intake, insulin stimulates the synthesis and secretion of leptin from adipose tissue. Conversely, leptin increases the synthesis and secretion of insulin, but also antagonises its actions; thus, excessively high levels of leptin, associated with obesity, lead to hyperinsulinaemia and insulin resistance—part of the metabolic syndrome associated with obesity (Section 7.2.3).

There is a circadian variation in leptin secretion, with an increase during the night. This is in response to glucocorticoid hormones, which are secreted in increased amount during the night. It is likely that the loss of appetite and weight loss associated with chronic stress, when there is increased secretion of glucocorticoids, is mediated by the effect of these hormones on leptin synthesis and secretion.

When leptin was first discovered, there was great excitement that, as in the obese mouse, human obesity (Chapter 7) might be due to a failure of leptin synthesis or secretion and that administration of leptin might be a useful treatment for severe obesity. However, most obese people secrete more leptin than lean people (because they have more adipose tissue), and it is likely that the problem is not due to lack of leptin, but rather to a loss of sensitivity of the leptin receptors. Only a very small number of people have been found in whom genetically determined obesity is due to a mutation in the gene for leptin, the leptin receptor, or a component of the downstream signalling pathway.

1.4.3   Appetite

In addition to hunger and satiety, which are basic physiological responses, food intake is controlled by appetite, which is related not only to physiological need but also to the pleasure of eating—flavour, texture, and a variety of social and psychological factors. The phenomenon of sensory-specific satiety, when there is satiety toward one food, but others may still be tempting, is the result of stimulation of individual neurons that respond to different combinations of taste, flavour, aroma, texture, and the sight of food.

1.4.3.1   Taste and flavour

Taste buds on the tongue can distinguish five basic tastes: salt, savoury, sweet, bitter, and sour as well as a less well understood ability to taste fat. The ability to taste salt, sweetness, savouriness, and fat permits detection of nutrients; the ability to taste sourness and bitterness permits avoidance of toxins in foods. There is some evidence that hormones such as leptin (Section 1.4.2) and ghrelin (Section 1.4.1.2) may affect the sensitivity of sweetness taste buds and possibly others as well. In addition, there is sensitivity, not due to taste buds, to chemical irritants such as the tingle of carbon dioxide in carbonated beverages, the cooling effect of menthol, and the burning and pungency of peppers and spices.

Altogether, there are some 6000 taste buds on the tongue and soft palate. Each one contains 30–50 sensory cells with microvilli, but not all sensory cells are exposed at the same time; thus, there is scope to alter the sensitivity to different tastes by changing the number of sensory cells exposed as well as by modification of the intracellular responses to stimulation of the receptors on the microvilli or transported ions.

Salt (correctly the mineral sodium) is essential to life, and wild animals will travel great distances to a salt lick. Like other animals, human beings have evolved a pleasurable response to salty flavours—this ensures that physiological needs are met. There is evidence that sensitivity to salt changes in response to the state of sodium balance in the body, with an increased number of active salt receptors on the tongue at times of sodium depletion. However, there is no shortage of salt in developed countries; indeed, average intakes of salt are considerably greater than requirements, and pose a hazard to health (Section 6.3.4).

The sensation of savouriness is distinct from that of saltiness and is sometimes called *umami* (the Japanese for savoury). It is largely due to the presence of free amino acids in foods, and permits detection of protein-rich foods. Stimulation of the umami receptors of the tongue is the basis of flavour enhancers such as monosodium glutamate, an important constituent of traditional oriental condiments that is widely used in manufactured foods.

The other instinctively pleasurable taste is sweetness, which permits detection of carbohydrates, and hence energy sources. Whilst it is only sugars (Section 4.2.1) and artificial sweeteners (Section 7.3.4.9) that have a sweet taste, human beings (and a few other animals) secrete the enzyme amylase in saliva, which catalyses the hydrolysis of starch, the major dietary carbohydrate, to sweet-tasting sugars whilst the food is being chewed (Section 4.2.2.1).

The tongue is not sensitive to the taste of triacylglycerols, but rather to free fatty acids, and especially polyunsaturated fatty acids (Section 4.3.1.1). This suggests that the lipase secreted by the tongue has a role in permitting the detection of fatty foods as an energy source, in addition to a very minor role in fat digestion (Section 4.3).

Sourness and bitterness are instinctively unpleasant sensations; many of the toxins that occur in foods have a bitter or sour flavour. Learnt behaviour will overcome the instinctive aversion, but this is a process of learning or acquiring tastes, not an innate or instinctive response.

The receptors for salt, sourness, and savouriness (umami) all act as ion channels, transporting sodium, hydrogen, or glutamate ions, respectively, into the cells of the taste buds.

The receptors for sweetness and bitterness act via cell surface receptors linked to intracellular formation second messengers. There is evidence that both cyclic adenosine monophosphate (cAMP, Section 10.3.2) and inositol trisphosphate (Section 10.3.3) mechanisms are involved, and more than one signal transduction pathway may be involved in the responses to sweetness or bitterness of different compounds. Some compounds may activate more than one subtype of receptor; there are at least 40–80 different cell surface bitterness receptors, all of which are linked to activation of the intracellular protein α-gustducin. Small changes in structure of compounds can affect whether they taste sweet or bitter; L-tryptophan is intensely bitter, whilst its stereoisomer D-tryptophan tastes very sweet.

In addition to the sensations of taste provided by the taste buds on the tongue, a great many flavours can be distinguished by the sense of smell. Some flavours and aromas (fruity flavours, fresh coffee, and, at least to a non-vegetarian, the smell of roasting meat) are pleasurable, tempting people to eat and stimulating appetite. Other flavours and aromas are repulsive, warning us not to eat the food. Again this can be seen as a warning of possible danger—the smell of decaying meat or fish tells us that it is not safe to eat.

Like the acquisition of a taste for bitter or sour foods, a taste for foods with what would seem at first to be an unpleasant aroma or flavour can also be acquired. Here things become more complex—a pleasant smell to one person may be repulsive to another. Some people enjoy the smell of cooked cabbage and Brussels sprouts, whilst others can hardly bear to be in the same room. The durian fruit is a highly prized delicacy in Southeast Asia, yet to the uninitiated, it has the unappetising aroma of sewage or faeces.

1.4.4   Why do people eat what they do?

People have different responses to the same taste or flavour. This may be explained in terms of childhood memories, pleasurable or otherwise. An aversion to the smell of a food may protect someone who has a specific allergy or intolerance (although sometimes people have a craving for the foods of which they are intolerant). Most often, we simply cannot explain why some people dislike foods that others eat with great relish. A number of factors influence why people choose to eat particular foods (Table 1.3).

1.4.4.1   The availability and cost of food

In developed countries, the simple availability of food is not a constraint on choice. There is a wide variety of foods available, and when fruits and vegetables are out of season at home, they are imported; frozen, canned, or dried foods are widespread. By contrast, in developing countries, the availability of food may be a major constraint on what people

Table 1.3 Factors that Influence the Choice of Foods

Availability of foods
Cost of foods
Time for preparation and consumption
Disability and infirmity
Personal likes and dislikes
Intolerance or allergy
Eating alone or in company
Marketing pressure and advertising
Religious and ethical taboos
Perceived or real health benefits and risks
Modified diet for control of disease
Illness or medication

choose. Little food is imported, and what is available will depend on the local soil and climate. In normal times, the choice of foods may be limited, whilst in times of drought, there may be little or no food available at all, and what little is available will be more expensive than what most people can afford. Even in developed countries, the cost of food is important, and for the most disadvantaged members of the community, poverty may impose severe constraints on their choice of foods.

1.4.4.2 Religion, habit, and tradition

Religious and ethical considerations are important in determining the choice of foods. Observant Jews and Muslims will only eat meat from animals that have cloven hooves and chew the cud. The terms *kosher* in Jewish law and *hallal* in Islamic law both mean clean; the meat of other animals, which are scavenging animals, birds of prey, and detritus-feeding fish, is regarded as unclean (*traife* or *haram*). We now know that many of these forbidden animals carry parasites that can infect human beings; thus, these ancient prohibitions are based on food hygiene.

Hindus will not eat beef. The reason for this is that the cow is far too valuable, as a source of milk and dung (as manure and fuel) and as a beast of burden, for it to be killed as a source of meat.

Many people refrain from eating meat as a result of humanitarian concern for the animals involved or because of real or perceived health benefits. Vegetarians can be divided into various groups, according to the strictness of their diet:

- Some avoid red meat, but will eat poultry and fish
- Some specifically avoid beef because of the potential risk of contracting variant Creutzfeld–Jacob disease from bovine spongiform encephalopathy-infected animals
- Pescetarians eat fish, but not meat or poultry
- Ovo-lacto-vegetarians will eat eggs and milk, but not meat or fish
- Lacto-vegetarians will eat milk, but not eggs
- Vegans will eat only plant foods and no foods of animal origin

Foods that are commonly eaten in one area may be little eaten elsewhere, even though they are available, simply because people have not been accustomed to eating them. To a very great extent, eating habits as adults continue the habits learnt as children.

Haggis and oat cakes travel south from Scotland as specialty items; black pudding is a staple of northern British breakfasts, but is rare in the southeast of England. Until the 1960s, yoghurt was almost unknown in Britain, apart from a few health food 'cranks' and immigrants from Eastern Europe; many British children believe that fish comes as rectangular fish fingers, whilst children in inland Spain may eat fish and other seafood three or four times a week. The French mock the British habit of eating lamb with mint sauce—and the average British reaction to such French delicacies as frogs' legs and snails in garlic is one of horror. The British eat their cabbage well boiled; the Germans and Dutch ferment it to produce sauerkraut.

This regional and cultural diversity of foods provides one of the pleasures of travel. As people travel more frequently they become (perhaps grudgingly) more adventurous in their choice of foods; thus, they create a demand for different foods at home, and there is an increasing variety of foods available in shops and restaurants.

A further factor that has increased the range of foods available has been immigration of people from a variety of different backgrounds, all of whom have, as they have become established, introduced their traditional foods to their new homes. It is difficult to realise that, in the 1960s, there was only a handful of tandoori restaurants in the whole of Britain, that pizza was something seen only in southern Italy and a few specialist restaurants, or that Balti cooking, Thai food, and sushi were unknown until the 1990s.

Some people are naturally adventurous and will try a new food just because they have never eaten it before. Others are more conservative and will try a new food only when they see someone else eating it safely and with enjoyment. Others are yet more conservative in their food choices; the most conservative eaters 'know' that they do not like a new food because they have never eaten it before.

1.4.4.3   Organic foods

Many people choose to eat organically produced foods in preference to those produced by conventional or intensive farming methods. Organic foods are plants grown without the use of (synthetic) pesticides, fungicides, or inorganic fertilisers and prepared without the use of preservatives. Foodstuffs must be grown on land that has not been treated with chemical fertilisers, herbicides, or pesticides for at least 3 years. Organic meat is from animals fed on organically grown crops without the use of growth promoters, with only a limited number of medicines to treat disease, and commonly maintained under traditional, non-intensive, or free-range conditions. Within the European Union, foods may be labelled as 'organic' if they contain at least 95% organic ingredients and not more than 0.9% genetically modified ingredients.

People who wish to avoid pesticide, fungicide, and other chemical residues in their food, or genetically modified crops, will choose organic produce. Other people will choose organic foods because they believe they are nutritionally superior to conventional produce or because they have a better flavour. There is little evidence that organic produce is nutritionally superior to that produced by conventional farming, although if organic fruits and vegetables are also slower-growing and possibly lower-yielding varieties, they may have a higher nutrient content. Many of the older, slower-growing, and lower-yielding fruits and vegetables have a better flavour than more recently introduced varieties that are grown for their rapid yield of a large crop of uniform size and shape. Flavour does not depend on whether or not they are grown organically, but many organic farmers do indeed grow traditional, more flavourful varieties.

The nutrient content of the same variety of a fruit or vegetable may vary widely, depending not only on the soil (and any fertilisers used) but also on how much sunlight the plant has received and how frequently it has been watered. The apples from one side of a tree may vary in nutrient content from those on the other side of the same tree. The yield, flavour, and nutrient content of the same crop may vary along the field.

Whilst organic produce is indeed free from chemical residues that may be harmful, there is a potential hazard. Animal manure is used in organic farming to a very much greater extent than in conventional farming, and unless salad vegetables are washed well, there is a potential risk of food poisoning from bacteria in the manure that remains on the produce.

1.4.4.4   *Luxury status of scarce and expensive foods*

Foods that are scarce or expensive have a certain appeal of fashion or style; they are (rightly) regarded as luxuries for special occasions rather than everyday meals. Conversely, foods that are widespread and inexpensive have less appeal.

In the 19th century, salmon and oysters were so cheap that the articles of apprentices in London specified that they should not be given salmon more than three times a week, whilst oysters were eaten by the poor. Through much of the 20th century, salmon was scarce, and a prized luxury food; fish farming has increased the supply of salmon to such an extent that it is again an inexpensive food. Chicken, turkey, guinea fowl, and trout, which were expensive luxury foods in the 1950s, are now widely available, as a result of changes in farming practice, and they form the basis of inexpensive meals. By contrast, fish such as cod, herring, and skate, once the basis of cheap meals, are now becoming scarce and expensive as a result of depletion of fish stocks by overexploitation.

1.4.4.5   *The social functions of food*

Human beings are social animals, and meals are important social functions. People eating in a group are likely to eat better or at least have a wider variety of foods and a more lavish and luxurious meal than people eating alone. Entertaining guests may be an excuse to eat foods that we know to be nutritionally undesirable and perhaps to eat to excess. The greater the variety of dishes offered, the more people are likely to eat. As we reach satiety with one food, so another, different, flavour is offered to stimulate appetite. A number of studies have shown that, faced with only one food, people tend to reach satiety sooner than when a variety of foods is on offer. This is the difference between hunger and appetite—even when we are satiated, we can still 'find room' to try something different.

Conversely, and more importantly, many lonely single people (and especially the bereaved elderly) have little incentive to prepare meals, and no stimulus to appetite. Whilst poverty may be a factor, apathy (and frequently, in the case of widowed men, ignorance) severely limits the range of foods eaten, possibly leading to undernutrition. When these problems are added to the problems of ill-fitting dentures (which make eating painful), arthritis (which makes handling many foods difficult), and the difficulty of carrying food home from the shops, it is not surprising that we include the elderly amongst the vulnerable groups of the population who are at risk of undernutrition (Section 8.3.1).

In hospitals and other institutions, there is a further problem. People who are unwell may have low physical activity, but they have higher than normal requirements for energy and nutrients as a part of the process of replacing tissue in convalescence (Section 9.1.2.3) or as a result of fever or the metabolic effects of cancer and other chronic diseases (Section 8.4). At the same time, illness impairs appetite, and a side effect of many drugs is to distort the sense of taste, depress appetite, or cause nausea. It is difficult to provide a range of exciting and attractive foods under institutional conditions, yet this is what is needed to tempt the patient's appetite.

1.4.5   *Disorders of appetite: anorexia nervosa and bulimia nervosa*

Whilst obesity is a major public health problem (Section 7.2), one effect of the publicity about obesity is to put pressure on people to reduce their body weight, even if they are within the desirable, healthy weight range. In some cases the pressure for slimness may be a factor in the development of anorexia nervosa, bulimia, and other eating disorders, although the evidence suggests that media and peer pressure activates the desire for thinness in people who are vulnerable because of low self-esteem and dissatisfaction with their body image but do not cultivate it otherwise. Anorexia nervosa and bulimia are due to interactions between higher brain centres and the hunger and satiety centres of the hypothalamus, so that a variety of psychological factors can override the normal sensations of hunger. The diagnostic criteria for anorexia nervosa and bulimia nervosa are shown in Table 1.4.

Those most at risk are adolescent girls; at any time, some 25% are dieting to lose weight, whether they need to or not, and 50% think they are too fat. Similar disturbances of eating behaviour can occur in older women and, more rarely, in adolescent boys and men. One cause of the problem in adolescent girls is a reaction to the physical changes of puberty. By refusing food, the girl believes that she can delay or prevent these changes. To a considerable extent, this is so. Breast development slows down or ceases as energy balance becomes more negative. When body weight falls below about 45 kg, menstruation ceases because of the lower secretion of leptin from the reduced amount of adipose tissue (Section 1.4.2).

The main feature of anorexia nervosa is a very severe restriction of food intake—with the obvious result of very considerable weight loss. Despite all evidence and arguments to the contrary, the anorectic subject is convinced that she is overweight and restricts her eating very severely. Dieting becomes the primary focus of her life. She has a preoccupation with, and often a considerable knowledge of, food and frequently has a variety of stylised compulsive behaviour patterns associated with food. As a part of her pathological obsession with thinness, the anorectic person frequently takes a great deal of strenuous exercise, often exercising to exhaustion in solitude. She will go to extreme lengths to avoid eating, and frequently, when forced to eat, will induce vomiting soon afterward. Many anorectics also make excessive use of laxatives.

Surprisingly, many anorectic people are adept at hiding their condition, and it is not unknown for the problem to remain unnoticed, even in a family setting. Food is played with, but little or none is actually eaten; excuses are frequently made to leave the table in the middle of the meal, perhaps on the pretext of going into the kitchen to prepare the next course.

Some anorectic subjects also exhibit a further disturbance of eating behaviour—bulimia or binge eating. After a period of eating very little, they suddenly eat an extremely large amount of food (40 MJ or more in a single meal, compared with an average daily requirement of 8–12 MJ), frequently followed by deliberate induction of vomiting and heavy doses of laxatives. This is followed by a further prolonged period of anorexia.

Bulimia also occurs in the absence of anorexia nervosa—a person of normal weight will consume a very large amount of food (commonly 40–80 MJ over a period of a few hours), again followed by induction of vomiting and excessive use of laxatives. In severe cases, such binges may occur five or six times a week.

It is estimated that about 2% of adolescent girls go through at least a short phase of anorexia, and another 3% have a borderline eating disorder. In most cases, anorexia is self-limiting, and normal eating patterns are re-established as the emotional crises of adolescence resolve. Other people may require specialist counselling and treatment, and in an unfortunate few, problems of eating behaviour persist into adult life.

Table 1.4 Diagnostic Criteria for the Classification of Eating Disorders

Anorexia nervosa

- Refusal to maintain body weight at or above a minimally normal weight for age and height; weight loss leading to maintenance of body weight less than 85% of that expected or failure to make expected weight gain during period of growth, leading to body weight less than 85% of that expected.
- Intense fear of gaining weight or becoming fat, even though underweight.
- Disturbance in the way one's body weight or shape are experienced, undue influence of body weight or shape on self-evaluation, or denial of the seriousness of the current low body weight.
- Amenorrhoea (for at least three consecutive cycles) in postmenarchal girls and (premenopausal) women when not pregnant.

Types of anorexia nervosa

Restricting type: During the current episode of anorexia nervosa, the person has not regularly engaged in binge-eating or purging behaviour (self-induced vomiting or misuse of laxatives, diuretics, or enemas).

Binge-eating–purging type: During the current episode of anorexia nervosa, the person has regularly engaged in binge-eating or purging behaviour (self-induced vomiting or the misuse of laxatives, diuretics, or enemas).

Bulimia nervosa

- Recurrent episodes of binge eating characterised by both

Eating, in a discrete period of time (e.g., within any 2-h period), an amount of food that is significantly larger than most people would eat during a similar period and under similar circumstances.

A sense of lack of control over eating during the episode, defined by a feeling that one cannot stop eating or control what or how much one is eating.

- Recurrent inappropriate compensatory behaviour to prevent weight gain

Self-induced vomiting

Misuse of laxatives, diuretics, enemas, or other medications

Fasting

Excessive exercise

- The binge eating and inappropriate compensatory behaviour both occur, on average, at least twice a week for 3 months.
- Self-evaluation is unduly influenced by body shape and weight.
- The disturbance does not occur exclusively during episodes of anorexia nervosa.

Types of bulimia nervosa

Purging type: During the current episode of bulimia nervosa, the person has regularly engaged in self-induced vomiting or the misuse of laxatives, diuretics, or enemas.

Nonpurging type: During the current episode of bulimia nervosa, the person has used inappropriate compensatory behaviour but has not regularly engaged in self-induced vomiting or misused laxatives, diuretics, or enemas.

Eating disorder not otherwise specified[a]

1. For female patients, all of the criteria for anorexia nervosa are met except that the patient has regular menses.
2. All of the criteria for anorexia nervosa are met except that, despite significant weight loss, the patient's current weight is in the normal range.

(Continued)

Table 1.4 Diagnostic Criteria for the Classification of Eating Disorders (*Continued*)

3. All of the criteria for bulimia nervosa are met except that the binge eating and inappropriate compensatory mechanisms occur fewer than twice a week or for less than 3 months.
4. The patient has normal body weight and regularly uses inappropriate compensatory behaviour after eating small amounts of food (e.g. self-induced vomiting).
5. Repeatedly chewing and spitting out, but not swallowing, large amounts of food.
6. Binge-eating disorder is recurrent episodes of binge eating in the absence of the regular inappropriate compensatory behaviour characteristic of bulimia nervosa.

Source: Adapted from American Psychiatric Association: Diagnostic and Statistical Manual of Mental Disorders, 4th edition, Washington, DC, American Psychiatric Association, 2000.
[a] Disorders of eating that do not meet the criteria for either anorexia nervosa or bulimia nervosa.

Key points

- The first need of the body is for water. In addition to obvious water in beverages, there is water in most foods, and water formed in the metabolism of metabolic fuels makes a significant contribution to fluid balance.
- There is a relationship between energy intake from food, energy expenditure in physical activity, and body weight, but two thirds of total energy expenditure is required to maintain nerve and muscle tone, circulation, breathing, and metabolic homeostasis.
- The main metabolic fuels are carbohydrate and fat; there is no absolute requirement for either (apart from small amounts of essential fatty acids). It is difficult to achieve an adequate energy intake on a very low fat diet, and fat is essential for the absorption of vitamins A, D, E, and K.
- There is a requirement for protein in addition to its role as a metabolic fuel.
- There is a requirement for minerals that have a function in the body, and for vitamins.
- Centres in the brain control hunger and satiety, in response to circulating concentrations of metabolic fuels and hormones secreted by the gastrointestinal tract and pancreas. Ghrelin stimulates appetite, whilst the other gastrointestinal hormones signal satiety.
- Long-term control of food intake and energy expenditure is largely by the hormone leptin, which is secreted mainly by adipose tissue; circulating concentrations of leptin reflect the adequacy (or otherwise) of body fat reserves. Leptin acts on the hypothalamus to regulate food intake and on muscle and adipose tissue to regulate energy expenditure.
- The sense of taste on the tongue permits detection of nutrients and avoidance of potential toxins.
- Food choices are complex; in addition to the cost and availability of foods, a variety of religious and ethical beliefs and social and individual factors affect what people choose to eat.
- Higher brain centres and psychological factors can override the physiological signals for hunger and satiety, leading to eating disorders including anorexia nervosa and bulimia nervosa.

chapter two

Enzymes and metabolic pathways

All metabolic processes depend on reaction between molecules, with breaking of some covalent bonds and the formation of others, yielding compounds that are different from the starting materials. To understand nutrition and metabolism, it is therefore essential to understand how chemical reactions occur, how they are catalysed by enzymes and how enzyme activity can be regulated and controlled.

Objectives

After reading this chapter, you should be able to

- Explain how covalent bonds are broken and formed; what is meant by thermoneutral, endothermic, and exothermic reactions, and how reactions come to equilibrium.
- Explain how a catalyst increases the rate at which a reaction comes to equilibrium and how enzymes act as catalysts.
- Explain how an enzyme exhibits specificity for both the substrates bound and the reaction catalysed.
- Define a unit of enzyme activity.
- Explain how pH, temperature, and the concentration of enzyme affect the rate of reaction.
- Describe and explain the dependence of the rate of reaction on the concentration of substrate, define the kinetic parameters K_m and V_{max} and explain how they are determined experimentally.
- Explain how enzymes may show cooperative binding of substrate, and how this affects the substrate dependence of activity.
- Describe the difference between reversible and irreversible inhibitors of enzymes, their clinical relevance, and how they may be distinguished experimentally.
- Describe the difference between competitive, non-competitive, and uncompetitive reversible inhibitors of enzymes, their clinical relevance, and how they may be distinguished experimentally.
- Explain what is meant by the terms coenzyme and prosthetic group, apoenzyme and holoenzyme; describe the roles of coenzymes in oxidation and reduction reactions.
- Describe the classification of enzymes on the basis of the reaction catalysed.
- Describe and explain what is meant by a metabolic pathway, and by linear, branched, spiral (looped), and cyclic pathways.

2.1   Chemical reactions: breaking and making covalent bonds

Breaking a covalent bond requires an initial input of energy in some form—normally as heat, but in some cases also light or other radiation. This is the activation energy of the reaction. The process of breaking a bond requires activation of the electrons forming the bond—a temporary movement of electrons from orbitals in which they have a stable configuration to orbitals further from the nucleus. Electrons that have been excited in this way have an unstable configuration, and the covalent bonds they contributed to are weakened and broken. Electrons cannot remain in this excited state for more than a fraction of a second. Sometimes, they simply return to their original unexcited state, emitting the same energy as was taken up to excite them, but usually as a series of small steps, rather than as a single step. Overall, there is no change when this occurs.

More commonly, the excited electrons adopt a different stable configuration, by interacting with electrons associated with different atoms and molecules. The result is the formation of new covalent bonds, and hence the formation of new compounds. In this case, there are three possibilities, as shown in Figure 2.1:

1. There may be an output of energy equal to the activation energy of the reaction, so that the energy level of the products is the same as that of the starting materials. Such a reaction is energetically neutral (thermoneutral).
2. There may be an output of energy greater than the activation of the reaction, so that the energy level of the products is lower than that of the starting materials. This is an exothermic reaction—it proceeds with the output of heat. An exothermic reaction will proceed spontaneously once the initial activation energy has been provided.
3. There may be an output of energy less than the activation energy, so that the energy level of the products is higher than that of the starting materials. The solution will take up heat from its surroundings and will have to be heated for the reaction to proceed. This is an endothermic reaction.

In general, reactions in which relatively large complex molecules are broken down to smaller molecules (catabolic reactions) are exothermic, whilst reactions that involve the

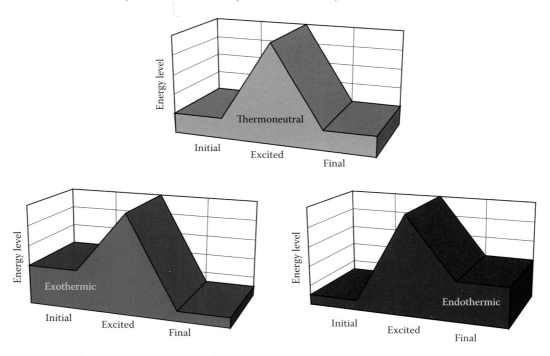

Figure 2.1 Energy changes in chemical reactions: thermoneutral, exothermic, and endothermic reactions.

synthesis of larger molecules from smaller ones (anabolic or biosynthetic reactions) are endothermic.

2.1.1   Equilibrium

Some reactions, such as the burning of ethanol (see Figure 2.21) or a hydrocarbon in air to form carbon dioxide and water, are highly exothermic, and the products of the reaction are widely dispersed. Such reactions proceed essentially in one direction only. However, most reactions do not proceed in only one direction. If two compounds, A and B, can react together to form X and Y, then X and Y can react to form A and B. The reactions can be written as

$$(1)\ A + B \rightarrow X + Y$$

$$(2)\ X + Y \rightarrow A + B.$$

Starting with only A and B in the solution, at first, only reaction (1) will occur, forming X and Y. However, as X and Y accumulate, they will undergo reaction (2), forming A and B. Similarly, starting with X and Y, at first, only reaction (2) will occur, forming A and B. As A and B accumulate, they will undergo reaction (1), forming X and Y.

In both cases, the final result will be a solution containing A, B, X, and Y. The relative amounts of [A + B] and [X + Y] will be the same regardless of whether the starting compounds (substrates) were A and B or X and Y. At this stage, the rate of reaction (1) forming X and Y and reaction (2) forming A and B will be equal. This is equilibrium, and the reaction can be written as

$$A + B \rightleftharpoons X + Y.$$

If there is a large difference in energy level between [A + B] and [X + Y] (i.e., if the reaction is exothermic in one direction, and therefore endothermic in the other), the position of the equilibrium will reflect this. If reaction (1) above is exothermic, then at equilibrium, there will be very little A and B remaining, most will have been converted to X and Y. Conversely, if reaction (1) is endothermic, then at equilibrium, relatively little of A and B will be converted to X and Y.

At equilibrium, the ratio of [A + B] to [X + Y] is constant for any given reaction. Therefore, if there is a constant addition of substrates, this will disturb the equilibrium and increase the amount of product formed. Similarly, continual removal of the products will increase the rate at which substrate is utilised.

A metabolic pathway is a sequence of reactions, and *in vivo*, very few reactions actually come to equilibrium. The product of one reaction is the substrate for the next; thus, there is a continual supply of substrate and removal of products, for each reaction, and there is a constant flux through the pathway—a dynamic steady state rather than equilibrium.

2.1.2   Catalysis

A catalyst increases the rate at which a reaction comes to equilibrium, without itself being consumed in the reaction; thus, a small amount of catalyst can effect the reaction of many thousands of molecules of substrate. Whilst a catalyst increases the rate at which a reaction comes to equilibrium, it does not affect the position of the equilibrium.

Catalysts affect the rate of reaction in three main ways:

1. By providing a surface on which the molecules that are to undergo reaction can come together at a higher concentration than would be possible in free solution, thus increasing the probability of them colliding and reacting. This also aligns the reactants in the correct orientation to undergo reaction.
2. By providing a microenvironment for the reactants that is different from the solution as a whole.
3. By participating in the reaction by withdrawing electrons from, or donating electrons to, covalent bonds. This enhances the breaking of bonds that is the essential prerequisite for chemical reaction, and lowers the activation energy of the reaction.

2.2   Enzymes

Enzymes are proteins that catalyse metabolic reactions. There are also a number of enzymes that are not proteins, but are catalytic molecules of RNA (Section 9.2.2)—these are sometimes referred to as ribozymes.

Proteins are linear polymers of amino acids (Section 4.4.2). Any protein adopts a characteristic pattern of folding, determined largely by the amino acids in its sequence, and their interactions with each other and the surrounding environment. This folding of the protein chain results in reactive groups from amino acids that may be widely separated in the primary sequence coming together at the surface and creating a site that has a defined shape and array of chemically reactive groups. This is the active site of the enzyme, which can be divided into two distinct domains: the binding site for the compounds that are to undergo reaction (the substrates) and the catalytic site. Figure 2.2 shows how three amino

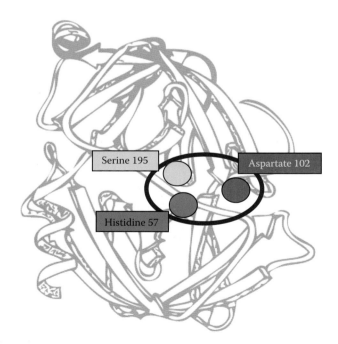

Figure 2.2 The formation of an active site in an enzyme as a result of folding of the protein chain.

acids that are widely separated in the primary sequence of the enzyme trypsin come together to form a catalytic triad as a result of folding of the protein chain.

Many enzymes also have a non-protein component of the catalytic site; this may be a metal ion, an organic compound that contains a metal ion (e.g., haem, Section 3.3.1.2), or an organic compound, which may be derived from a vitamin (Table 2.1 and Chapter 11) or may be a compound that is readily synthesised in the body. This non-protein part of the active site may be covalently bound, when it is generally referred to as a prosthetic group, or may be tightly, but not covalently, bound, when it is usually referred to as a coenzyme (Section 2.4).

Reactive groups in amino acid side-chains and coenzymes or prosthetic groups at the active site facilitate the making or breaking of specific chemical bonds in the substrate by donating or withdrawing electrons. In this way, the enzyme lowers the activation energy of a chemical reaction (Figure 2.3) and increases the rate at which the reaction attains equilibrium, under much milder conditions than are required for a simple chemical catalyst. To hydrolyse a protein into its constituent amino acids in the laboratory, it is necessary to use concentrated acid as a catalyst and heat the sample in a sealed tube at 105°C overnight to

Table 2.1 The Major Coenzymes

		Source	Functions
CoA	Coenzyme A	Pantothenic acid	Acyl transfer reactions
FAD	Flavin adenine dinucleotide	Vitamin B_2	Oxidation reactions
FMN	Flavin mononucleotide (riboflavin phosphate)	Vitamin B_2	Oxidation reactions
NAD	Nicotinamide adenine dinucleotide	Niacin	Oxidation and reduction reactions
NADP	Nicotinamide adenine Dinucleotide phosphate	Niacin	Oxidation and reduction reactions
PLP	Pyridoxal phosphate	Vitamin B_6	Amino acid metabolism

Note: There are a number of other coenzymes that are discussed where they are relevant to specific metabolic pathways. In addition to those shown in this table, most of the other vitamins also function as coenzymes (see Chapter 11).

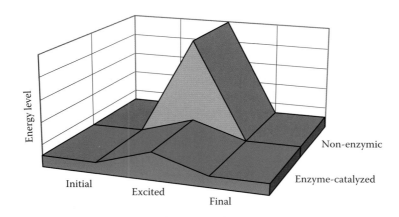

Figure 2.3 The effect of enzyme catalysis on the activation energy of a reaction. The enzyme does not affect the initial or final energy level, only the activation energy.

provide the activation energy of the hydrolysis. This is the process of digestion of proteins, which occurs under relatively mild acid or alkaline conditions, at 37°C, and is complete within a few hours of eating a meal (Section 4.4).

2.2.1   *Specificity of enzymes*

The binding of substrates to enzymes involves interactions between the substrates and reactive groups of the amino acid side chains that make up the active site of the enzyme. This means that enzymes show a considerable specificity for the substrates they bind. Normally, several different interactions must occur before the substrate can bind in the correct orientation to undergo reaction, and binding of the substrate often causes a change in the conformation of the active site, bringing reactive groups closer to the substrate.

Figure 2.4 shows the active sites of three enzymes that catalyse the same reaction— hydrolysis of a peptide bond in a protein (Section 4.4.3); in all three enzymes, the catalytic site is the same as that shown for trypsin in Figure 2.2. The three enzymes show different specificity for the bond that they hydrolyse:

1. Trypsin catalyses cleavage of the esters of basic amino acids.
2. Chymotrypsin catalyses hydrolysis of the esters of aromatic amino acids.
3. Elastase catalyses hydrolysis of the esters of small neutral amino acids.

This difference in specificity for the bond to be hydrolysed is explained by differences in the substrate binding sites of the three enzymes. In all three, the substrate binds in a groove at the surface, bringing the bond to be cleaved over the serine residue that initiates the catalysis. The amino acid providing the carboxyl side of the peptide bond to be cleaved sits in a pocket below this groove, and it is the nature of the amino acids that line this pocket that determines the specificity of the enzymes:

- In trypsin, there is an acidic group (from aspartate) at the base of the pocket—this will attract a basic amino acid side chain.
- In chymotrypsin, the pocket is lined by small neutral amino acids; thus, a relatively large aromatic group can fit in.
- In elastase, there are two bulky amino acid side chains in the pocket; thus, only a small neutral side chain can fit in.

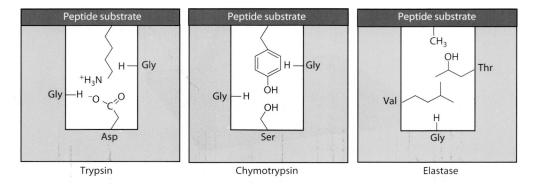

Figure 2.4 Enzyme specificity: the substrate binding sites of trypsin, chymotrypsin, and elastase.

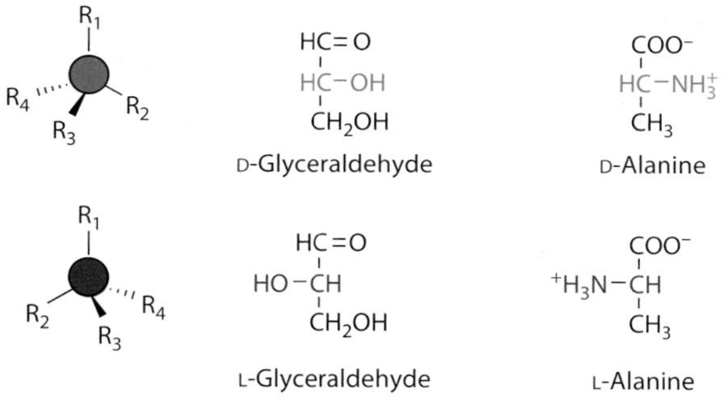

$$R_1$$
$$R_4 \cdots \bullet \: R_2$$
$$R_3$$

HC=O
HC−OH
CH₂OH

D-Glyceraldehyde

COO⁻
HC−NH₃⁺
CH₃

D-Alanine

$$R_1$$
$$R_2 \: \bullet \cdots R_4$$
$$R_3$$

HC=O
HO−CH
CH₂OH

L-Glyceraldehyde

COO⁻
⁺H₃N−CH
CH₃

L-Alanine

Figure 2.5 DL-Isomerism: the arrangement of substituent groups around an asymmetric carbon atom.

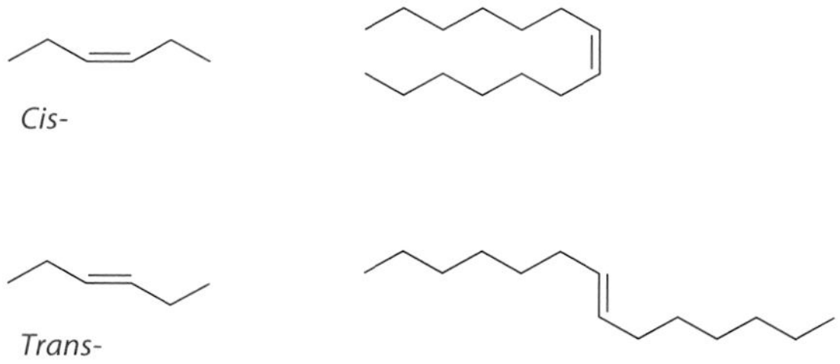

Cis-

Trans-

*Figure 2.6 Cis–trans-*isomerism: the continuation of the carbon chain on one side or the other of a carbon–carbon double bond.

Chemically, D- and L-isomers of a compound (Figure 2.5) and *cis-* and *trans-*isomers (Figure 2.6) behave identically, and it can often be difficult to distinguish between isomers. However, the isomers have different shapes, and enzymes readily discriminate between them—the shape and conformation of the substrate are critically important for binding to an enzyme. (Most of the naturally occurring and physiologically relevant sugars are D-isomers, and most amino acids are L-isomers; the nutritional and heath importance of *trans-*isomers of unsaturated fatty acids is discussed in Section 6.3.2.1.)

The participation of reactive groups at the active site of the enzyme provides not only specificity for the substrates that will bind but also for the reaction that will be catalysed. For example, in a non-enzymic model system, an amino acid may undergo α-decarboxylation to yield an amine, transfer of the α-amino group and replacement with an oxo-group (Section 9.3.1.2), isomerisation between the D- and L-isomers, or a variety of reactions involving elimination or replacement of the side chain. In an enzyme-catalysed reaction, only one of the possible reactions will normally be catalysed by a given enzyme.

2.2.2   The stages in an enzyme-catalysed reaction

An enzyme-catalysed reaction can be considered to occur in three distinct steps, each of which is reversible:

1. Binding of the substrate (S) to the enzyme (Enz) to form the enzyme-substrate complex: Enz + S ⇌ Enz-S
2. Reaction of the enzyme–substrate complex to form the enzyme-product complex: Enz-S ⇌ Enz-P

3. Breakdown of the enzyme–product complex, with release of the product (P): Enz-P ⇌ Enz + P

Overall, the process can be written as: Enz + S ⇌ Enz-S ⇌ Enz-P ⇌ Enz + P

There are two models for the binding of a substrate to an enzyme:

1. The lock and key model, in which the reactive groups at the substrate-binding site and the catalytic site are perfectly aligned to permit substrate binding and catalysis.
2. The induced fit model, in which binding of the substrate causes a conformational change in the catalytic site, bringing the reactive groups into the correct alignment with the substrate to catalyse the reaction. An extreme form of induced fit is seen in multi-subunit enzymes (allosteric enzymes, Section 2.3.3.3) that show cooperative binding of the substrate. Binding the substrate at one of the binding sites affects the conformation at the other active sites, enhancing the binding of further molecules of the substrate.

2.2.3 Units of enzyme activity

In the relatively rare cases when an enzyme has been purified, it is possible to express the amount of enzyme in tissues or plasma as the number of moles of enzyme protein present, for example, by raising antibodies against the purified protein for use in an immunoassay. However, what is more important is not how much of the enzyme protein is present in the cell, but how much catalytic activity there is—how much substrate can be converted to product in a given time. Therefore, amounts of enzymes are usually expressed in units of activity.

The SI unit of catalysis is the katal = 1 mol of substrate converted per second. However, enzyme activity is usually expressed as the number of micromoles (μmol) of substrate converted (or of product formed) per minute. This is the standard unit of enzyme activity, determined under specified optimum conditions for that enzyme at 30°C. This temperature is a compromise between mammalian biochemists, who would work at body temperature (37°C for human beings), and microbiological biochemists, who would normally work at 20°C.

2.3 Factors affecting enzyme activity

Any given enzyme has an innate activity—for many enzymes, the catalytic rate constant is of the order of 1000–5000 mol of substrate converted per mole of enzyme per second or higher. However, a number of factors affect the activity of enzymes.

2.3.1 The effect of pH

Both the binding of the substrate to the enzyme and catalysis of the reaction depend on interactions between the substrates and reactive groups in the amino acid side chains that make up the active site. They have to be in the appropriate ionisation state for binding and reaction to occur—this depends on the pH of the medium. Any enzyme will have maximum activity at a specific pH—the optimum pH for that enzyme. As the pH increases or decreases away from the optimum, the activity of the enzyme decreases. Most enzymes have little or no activity 2–3 pH units away from their pH optimum. Although the average pH of cell contents (and plasma) is around 7.4, individual subcellular compartments and organelles may be very acidic or alkaline.

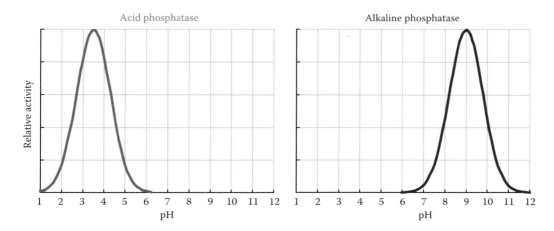

Figure 2.7 The effect of pH on enzyme activity.

Figure 2.7 shows the activity of two enzymes that are found in plasma and catalyse the same reaction, hydrolysis of a phosphate ester: acid phosphatase (released from the prostate gland) has a pH optimum around 3.5 whilst alkaline phosphatase (released from liver and bone) has a pH optimum around 9.0. Neither has any significant activity at pH 7.35–7.45, which is the normal range in plasma. However, alkaline phosphatase is significantly active in the alkaline microenvironment at cell surfaces and is important, for example, in the hydrolysis of pyridoxal phosphate (the main form of vitamin B_6 in plasma, Section 11.9.1) to free pyridoxal for uptake into tissues.

2.3.2   *The effect of temperature*

Chemical reactions proceed faster at higher temperatures, for two reasons:

1. Molecules move faster at higher temperatures and hence have a greater chance of colliding to undergo reaction.
2. At a higher temperature, it is easier for electrons to gain activation energy and hence be excited into unstable orbitals to undergo reaction.

With enzyme-catalysed reactions, although the rate at which the reaction comes to equilibrium increases with temperature, there is a second effect of temperature—denaturation of the enzyme protein (Section 4.4.2.3), leading to irreversible loss of activity. As the temperature increases, the movement of parts of the protein molecules relative to each other increases, leading to disruption of the hydrogen bonds that maintain the folded structure of the protein. When this happens, the protein chain unfolds, and the active site is lost. As the temperature increases further, the denatured protein becomes insoluble and precipitates out of solution.

Temperature thus has two opposing effects on enzyme activity (Figure 2.8). At relatively low temperatures (up to about 50°C–55°C), increasing temperature results in an increase in the rate of reaction. However, as the temperature increases further, denaturation of the enzyme protein becomes increasingly important, resulting in a rapid fall in activity at higher temperatures. The rate of increase in the rate of reaction with increasing

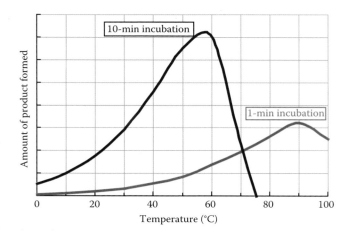

Figure 2.8 The temperature dependence of enzyme activity. In a short incubation (1 min), the enzyme may have an optimum temperature as high as 90°C, but in longer incubations, this falls because of denaturation of the enzyme; thus, in a 10-min incubation, the optimum temperature is about 55°C.

temperature depends on the activation energy of the reaction being catalysed; the rate of decrease in activity at higher temperatures is a characteristic of the enzyme itself.

The apparent temperature optimum of an enzyme-catalysed reaction depends on the time for which the enzyme is incubated. During a short incubation (e.g., 1 min), there is negligible denaturation, and so the apparent optimum temperature is relatively high, whilst during a longer incubation, denaturation is important, and so the apparent optimum temperature is lower.

The effect of temperature is not normally physiologically important, since body temperature is maintained close to 37°C. However, some of the effects of fever (when body temperature may increase to 40°C) or hypothermia may be due to changes in the rates of enzyme-catalysed reactions. Because different enzymes respond differently to changes in temperature, there may be a loss of the normal integration between different reactions and metabolic pathways.

2.3.3 *The effect of substrate concentration*

In a simple chemical reaction involving a single substrate, the rate at which product is formed increases linearly as the concentration of the substrate increases. When more substrate is available, more will undergo reaction.

With enzyme-catalysed reactions, the change in the rate of formation of product with increasing concentration of substrate is not linear but hyperbolic (Figure 2.9). At relatively low concentrations of substrate (region A in Figure 2.9), the catalytic site of the enzyme will be empty at times, until more substrate binds to undergo reaction. Under these conditions, the rate of product formation is limited by the time taken for another molecule of substrate to bind to the enzyme. A relatively small change in the concentration of substrate has a large effect on the rate at which product is formed in this region of the curve.

At high concentrations of substrate (region B in Figure 2.9), as the product leaves the catalytic site, another molecule of substrate binds more or less immediately, and the enzyme is saturated with substrate. The limiting factor in the formation of product is now

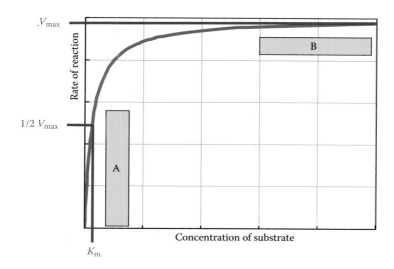

Figure 2.9 The substrate dependence of an enzyme-catalysed reaction. In region A, the enzyme is very unsaturated with substrate, and the rate of reaction increases sharply with increasing concentration of the substrate. In region B, the enzyme is almost saturated with substrate, and there is little change in the rate of reaction with increasing substrate concentration.

the rate at which the enzyme can catalyse the reaction and not the availability of substrate. The enzyme is acting at or near its maximum rate (or maximum velocity, abbreviated to V_{max}). Even a relatively large change in the concentration of substrate has little effect on the rate of formation of product in this region of the curve.

From a graph of the rate of formation of product versus the concentration of substrate (Figure 2.9), it is easy to estimate the maximum rate of reaction that an enzyme can achieve (V_{max}) when it is saturated with substrate. However, it is not possible to determine from this graph the concentration of substrate required to achieve saturation because the rate of reaction gradually approaches V_{max} as the concentration of substrate increases and only really achieves its true V_{max} at an infinite concentration of substrate.

It is easy to estimate the concentration of substrate at which the enzyme has achieved half its maximum rate of reaction. The concentration of substrate to achieve half V_{max} is called the Michaelis constant of the enzyme (abbreviated to K_m), to commemorate Michaelis, who, together with Menten, first formulated a mathematical model of the dependence of the rate of enzymic reactions on the concentration of substrate.

The K_m of an enzyme is not affected by the amount of the enzyme protein that is present. It is an (inverse) index of the affinity of the enzyme for its substrate. An enzyme that has a high K_m has a lower affinity for its substrate than an enzyme with a lower K_m. The higher the value of K_m, the greater is the concentration of substrate required to achieve half-saturation of the enzyme.

In general, enzymes that have a low K_m compared with the normal concentration of substrate in the cell are likely to be acting at or near their maximum rate and hence have a more or less constant rate of reaction despite (modest) changes in the concentration of substrate. By contrast, an enzyme that has a high K_m compared with the normal concentration of substrate in the cell will show a large change in the rate of reaction with relatively small changes in the concentration of substrate.

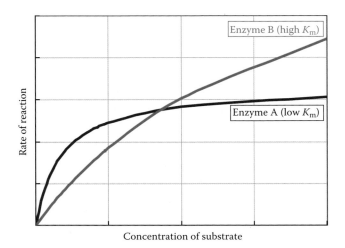

Figure 2.10 Two enzymes competing for the same substrate. Enzyme A has a relatively low K_m (a high affinity for the substrate) and reaches saturation (and hence its V_{max}) at a low concentration of substrate. Enzyme B has a higher K_m, and its rate of reaction continues to increase with increasing concentration of substrate after enzyme A has reached saturation. At low concentrations of substrate, most undergoes the reaction catalysed by enzyme A; at higher concentrations of substrate, the reaction catalysed by enzyme B predominates.

If two enzymes in a cell can both act on the same substrate, catalysing different reactions, the enzyme with the lower K_m will be able to bind more substrate, and therefore its reaction will be favoured at relatively low concentrations of substrate. Thus, knowing the values of K_m and V_{max} for two enzymes, for example, at a branch point in a metabolic pathway (Figure 2.22), it is possible to predict which branch will predominate in the presence of different concentrations of the substrate. As shown in Figure 2.10, at low concentrations of substrate, the reaction catalysed by the enzyme with the lower K_m predominates, but as the concentration of substrate increases, this enzyme becomes saturated and acts at a more or less constant rate, whilst the rate of the reaction catalysed by the enzyme with the higher K_m continues to increase.

2.3.3.1   *Experimental determination of* K_m *and* V_{max}

Plotting the graph of rate of reaction against substrate concentration, as in Figure 2.9, permits only a very approximate determination of the values of K_m and V_{max}, and a number of methods have been developed to convert this hyperbolic relationship into a linear relationship, to permit more precise fitting of a line to the experimental points, and hence more precise estimation of K_m and V_{max}.

The most widely used such linearisation of the data is the Lineweaver–Burk double reciprocal plot of 1/rate of reaction versus 1/[substrate], shown in Figure 2.11. This has an intercept on the *y* (1/*v*) axis = $1/V_{max}$ when 1/s = 0 (i.e., at an infinite concentration of substrate) and an intercept on the *x* (1/s) axis = $-1/K_m$. There are notes on other ways of linearising the data in the theory screens for the enzyme assay program in the Virtual Laboratory on the CD.

Experimentally, the values of K_m and V_{max} are determined by incubating the enzyme (at optimum pH) with different concentrations of substrate, plotting the graph shown

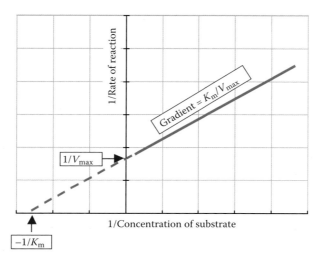

Figure 2.11 The Lineweaver–Burk double reciprocal plot to determine K_m and V_{max}.

in Figure 2.11, and extrapolating back from the experimental points to determine the intercepts.

The Michaelis–Menten equation that describes the dependence of rate of reaction on concentration of substrate is

$$\text{Rate of reaction } v = (V_{max} \times [S])/([S] + K_m)$$

where [S] is the concentration of substrate.

One of the underlying assumptions of the Michaelis–Menten model is that there is no change in the concentration of substrate—this means that what should be measured is the initial rate of reaction. This is usually estimated by determining the amount of product formed at a series of short time intervals after the initiation of the reaction, then plotting a rate curve (product formed against time incubated) and estimating the tangent to this curve as the initial rate of reaction.

2.3.3.2   Enzymes with two substrates
Most enzyme catalysed reactions involve two substrates; it is only enzymes catalysing lysis of a molecule or an isomerisation reaction that have only a single substrate.

For a reaction involving two substrates (and two products),

$$A + B \rightleftharpoons C + D,$$

the enzyme may act by either

1. An ordered mechanism, in which each substrate binds in turn,

$$A + \text{Enz} \rightleftharpoons A\text{-Enz}$$

$$A\text{-Enz} + B \rightleftharpoons A\text{-Enz-B} \rightleftharpoons C\text{-Enz-D} \rightleftharpoons C\text{-Enz} + D$$

$$C\text{-Enz} \rightleftharpoons \text{Enz} + C$$

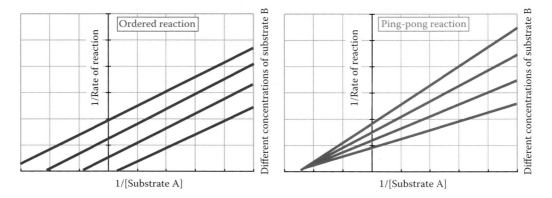

Figure 2.12 The Lineweaver–Burk double reciprocal plots for ordered and ping-pong two-substrate reactions.

2. A ping-pong mechanism in which one substrate undergoes reaction, modifying the enzyme and releasing product, then the second substrate binds, reacts with the modified enzyme, and restores it to the original state:

$$A + Enz \rightleftharpoons A\text{-}Enz \rightleftharpoons C\text{-}Enz^* \rightleftharpoons C + Enz^*$$

$$B + Enz^* \rightleftharpoons B\text{-}Enz^* \rightleftharpoons D\text{-}Enz \rightleftharpoons D + Enz.$$

These two different mechanisms can be distinguished by plotting $1/v$ against 1[substrate A] at several different concentrations of substrate B; as shown in Figure 2.12, the lines are parallel if the mechanism is ordered but converge for a ping-pong reaction.

2.3.3.3 *Cooperative (allosteric) enzymes*

Not all enzymes show the simple hyperbolic dependence of rate of reaction on substrate concentration shown in Figure 2.9. Some enzymes consist of several separate protein chains, each with an active site. In many such enzymes, the binding of substrate to one active site changes the conformation not only of that active site but of the whole multi-subunit array. This change in conformation affects the other active sites, altering the ease with which substrate can bind. This is cooperativity—the different subunits of the complete enzyme cooperate with each other. Because there is a change in the conformation (or shape) of the enzyme molecule, the phenomenon is also called allostericity (from the Greek for *different shape*), and such enzymes are called allosteric enzymes.

Figure 2.13 shows the change in rate of reaction with increasing concentration of substrate for an enzyme that displays substrate cooperativity. At low concentrations of substrate, the enzyme has little activity. As one of the binding sites is occupied, this causes a conformational change and increases the ease with which the other sites can bind substrate. Therefore, there is a steep increase in the rate of reaction with increasing concentration of substrate. Of course, as all the sites become saturated, the rate of reaction cannot increase any further with increasing concentration of substrate; the enzyme achieves its maximum rate of reaction.

Enzymes that display substrate cooperativity are often important in controlling the overall rate of metabolic pathways (Section 10.2.1). Their rate of reaction is extremely sensitive to the concentration of substrate. Furthermore, this sensitivity can readily be modified by a variety of compounds that bind to specific regulator sites on the enzyme and affect its

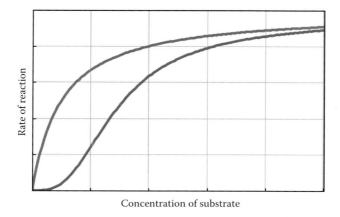

Figure 2.13 The substrate dependence of an enzyme showing subunit cooperativity—a sigmoid curve. For comparison, the hyperbolic substrate dependence of an enzyme not showing substrate cooperativity is shown in grey.

conformation, thus affecting the conformation of all of the active sites of the multi-subunit complex, either activating the enzyme at low concentrations of substrate by decreasing cooperativity or inhibiting it by increasing cooperativity (Figure 10.3).

2.3.4 Inhibition of enzyme activity

Inhibition of the activity of key enzymes in metabolic pathways by end products or metabolic intermediates is an important part of metabolic integration and control (Section 10.1). In addition, many of the drugs used to treat diseases act by inhibiting enzymes. Some inhibit the patient's enzyme, thus altering metabolic regulation; others act by preferentially inhibiting enzymes in the organisms that are causing disease.

Inhibitors may either act reversibly, i.e., inhibition wears off as the inhibitor is metabolised, or irreversibly, causing chemical modification of the enzyme protein, i.e., the effect of the inhibitor is prolonged and only diminishes gradually as the enzyme protein is catabolised and replaced (Section 9.1.1). When designing drugs, it is important to know whether they act as reversible or irreversible inhibitors. An irreversible inhibitor may only need to be administered every few days; however, it is more difficult to adjust the dose to match the patient's needs because of the long duration of action. By contrast, it is easy to adjust the dose of a reversible inhibitor to produce the desired effect, but such a compound may have to be taken several times a day, depending on the rate at which it is metabolised or excreted.

2.3.4.1 Irreversible inhibitors

Irreversible inhibitors are commonly chemical analogues of the substrate and bind to the enzyme in the same way as does the substrate, then undergo part of the normal reaction sequence. However, at some stage they form a covalent bond to a reactive group in the active site, resulting in inactivation of the enzyme. Such inhibitors are sometimes called mechanism-dependent inhibitors, or suicide inhibitors because they cause the enzyme to 'commit suicide'.

Experimentally, it is easy to distinguish between irreversible and reversible inhibitors by dialysis—placing the mixture of enzyme and inhibitor inside a sac of semi-permeable membrane with pores that will permit small molecules, such as the inhibitor, to cross, but

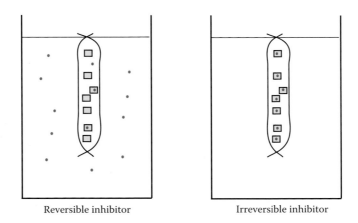

Reversible inhibitor   Irreversible inhibitor

Figure 2.14 Differentiating between reversible and irreversible inhibition by dialysis. The enzyme plus inhibitor is placed in a tube of semi-permeable membrane that will allow small molecules (e.g., the inhibitor) but not large ones (e.g., the enzyme) to cross. The reversible inhibitor is not covalently bound to the enzyme, and so can equilibrate across the membrane into the larger volume of buffer outside as the inhibitor is removed; thus, enzyme activity is restored. The irreversible inhibitor remains covalently bound to the enzyme and cannot be removed.

not large molecules such as the enzyme (Figure 2.14). A reversible inhibitor is not covalently bound to the enzyme and so can equilibrate across the membrane into the larger volume of buffer outside. Incubation of the enzyme with substrate after a period of dialysis will show that activity has been restored as the inhibitor is removed. By contrast, an irreversible inhibitor is covalently bound to the enzyme and cannot be removed by dialysis; thus, activity is not restored.

2.3.4.2 Competitive reversible inhibitors

A competitive inhibitor is a compound that binds to the active site of the enzyme in competition with the substrate. Often, but not always, such compounds are chemical analogues of the substrate. Although a competitive inhibitor binds to the active site, it does not undergo reaction, or, if it does, not to yield the product that would have been obtained by reaction of the normal substrate.

A competitive inhibitor reduces the rate of reaction because at any time some molecules of the enzyme have bound the inhibitor, and therefore are not free to bind the substrate. However, the binding of the inhibitor to the enzyme is reversible, and therefore, there is competition between the substrate and the inhibitor for the enzyme. This means that the sequence of the reaction in the presence of a competitive inhibitor can be shown as

$$Enz + S + I \rightleftharpoons Enz\text{-}I$$

$$Enz + S + I \rightleftharpoons Enz\text{-}S \rightleftharpoons Enz\text{-}P \rightleftharpoons Enz + P.$$

Figure 2.15 shows the s/v and double reciprocal plots for an enzyme incubated with various concentrations of a competitive inhibitor. If the concentration of substrate is increased, it will compete more effectively with the inhibitor for the active site of the enzyme. This means that at high concentrations of substrate the enzyme will achieve the same maximum rate of reaction (V_{max}) in the presence or absence of inhibitor. It is simply

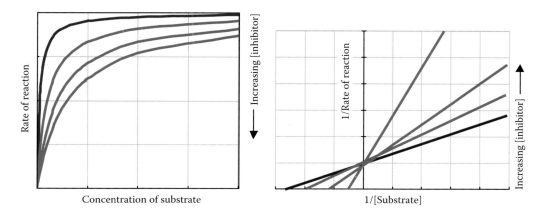

Figure 2.15 Substrate/velocity and Lineweaver–Burk double reciprocal plots for an enzyme incubated with varying concentrations of a competitive inhibitor. V_{max} is unchanged, but K_m increases with increasing concentrations of inhibitor.

that in the presence of inhibitor the enzyme requires a higher concentration of substrate to achieve saturation—in other words, the K_m of the enzyme is higher in the presence of a competitive inhibitor.

The effect of a competitive inhibitor as a drug that is that the final rate at which product is formed is unchanged, but there is an increase in the concentration of the substrate of the inhibited enzyme in the cell. As the inhibitor acts, the concentration of substrate increases, eventually becoming high enough for the enzyme to reach a more or less normal rate of reaction. This means that a competitive inhibitor is appropriate for use as a drug when the aim is to increase the available pool of substrate (perhaps to allow an alternative reaction to proceed) but inappropriate if the aim is to reduce the amount of product formed.

2.3.4.3 *Non-competitive reversible inhibitors*

Compounds that are non-competitive inhibitors bind to the enzyme–substrate complex rather than to the free enzyme. The enzyme–substrate–inhibitor complex only reacts slowly to form enzyme–product–inhibitor; thus, the effect of a non-competitive inhibitor is to slow down the rate at which the enzyme catalyses the formation of product. The reaction sequence can be written as

$$\text{Enz} + \text{S} + \text{I} \rightleftharpoons \text{Enz-S} + \text{I} \rightleftharpoons \text{Enz-S-I} (\rightleftharpoons) \text{Enz-P-I} \rightleftharpoons \text{Enz} + \text{P} + \text{I}.$$

Because there is no competition between the inhibitor and the substrate for binding to the enzyme, increasing the concentration of substrate has no effect on the activity of the enzyme in the presence of a non-competitive inhibitor. The K_m of the enzyme is unaffected by a non-competitive inhibitor, but the V_{max} is reduced. Figure 2.16 shows the s/v and double reciprocal plots for an enzyme incubated with several concentrations of a non-competitive inhibitor.

A non-competitive inhibitor would be appropriate for use as a drug when the aim is either to increase the concentration of substrate in the cell or to reduce the rate at which the product is formed, since, unlike a competitive inhibitor, the accumulation of substrate has no effect on the degree of inhibition.

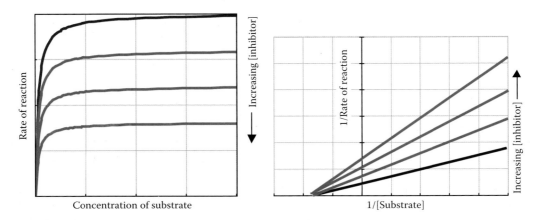

Figure 2.16 Substrate/velocity and Lineweaver–Burk double reciprocal plots for an enzyme incubated with varying concentrations of a non-competitive inhibitor. K_m is unchanged, but V_{max} decreases with increasing concentrations of inhibitor.

2.3.4.4   *Uncompetitive reversible inhibitors*

Compounds that are uncompetitive inhibitors bind to the enzyme, but unlike competitive inhibitors (Section 2.3.4.2), they enhance the binding of substrate (i.e., they lower K_m). However, as with non-competitive inhibitors (Section 2.3.4.3), the enzyme–inhibitor–substrate complex only undergoes reaction slowly; thus, the V_{max} of the reaction is reduced. The reaction sequence can be written as

$$\text{Enz} + \text{S} + \text{I} \rightleftharpoons \text{Enz-I} + \text{S} \rightleftharpoons \text{Enz-I-S} (\rightleftharpoons) \text{Enz-I-P} \rightleftharpoons \text{Enz} + \text{P} + \text{I}.$$

Figure 2.17 shows the *s/v* and double reciprocal plots for an enzyme incubated with several concentrations of an uncompetitive inhibitor. Because the binding of the inhibitor enhances the binding of substrate, addition of more substrate does not overcome the effect of the inhibitor.

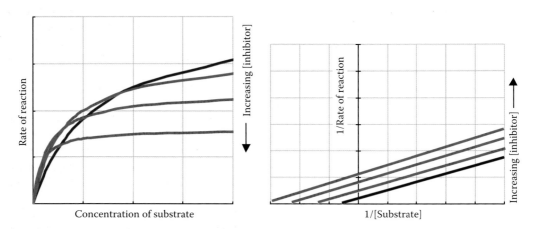

Figure 2.17 Substrate/velocity and Lineweaver–Burk double reciprocal plots for an enzyme incubated with varying concentrations of an uncompetitive inhibitor. Both K_m and V_{max} are decreased with increasing concentrations of inhibitor.

Uncompetitive inhibition is rare; like a non-competitive inhibitor, an uncompetitive inhibitor would be appropriate for use as a drug when the aim is either to increase the concentration of substrate in the cell or to reduce the rate at which the product is formed, since the accumulation of substrate has no effect on the degree of inhibition.

2.4   Coenzymes and prosthetic groups

Although most enzymes are proteins, many contain small non-protein molecules as an integral part of their structure. These may be organic compounds or metal ions. In either case, they are essential to the function of the enzyme, and the enzyme has no activity in the absence of the metal ion or coenzyme.

When an organic compound or metal ion is covalently bound to the active site of the enzyme it is referred to as a prosthetic group; compounds that are tightly but not covalently bound are referred to as coenzymes. Like the enzyme itself, the coenzyme or prosthetic group participates in the reaction, but at the end of the reaction sequence, it is unchanged. Sometimes, the coenzyme is chemically modified in the reaction with the first substrate then restored to its original state by reaction with the second substrate. This would be a ping-pong reaction (Section 2.3.3.2); transaminases (Section 9.3.1.2) catalyse a ping-pong reaction in which the amino group from the first substrate forms an amino derivative of the coenzyme as an intermediate step in the reaction.

Some compounds that were historically considered to be coenzymes do not remain bound to the active site of the enzyme but bind and leave in the same way as other substrates. Such compounds include the nicotinamide nucleotide coenzymes (NAD and NADP) and coenzyme A. Although they are not strictly coenzymes, they are present in the cell in very much smaller concentrations than most substrates, and are involved in a relatively large number of reactions; thus, they turn over rapidly.

Table 2.1 shows the major coenzymes, the vitamins they are derived from, and their principal metabolic functions.

2.4.1   Coenzymes and metal ions in oxidation and reduction reactions

Oxidation is the process of removing electrons from a molecule, either alone or together with hydrogen ions (protons, H^+). For example, Fe^{3+} is formed by removal of an electron from Fe^{2+}, whilst in the oxidation of a hydrocarbon such as ethane (C_2H_6) to ethene (C_2H_4) two hydrogen atoms are transferred onto a carrier: $CH_3\text{-}CH_3 + \text{carrier} \rightleftharpoons CH_2 = CH_2 + \text{carrier-}H_2$. In some oxidation reactions, oxygen is reduced to water or hydrogen peroxide by the hydrogen removed from the substrate being oxidised, as in the oxidation of glucose to carbon dioxide: $C_6H_{12}O_6 + 6O_2 \rightarrow 6CO_2 + 6H_2O$.

Reduction is the reverse of oxidation; the addition of hydrogen, or electrons, or the removal of oxygen, are all reduction reactions. In the reaction above, ethane was oxidised to ethene at the expense of a carrier, which was reduced in the process. The addition of hydrogen to the carrier is a reduction reaction. Similarly, the addition of electrons to a molecule is a reduction; thus, just as the conversion of Fe^{2+} to Fe^{3+} is an oxidation reaction, the reverse reaction, the conversion of Fe^{3+} to Fe^{2+}, is a reduction.

Most of the catabolic reactions involved in energy metabolism involve the oxidation of metabolic fuels, whilst many of the biosynthetic reactions involved in the formation of metabolic fuel reserves and the synthesis of body components are reduction reactions.

In some metabolic oxidation and reduction reactions, the hydrogen acceptor or donor is a prosthetic group, e.g., haem (Section 2.4.1.1) or riboflavin (Section 2.4.1.2). In other cases, the hydrogen acceptor or donor acts as a substrate of the enzyme (e.g., the nicotinamide nucleotide coenzymes, Section 2.4.1.3).

2.4.1.1   Metal ions

The electron acceptor or donor may be a transition metal ion that can have two different stable electron configurations. Commonly, iron (which can form Fe^{2+} or Fe^{3+} ions) and copper (which can form Cu^+ or Cu^{2+} ions) are involved.

In some enzymes, the metal ion is bound to the enzyme protein; in others, it is incorporated in an organic molecule, which in turn is attached to the enzyme. For example, haem is an organic compound containing iron, which is the coenzyme for a variety of enzymes collectively known as the cytochromes (Section 3.3.1.2). Haem is also the prosthetic group of haemoglobin, the protein in red blood cells that binds and transports oxygen between the lungs and other tissues, and myoglobin in muscle. However, in haemoglobin and myoglobin, the iron of haem does not undergo oxidation; it binds oxygen but does not react with it.

2.4.1.2   Riboflavin and flavoproteins

Vitamin B_2 (riboflavin, Section 11.7) is important in a wide variety of oxidation and reduction reactions. A few enzymes contain riboflavin itself, whilst others contain a riboflavin derivative: either riboflavin phosphate (sometimes called flavin mononucleotide) or flavin adenine dinucleotide (FAD, Figure 2.18). When an enzyme contains riboflavin, it is

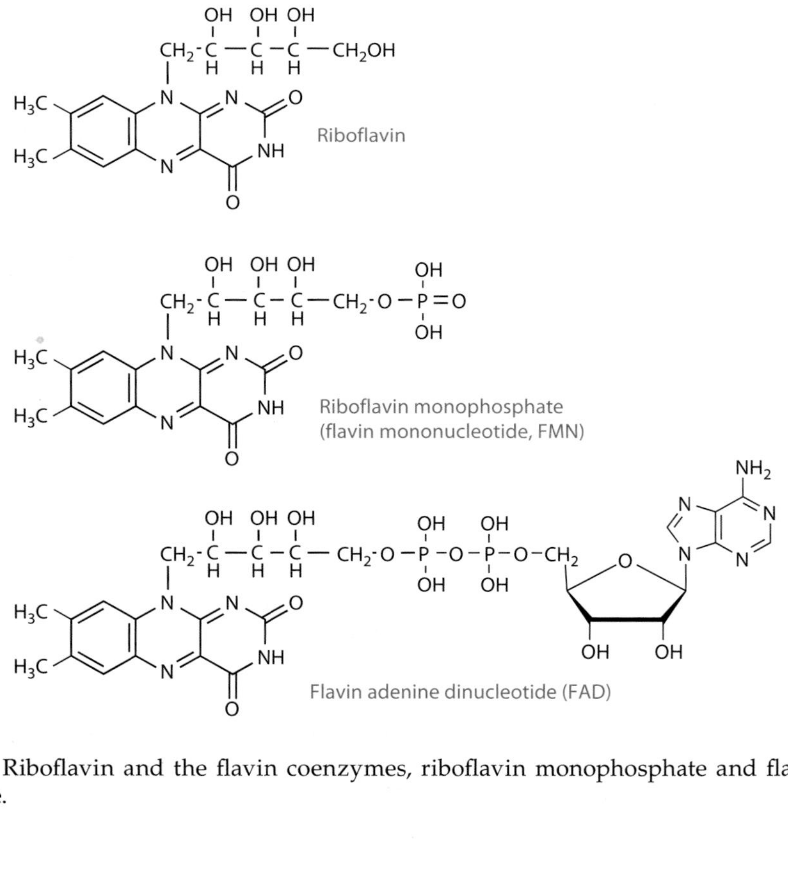

Figure 2.18 Riboflavin and the flavin coenzymes, riboflavin monophosphate and flavin adenine dinucleotide.

usually covalently bound at the active site. Although riboflavin phosphate and FAD are not normally covalently bound to the enzyme, they are very tightly bound, and can be regarded as prosthetic groups. The resultant enzymes with attached riboflavin are collectively known as flavoproteins.

The riboflavin moiety of flavoproteins can be reduced in a single step in which two hydrogen atoms are transferred at the same time forming fully reduced flavin-H$_2$ or in two separate steps in which one hydrogen is transferred to form the flavin radical (generally written as flavin-H), followed by transfer of a second hydrogen to form the fully reduced flavin-H$_2$ (Figure 2.19).

In some reactions, a single hydrogen is transferred to form flavin-H, which is then recycled in a separate reaction; in other reactions two molecules of flavin each accept one hydrogen atom from the substrate to be oxidised, forming two mol of flavin-H. Other reactions involve the sequential transfer of two hydrogens onto the flavin, forming first the flavin-H radical, then fully reduced flavin-H$_2$. Flavins can thus act as intermediates between obligatory single-electron reactions (for example, haem and obligatory two-electron reactions involving NAD) (Section 3.3.1.2).

The reoxidation of reduced flavins in enzymes that react with oxygen is a major source of potentially damaging oxygen radicals (Section 6.5.2.1).

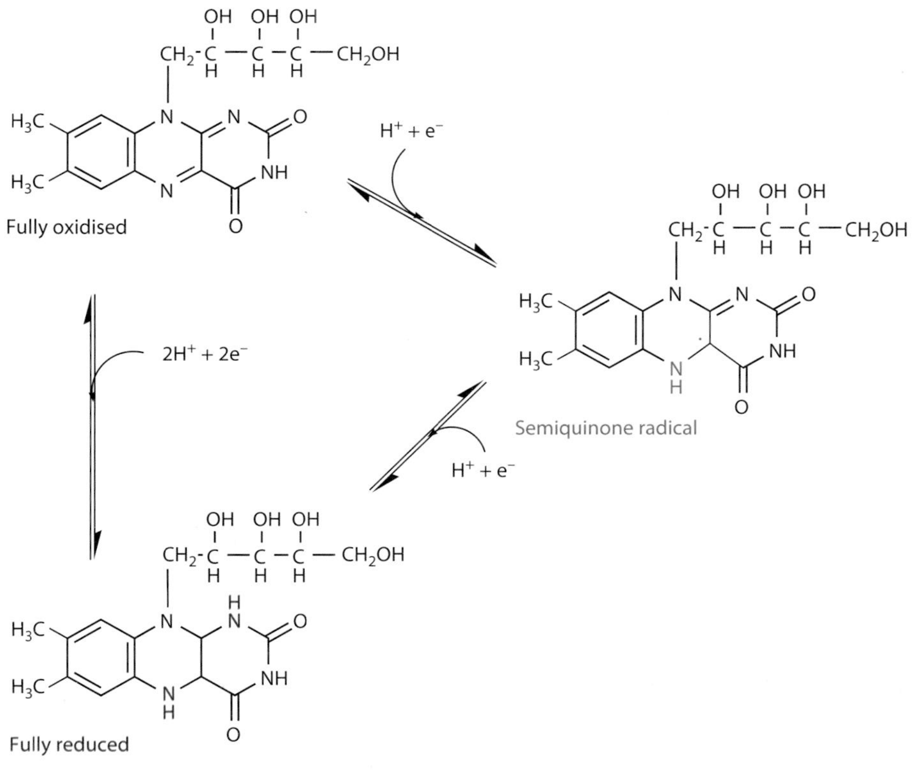

Figure 2.19 Oxidation and reduction of the flavin coenzymes. The reaction may proceed as either a single two-electron reaction or as two single-electron steps with intermediate formation of the riboflavin semiquinone radical.

2.4.1.3   The nicotinamide nucleotide coenzymes: NAD and NADP

The vitamin niacin (Section 11.8) is important for the formation of two related compounds, the nicotinamide nucleotide coenzymes, nicotinamide adenine dinucleotide (NAD) and nicotinamide adenine dinucleotide phosphate (NADP, Figure 2.20). They differ only in that NADP has an additional phosphate group esterified to the ribose. The whole of the coenzyme molecule is essential for binding to enzymes, and most enzymes can bind and use only one of these two coenzymes, either NAD or NADP, despite the overall similarity in their structures.

The functionally important part of these coenzymes is the nicotinamide ring, which undergoes a two-electron reduction. In the oxidised coenzymes, there is a positive charge associated with the nitrogen atom in the nicotinamide ring, and the oxidised forms of the coenzymes are usually shown as NAD^+ and $NADP^+$. Reduction involves the transfer of two electrons and two hydrogen ions (H^+) from the substrate to the coenzyme. One electron neutralises the positive charge on the nitrogen atom. The other, with its associated H^+ ion, is incorporated into the ring as a second hydrogen at carbon 2.

The second H^+ ion removed from the substrate remains associated with the coenzyme. This means that the reaction can be shown as

$$X\text{-}H_2 + NAD^+ \rightleftharpoons X + NADH + H^+$$

where $X\text{-}H_2$ is the substrate and X is the product (the oxidised form of the substrate).

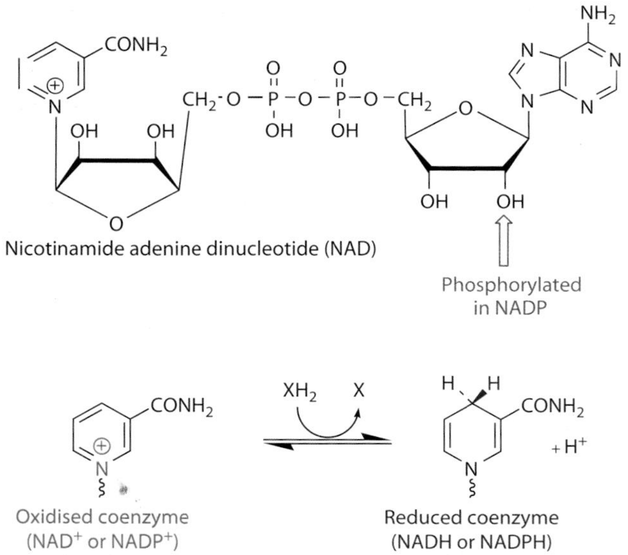

Nicotinamide adenine dinucleotide (NAD)

Phosphorylated
in NADP

Oxidised coenzyme
(NAD^+ or $NADP^+$)

Reduced coenzyme
(NADH or NADPH)

Figure 2.20 The nicotinamide nucleotide coenzymes, NAD and NADP. In the oxidised coenzyme, there is one hydrogen at carbon 4, but by convention, this is not shown when the ring is drawn. In the reduced coenzymes, both hydrogens are shown, with a dotted bond to one hydrogen and a bold bond to the other, to show that the ring as a whole is planar, with one hydrogen at carbon 4 above the plane of the ring, and the other below.

Note that the reaction is reversible, and NADH can act as a reducing agent:

$$X + NADH + H^+ \rightleftharpoons X\text{-}H_2 + NAD^+$$

where X is now the substrate and X-H$_2$ is the product (the reduced form of the substrate).

The usual notation is that NAD and NADP are used when the oxidation state is not relevant, and NAD(P) when either NAD or NADP is being discussed. The oxidised coenzymes are shown as NAD(P)$^+$, and the reduced forms as NAD(P)H.

Unlike flavins and metal coenzymes, the nicotinamide nucleotide coenzymes do not remain bound to the enzyme but act as substrates, binding to the enzyme, undergoing reduction, and then leaving. The reduced coenzyme is then reoxidised either by reaction with another enzyme, for which it acts as a hydrogen donor, or by way of the mitochondrial electron transport chain (Section 3.3.1.2). Cells contain only a small amount of NAD(P) (of the order of 400 nmol/g in liver), which is rapidly cycled between the oxidised and reduced forms by different enzymes.

In general, NAD$^+$ is the coenzyme for oxidation reactions, with most of the resultant NADH being reoxidised directly or indirectly via the mitochondrial electron transport chain (Section 3.3.1.2), whilst NADPH is the main coenzyme for reduction reactions (e.g., the synthesis of fatty acids, Section 5.6.1).

2.5   The classification and naming of enzymes

There is a formal system of enzyme nomenclature, in which each enzyme has a number, and the various enzymes are classified according to the type of reaction catalysed and the substrates, products, and coenzymes of the reaction. This is used in research publications, when there is a need to identify an enzyme unambiguously, but for general use, there is a less formal system of naming enzymes. Almost all enzyme names end in *-ase*, and many are derived simply from the name of the substrate acted on, with the suffix *-ase*. In some cases, the type of reaction catalysed is also included.

Altogether, there are some 5–10,000 enzymes in human tissues. However, they can be classified into only six groups, depending on the types of chemical reaction they catalyse:

1. Oxidation and reduction reactions
2. Transfer of a reactive group from one substrate onto another
3. Hydrolysis of bonds
4. Addition across carbon–carbon double bonds
5. Rearrangement of groups within a single molecule of substrate
6. Formation of bonds between two substrates, frequently linked to the hydrolysis of ATP → ADP + phosphate

This classification of enzymes is expanded in Table 2.2, to give some examples of the types of reactions catalysed.

Each enzyme has a four-part number indicating the overall class of reaction (1–6 in the list above), then the subclass, sub-subclass, and finally the unique number for that enzyme within its sub-subclass. In formal nomenclature, this is shown as EC (for Enzyme Commission) xx.xx.xx.xx.

Table 2.2 Classification of Enzyme-Catalysed Reactions

1. Oxidoreductases	Oxidation and reduction reactions	
	Dehydrogenases	Addition or removal of H
	Oxidases	Two-electron transfer to O_2, forming H_2O_2
		Two-electron transfer to $1/2\ O_2$, forming H_2O
	Oxygenases	Incorporate O_2 into product
	Hydroxylases	Incorporate $1/2\ O_2$ into product as –OH and form H_2O
	Peroxidases	Use as H_2O_2 as oxygen donor, forming H_2O
2. Transferases	Transfer a chemical group from one substrate to the other	
	Kinases	transfer phosphate from ATP onto substrate
3. Hydrolases	Hydrolysis of C–O, C–N, O–P, and C–S bonds	
		(e.g., esterases, proteases, phosphatases, deamidases)
4. Lyases	Addition across a carbon–carbon double bond	
		(e.g., dehydratases, hydratases, decarboxylases)
5. Isomerases	Intramolecular rearrangements	
6. Ligases (synthetases)	Formation of bonds between two substrates	
		Frequently linked to utilisation of ATP, with intermediate formation of phosphorylated enzyme or substrate

2.6 *Metabolic pathways*

A simple reaction such as the oxidation of ethanol (alcohol) to carbon dioxide and water can proceed in a single step—for example, simply by setting fire to the alcohol in air. The reaction is exothermic, and the oxidation of ethanol to carbon dioxide and water has an output of 29 kJ/g.

When alcohol is metabolised in the body, although the overall reaction is the same, it does not proceed in a single step, but as a series of linked reactions, each resulting in a small change in the substrate. In general, any enzyme only catalyses a single simple change in the substrate, although there are enzymes that catalyse more complex reactions. The metabolic oxidation of ethanol (Figure 2.21) involves 11 enzyme-catalysed steps as well as the mitochondrial electron transport chain (Section 3.3.1.2). The energy yield is still 29 kJ/g, since the starting material (ethanol) and the end products (carbon dioxide and water) are the same, and the overall change in energy level is the same, regardless of the route taken. Such a sequence of linked enzyme-catalysed reactions is a metabolic pathway.

Metabolic pathways can be divided into three broad groups:

1. **Catabolic pathways** are involved in the breakdown of relatively large molecules, and oxidation of substrates, ultimately to carbon dioxide and water. These are the main energy-yielding metabolic pathways.
2. **Anabolic pathways** are involved in the synthesis of compounds from simpler precursors. These are the main energy-requiring metabolic pathways. Many are reduction reactions and many involve condensation reactions. Similar reactions are also involved in the metabolism of drugs and other foreign compounds, hormones, and neurotransmitters to yield products that are excreted in the urine or bile.

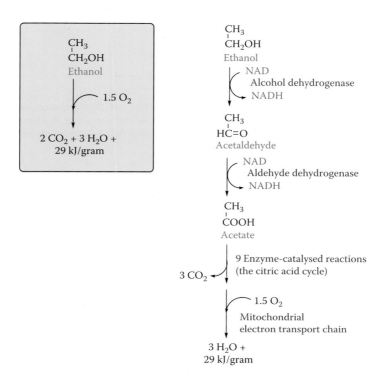

Figure 2.21 The oxidation of ethanol. The box shows the rapid non-enzymic reaction when ethanol is burnt in air; metabolic oxidation of ethanol involves 11 separate enzyme-catalysed steps as well as the mitochondrial electron transport chain. The final products, water and carbon dioxide, and the energy yield of 29 kJ/g are the same for burning ethanol in air or metabolising it.

   3. **Central pathways** are involved in interconversions of substrates that can be regarded as being both catabolic and anabolic and are sometimes called amphibolic. The principal such pathway is the citric acid cycle (Section 5.4.4).

   In some pathways, all the enzymes are free in solution, and intermediate products are released from one enzyme, equilibrate with the pool of intermediate in the cell, and then bind to the next enzyme. In other cases there is channelling of substrates; the product of one enzyme is passed directly to the active site of the next, without equilibrating with the pool of intermediate in the cell.

   Sometimes, this channelling of substrates is achieved by the assembly of the individual enzymes that catalyse a sequence of reactions into a multi-enzyme complex that is in free solution in the cytosol; examples of multi-enzyme complexes include pyruvate dehydrogenase (Section 5.4.3.1) and the very large multi-enzyme complex that catalyses the synthesis of fatty acids (Section 5.6.1). In some cases, enzymes that catalyse adjacent steps in a pathway have undergone gene fusion during evolution; thus, there is a single protein with two catalytic sites, the first of which passes its product directly onto the next.

   In other cases (e.g., the β-oxidation of fatty acids, Section 5.5.2), the enzymes involved in the pathway are arranged on a membrane in such a way that each passes its product to the next in turn, and none of the intermediates can be detected in solution. Such an array of enzymes is sometimes known as a metabolon.

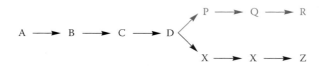

Figure 2.22 Linear and branched metabolic pathways. The relative amounts of intermediate D converted to end products R and Z will depend largely on the values of K_m for the two enzymes involved at the branch point, that forming intermediate P and that forming intermediate X (see also Figure 2.10).

2.6.1   Linear and branched pathways

The simplest type of metabolic pathway is a single sequence of reactions in which the starting material is converted to the end product with no possibility of alternative reactions or branches in the pathway.

Simple linear pathways are rare because many of the intermediate compounds in metabolism can be used in a variety of pathways, depending on the need for different products. Many metabolic pathways involve branch points (Figure 2.22), where an intermediate may proceed down one branch or another. The fate of an intermediate at a branch point will depend on the relative activities of the two enzymes that are competing for the same substrate. As discussed above (Section 2.3.3.1), if the enzymes catalysing the reactions from D → P and from D → X have different values of K_m, then it is possible to predict which branch will predominate at any given intracellular concentration of intermediate D.

Enzymes catalysing reactions at branch points are usually subject to regulation (Section 10.1), to direct substrates through one branch or the other, depending on the body's requirements at the time.

2.6.2   Spiral or looped reaction sequences

Sometimes, a metabolic pathway involves repeating a series of reactions several times over. For example, the oxidation of fatty acids (Section 5.5.2) proceeds by the sequential removal of two-carbon units. The removal of each two-carbon unit involves a repeated sequence of four reactions, and the end product of each cycle of the pathway is a fatty acid that is two carbons shorter than the one that entered. It then undergoes the same sequence of reactions (Figure 2.23).

Similarly, the synthesis of fatty acids (Section 5.6.1) involves the repeated addition of two-carbon units until the final chain length (16 carbon atoms) has been achieved. The addition of each two-carbon unit involves four separate reaction steps, which are repeated in each cycle of the pathway. The enzymes of this pathway form a large multi-enzyme complex in which the growing fatty acid chain is transferred from one active site to the next by a flexible carrier protein (the acyl carrier protein).

2.6.3   Cyclic pathways

The third type of metabolic pathway is cyclic; a product is assembled, or a substrate is catabolised, attached to a carrier molecule that is unchanged at the end of each cycle of reactions.

Figure 2.24 shows a cyclic biosynthetic pathway in cartoon form; the product is built up in a series of reactions, then released, regenerating the carrier molecule. An example of such a pathway is the urea synthesis cycle (Section 9.3.1.4).

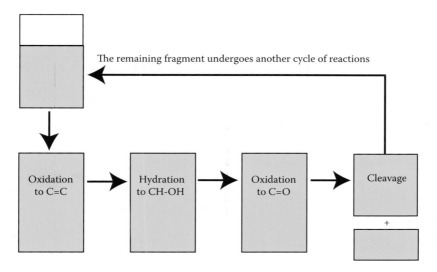

Figure 2.23 A spiral or looped (repeating) metabolic pathway. The product of the final reaction (cleavage) undergoes repeated cycles of reaction. An example of such a pathway is the β-oxidation of fatty acids (see Figure 5.24).

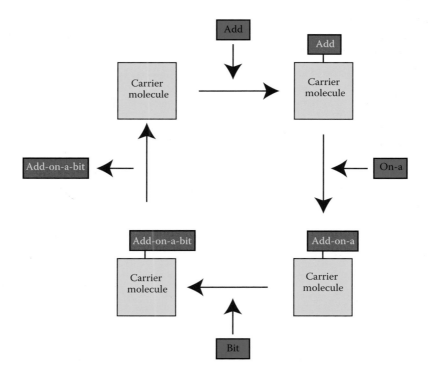

Figure 2.24 A biosynthetic cyclic metabolic pathway. The product is built up sequentially on a carrier molecule that is unchanged at the end of the reaction cycle. As long as sufficient amounts of the substrates are available, increasing the concentration of any of the intermediates of the cycle will lead to an increase in the amount of carrier molecule available, and hence an increased rate of formation of the final product. An example of such a pathway is the urea synthesis cycle (see Figure 9.16).

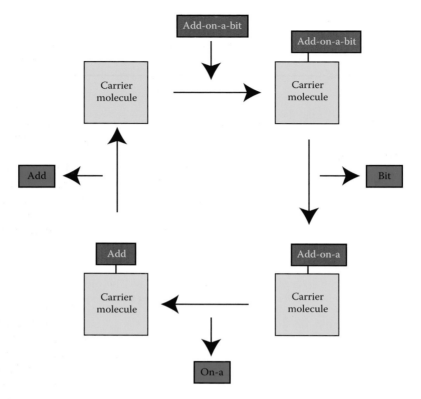

Figure 2.25 A catabolic cyclic metabolic pathway. The substrate to be catabolised is reacted with a carrier molecule and is then broken down sequentially, leaving the unchanged carrier molecule at the end of the reaction cycle. As long as a sufficient amount of the substrate is available, increasing the concentration of any of the intermediates of the cycle will lead to an increase in the amount of carrier molecule available and hence an increased rate of catabolism of the substrate. An example of such a pathway is the citric acid cycle (see Figure 5.18).

Figure 2.25 shows a cyclic catabolic pathway in cartoon form; the substrate is bound to the carrier molecule, then undergoes a series of reactions in which parts are removed, until at the end of the reaction sequence the original carrier molecule is left. An example of such a pathway is the citric acid cycle (Section 5.4.4).

The intermediates in a cyclic pathway can be considered to be catalysts, in that they participate in the reaction sequence, but at the end, they apparently emerge unchanged. Until all the enzymes in a cyclic pathway are saturated (and hence acting at V_{max}), as long as enough of the initial substrate is available, the addition of any one of the intermediates will result in an increase in the intracellular concentration of all intermediates, and hence an increase in the concentration of the carrier molecule. This leads to an increase in the rate at which the cycle runs, and either the substrate is catabolised or the product is formed (see the urea synthesis experiment in the Virtual Laboratory on the CD).

2.7   *Enzymes in clinical chemistry and medicine*

There are three areas in which enzymes can be exploited in clinical chemistry, measurement of metabolites, measurement of enzymes in plasma as a diagnostic tool, and assessment of vitamin nutritional status.

2.7.1 Measurement of metabolites in blood, urine, and tissue samples

Enzyme assays provide two advantages over conventional chemical assays: they have high sensitivity; thus, very small amounts of analyte can be detected (and therefore only small amounts of sample are needed), and because enzymes have a high degree of specificity for their substrates, they are very specific for the substance being measured. For example, the chemical measurement of glucose in urine depends on reduction of Cu^{2+} to Cu^+ in alkaline solution, and a variety of other compounds that may occur in urine will also reduce copper ions; by contrast, the enzyme glucose oxidase detects only glucose and not other reducing compounds.

Obviously, to measure the amount of a substrate in a sample, the limiting factor in the formation of the product must be the concentration of substrate available. The enzyme must be present in excess, and the sample must be diluted to ensure that the concentration of substrate is considerably lower than the K_m of the enzyme—i.e. the reaction conditions are such that the enzyme is operating in region A of Figure 2.9, and a small difference in substrate leads to a large difference in the amount of product formed.

2.7.2 Measurement of enzymes in blood samples

Many enzymes occur in blood plasma as a result of both normal turnover of cells and also pathological tissue damage; they are released into the bloodstream by the dying cells. Although these enzymes can be measured in plasma, they have no function in the bloodstream; they are simply markers of tissue turnover and damage. An abnormally high amount of one or more enzymes in a plasma sample is indicative of tissue damage, and the pattern of enzymes released is a useful diagnostic tool (Table 2.3). In a number of cases, there are different forms of the same enzyme in different tissues—isoenzymes that catalyse the same reaction but differ in their pH optimum, sensitivity to inhibitors or mild heat treatment, or some other readily measurable property; thus, it is possible to differentiate between, for example, alkaline phosphatase from the bone or liver, which would be useful in determining, for example, whether bone pain was due to primary bone disease or metastasis of a liver cancer into bone.

Figure 2.26 shows the pattern of enzymes released by damaged cardiac muscle cells after a myocardial infarction. The extent to which the enzymes are raised above the normal

Table 2.3 Diagnostically Useful Enzymes in Plasma

Enzyme	Elevated in
Acid phosphatase	Prostate cancer
Alanine aminotransferase	Liver disease
Alkaline phosphatase (different tissue-specific isoenzymes in bone and liver)	Cholestatic liver disease, bone disease, rickets, and osteomalacia (see Section 11.3.4)
Amylase	Acute pancreatitis
Aspartate aminotransferase	Liver disease, muscle disease, myocardiac infarction
Creatine kinase	Muscle disease, myocardiac infarction
γ-Glutamyl transpeptidase	Early liver disease
Lactate dehydrogenase (different tissue-specific isoenzymes in liver, skeletal, and cardiac muscle)	Liver disease, muscle disease, myocardiac infarction

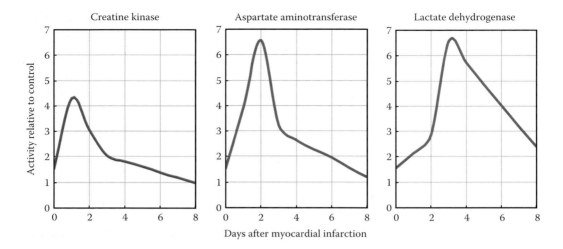

Figure 2.26 The time course and relative increases in the activity of plasma enzymes after a myocardial infarction. The enzymes are released from dying heart muscle cells and have no function in the bloodstream.

level indicates the severity of the tissue damage. If the activities of the enzymes do not fall in the expected way, this is an indication that the patient has suffered one or more further infarctions, suggesting a poor prognosis.

If the aim is to determine the activity of an enzyme in plasma, then obviously, the limiting factor must be the amount of enzyme present and not the amount of substrate provided in the assay medium. Ideally, the enzyme should be saturated with substrate; conventionally, the concentration of substrate added is some 10 to 20 times greater than the K_m of the enzyme; thus, it is acting at or near V_{max} (i.e., in region B of Figure 2.9), and a small change in the amount of substrate will have little or no effect on the activity of the enzyme.

2.7.3   Assessment of vitamin nutritional status

For enzymes that have a tightly bound cofactor that is derived from a vitamin, the extent to which red blood cells can compete with other tissues for the coenzyme provides a sensitive means of assessing nutritional status. Three such coenzymes are

1. Thiamin diphosphate (derived from vitamin B_1, Section 11.6), the coenzyme of transketolase
2. Flavin adenine dinucleotide (derived from vitamin B_2, Section 11.7), the coenzyme of glutathione reductase
3. Pyridoxal phosphate (derived from vitamin B_6, Section 11.9), the coenzyme of various transaminases

Tissue contains

- Enzyme protein with coenzyme (the holo-enzyme), which is catalytically active
- Enzyme protein without coenzyme (the apo-enzyme), which is catalytically inactive

Incubation of a red blood cell lysate with substrate *in vitro* without added coenzyme permits measurement of what was initially present as holo-enzyme, whilst incubation with substrate after the addition of coenzyme permits activation (and hence measurement) of the apo-enzyme as well. The increase in catalytic activity after addition of coenzyme is the activation coefficient; for someone whose vitamin status was good, the activation coefficient will be only slightly greater than 1.0; the higher the activation coefficient (meaning that there is more apo-enzyme without its coenzyme), the poorer the subject's vitamin status.

Key points

- Breaking covalent bonds involves an input of energy (the activation energy) to excite electrons to an unstable configuration.
- Exothermic reactions proceed with output of heat; endothermic reactions require an input of energy.
- Enzymes catalyse reactions by lowering the activation energy; they increase the rate at which equilibrium is reached, but do not affect the position of equilibrium. *In vivo*, reactions are not normally at equilibrium because there is constant flux through a pathway.
- The active site of an enzyme comprises a substrate binding site and a catalytic site; both are formed by reactive groups in the side chains of amino acids that may be some distance apart in the primary sequence of the protein.
- Enzymes show considerable specificity for the substrates bound, and the reaction catalysed.
- Enzymes may have non-protein components, coenzymes or prosthetic groups that may be covalently or non-covalently bound to the protein and are essential for activity.
- Most enzymes show a hyperbolic relation between the concentration of substrate and the rate of reaction; V_{max} is the maximum rate of reaction when the enzyme is saturated with substrate.
- K_m is an inverse measure of the affinity of an enzyme for its substrate; it is the concentration of substrate at which the enzyme achieves half V_{max}.
- A variety of compounds inhibit enzymes; irreversible inhibitors bind covalently to the active site, permanently inactivating a molecule of enzyme. Reversible inhibitors may be competitive with respect to substrate, non-competitive or uncompetitive.
- A metabolic pathway is a sequence of enzyme-catalysed reactions; pathways may be linear, branched, looped, or cyclic.
- Enzymes can be used to measure metabolites in blood, urine, and tissue samples; measurement of enzymes in plasma samples is useful diagnostically.

Further resources on the CD

The enzyme assay and enzyme purification computer simulations in the virtual laboratory on the CD.

chapter three

The role of ATP in metabolism

Adenosine triphosphate (ATP) acts as the central link between energy-yielding metabolic pathways and energy expenditure in physical and chemical work. The oxidation of metabolic fuels is linked to the phosphorylation of adenosine diphosphate (ADP) to ATP, whereas the expenditure of metabolic energy for the synthesis of body constituents, transport of compounds across cell membranes, and the contraction of muscle results in the hydrolysis of ATP to yield ADP and phosphate ions. The total body content of ATP + ADP is under 350 mmol (about 10 g), but the amount of ATP synthesised and used each day is about 100 mol—about 70 kg, an amount equal to body weight.

Objectives

After reading this chapter, you should be able to

- Explain how endothermic reactions can be linked to the overall hydrolysis of ATP → ADP and phosphate.
- Describe how compounds can be transported across cell membranes against a concentration gradient and explain the roles of ATP and proton gradients in active transport.
- Describe the role of ATP in muscle contraction and the role of creatine phosphate as a phosphagen.
- Describe the structure and functions of the mitochondrion and explain the processes involved in the mitochondrial electron transport chain and oxidative phosphorylation, explain how substrate oxidation is regulated by the availability of ADP, and how respiratory poisons and uncouplers act.

3.1   The adenine nucleotides

Nucleotides consist of a purine or pyrimidine base linked to the 5-carbon sugar ribose. The base plus sugar is a nucleoside; in a nucleotide the sugar is phosphorylated. Nucleotides may be mono-, di-, or triphosphates.

Figure 3.1 shows the nucleotides formed from the purine adenine—the adenine nucleotides, adenosine monophosphate (AMP), ADP, and ATP. Similar families of nucleotides that are important in metabolism are formed from the guanine and uracil. See also Section 10.3.2 for a discussion of the role of cyclic AMP in metabolic regulation and hormone action and Section 10.3.1 for the role of guanine nucleotides in response to hormone action.

In the nucleic acids (DNA and RNA, Sections 9.2.1 and 9.2.2), it is the purine or pyrimidine base that is important, carrying the genetic information. However, in the link between energy-yielding metabolism and the performance of physical and chemical work, what is important is the phosphorylation of the ribose of the nucleotides. Although most enzymic reactions are linked to utilisation of ATP, a small number are linked to guanosine triphosphate (GTP) or uridine triphosphate (UTP).

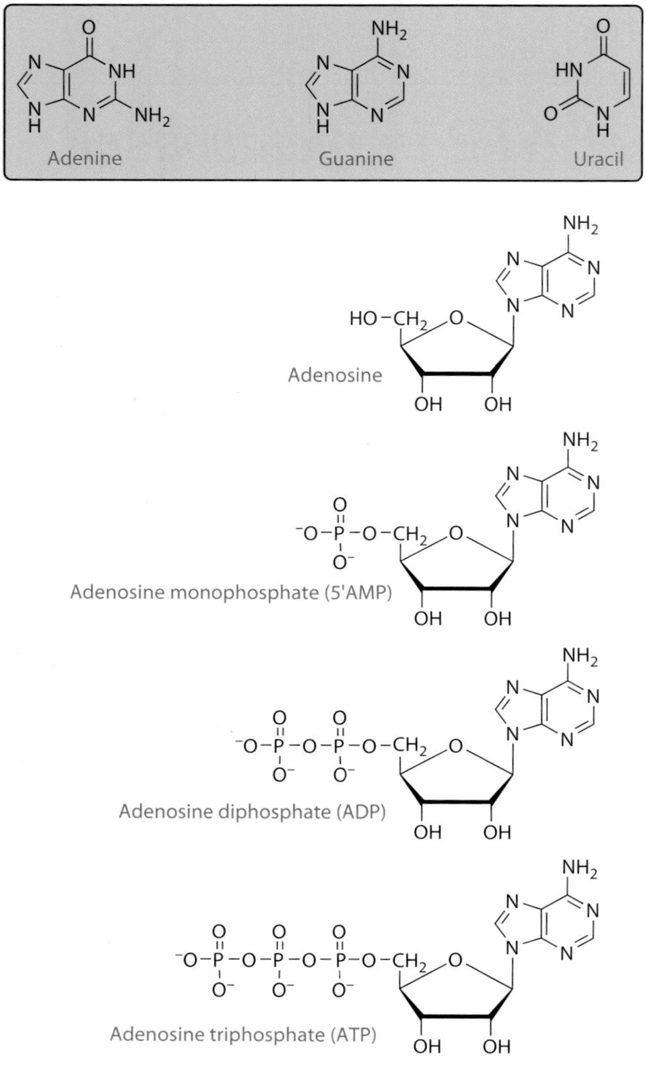

Figure 3.1 The adenine nucleotides (the box shows the structures of adenine, guanine, and uracil; guanine and uracil form a similar series of nucleotides).

3.2 Functions of ATP

Under normal conditions, the processes shown in Figure 3.2 are tightly coupled; thus, the oxidation of metabolic fuels is controlled by the availability of ADP, which, in turn, is controlled by the rate at which ATP is being utilised in performing physical and chemical work. Work output, or energy expenditure, thus controls the rate at which metabolic fuels are oxidised and hence the amount of food that must be eaten to meet energy requirements. Metabolic fuels in excess of immediate requirements are stored as reserves of glycogen in muscle and liver (Section 5.6.3) and fat in adipose tissue (Section 5.6.1).

In all of the reactions in which ATP is utilised, what is observed overall is hydrolysis of ATP → ADP and phosphate. However, although this is the overall reaction, simple

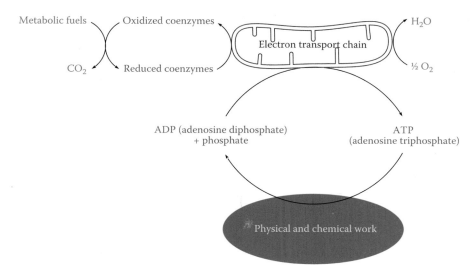

Figure 3.2 Linkage between ATP utilisation in physical and chemical work and the oxidation of metabolic fuels.

hydrolysis of ATP does not achieve any useful result; it is the intermediate steps in the reaction of ATP + H_2O → ADP + phosphate that are important.

3.2.1   The role of ATP in endothermic reactions

The equilibrium of an endothermic reaction A + B ⇌ C + D lies well to the left unless there is an input of energy (Section 2.1.1). The hydrolysis of ATP is exothermic, and the equilibrium of the reaction ATP + H_2O ⇌ ADP + phosphate lies well to the right. Linkage between the two reactions could thus ensure that the (unfavoured) endothermic reaction could proceed together with overall hydrolysis of ATP → ADP + phosphate.

Such linkage between two apparently unrelated reactions can easily be achieved in enzyme-catalysed reactions; there are three possible mechanisms:

1. Phosphorylation of the hydroxyl group of a serine, threonine, or tyrosine residue in the enzyme (Figure 3.3), thus altering the chemical nature of its catalytic site. Phosphorylation of the enzyme is also important in regulating metabolic pathways, especially in response to hormone action (Section 10.3).

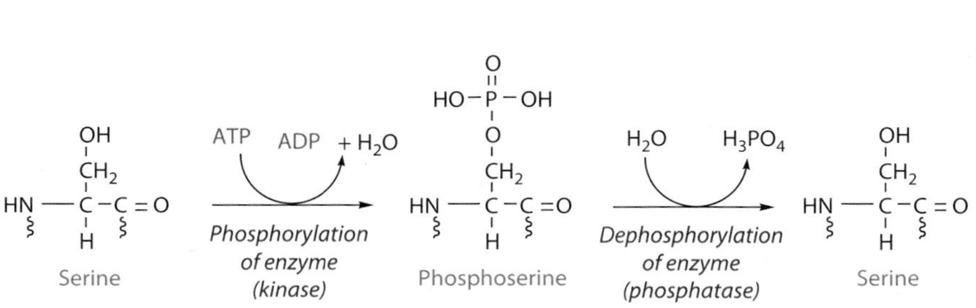

Figure 3.3 The role of ATP in endothermic reactions—phosphorylation of the enzyme.

2. Phosphorylation of one of the substrates. The synthesis of glutamine from glutamate and ammonia (Figure 3.4 and Section 9.3.1.3) involves the formation of a phosphorylated intermediate.

3. Transfer of the adenosyl group of ATP onto one of the substrates (Figure 3.5). The activation of the methyl group of the amino acid methionine in methyltransfer reactions involves formation of *S*-adenosyl methionine (Figure 6.22).

Not only is the hydrolysis of ATP → ADP + phosphate an exothermic reaction, but the concentration of ATP in cells is always very much higher than that of ADP (a ratio of about 500:1), again ensuring that the reaction will proceed in the direction of ATP hydrolysis. The concentration of ADP in the cell is kept low in two ways:

1. ADP is normally rapidly phosphorylated to ATP, which is linked to the oxidation of metabolic fuels (Section 3.3.1).

2. If ADP begins to accumulate, adenylate kinase catalyses the reaction: $2 \times \text{ADP} \rightleftharpoons \text{AMP} + \text{ATP}$. This not only removes ADP and provides (a small amount of) ATP, AMP also acts as a signal of the energy state of the cell and is a potent activator or inhibitor of a number of key enzymes that regulate metabolic pathways (Section 10.2.2.1).

In a number of cases, there is a further mechanism to ensure that the equilibrium of an ATP-linked reaction lies to the right, to such an extent that the reaction is essentially irreversible. The reaction shown in Figure 3.6 results in the hydrolysis of ATP → AMP + pyrophosphate. There is an active pyrophosphatase in cells, which catalyses the hydrolysis of pyrophosphate to yield 2 mol of phosphate, removing one of the products of the reaction; thus, the substrate for the reverse reaction is not available.

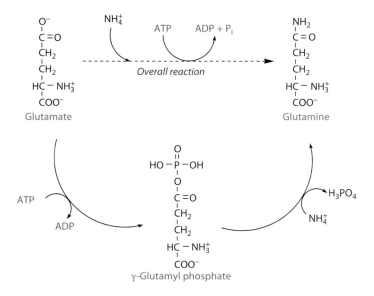

Figure 3.4 The role of ATP in endothermic reactions—phosphorylation of the substrate.

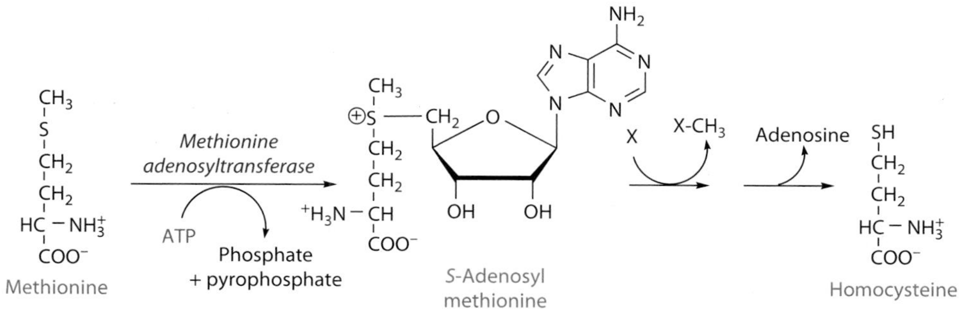

Figure 3.5 The role of ATP in endothermic reactions—adenylation of the substrate (see also Figure 6.22).

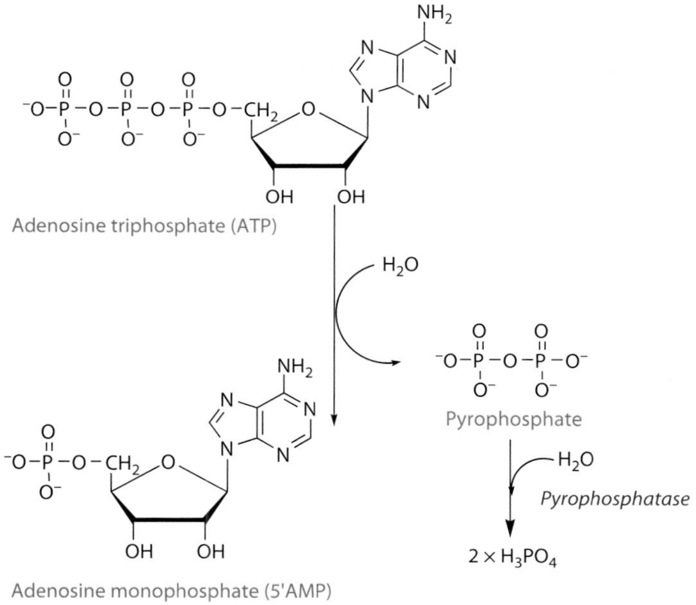

Figure 3.6 Hydrolysis of ATP → AMP and pyrophosphate and the action of pyrophosphatase.

3.2.2   *Transport of materials across cell membranes*

Lipid-soluble compounds will diffuse freely across cell membranes, since they can dissolve in the membrane—this is passive diffusion. However, because most lipid-soluble compounds are hydrophobic, they normally require to be bound to transport proteins in the extracellular fluid, and to binding proteins inside the cell. Hydrophilic compounds require a transport protein to cross the lipid membrane—this is facilitated or carrier-mediated diffusion. Neither passive nor facilitated diffusion alone can lead to a greater concentration of the material being transported inside the cell than that present outside.

Concentrative uptake of the material being transported may be achieved in three main ways: protein binding, metabolic trapping, and active transport. The latter two mechanisms are ATP-dependent.

3.2.2.1   *Protein binding for concentrative uptake*

Hydrophobic compounds are transported in plasma bound to transport proteins (e.g., serum albumin, the plasma retinol binding protein, Section 11.2.2.2, and steroid hormone binding proteins, or dissolved in the lipid core of plasma lipoproteins, Section 5.6.2). Accumulation to a higher concentration than in plasma depends on an intracellular binding protein that has a greater affinity for the ligand than does the plasma transport protein. The different isomers of vitamin E (Section 11.4.1) have very different biological activity (or potency); at least part of this is explained by the specificity of the intracellular vitamin E binding proteins for the different isomers.

For a hydrophilic compound that enters the cell by carrier-mediated diffusion, a net increase in concentration inside the cell can sometimes be achieved by binding it to an intracellular protein. Binding proteins are important in the intestinal absorption of calcium (Section 11.15.1) and iron (Section 11.15.2.3).

3.2.2.2   *Metabolic trapping*

Glucose enters and leaves liver cells by carrier-mediated diffusion, although in other tissues, there is (sodium-dependent) active transport of glucose. In the fed state, when there is a great deal of glucose to be stored as glycogen, it diffuses into the liver cells and is phosphorylated to glucose 6-phosphate, a reaction catalysed by the enzymes hexokinase and glucokinase, using ATP as the phosphate donor (Section 5.4.1). Glucose 6-phosphate does not cross cell membranes, and therefore, there is a net accumulation of [glucose plus glucose 6-phosphate] inside the cell, at the expense of 1 mol of ATP per 1 mol of glucose trapped in this way. Vitamins B_2 (riboflavin, Section 11.7) and B_6 (Section 11.9) are similarly accumulated inside cells by phosphorylation at the expense of ATP.

3.2.2.3   *Active transport*

Active transport is the accumulation of a higher concentration of a compound on one side of a cell membrane than the other, without chemical modification such as phosphorylation. The process is dependent on hydrolysis of ATP $\rightarrow$ ADP + phosphate, either directly, in the case of ion pumps, or indirectly, when metabolites are transported by proton- or sodium-dependent transporters.

3.2.2.4   *P-type transporters*

In the P-type transporters, which transport cations, the transport protein is phosphorylated as part of the cycle of activity. Figure 3.7 shows the role of ATP in the sodium–potassium transporter. When the protein has bound ATP, it has a high affinity for Na^+ ions inside the cell. Phosphorylation of the protein causes a conformational change; thus, the three bound Na^+ ions are expelled from the cell, and the transport now binds two K^+ ions at the outer surface of the membrane. Binding of K^+ ions causes a further conformational change, with dephosphorylation of the protein, which now binds ATP again, expels K^+ ions into the cytosol, and is ready to bind more Na^+ ions. There is an animation to show the action of a P-type transporter on the CD.

3.2.2.5   *ABC transporters*

Figure 3.8 shows the role of ATP in transport proteins that bind and hydrolyse ATP but are not phosphorylated. These proteins all have a similar ATP-binding motif and are known as ATP-binding cassette proteins (ABC transporters). Some ABC transporters act for uptake of molecules into the cell, others act to transport molecules out of the cell.

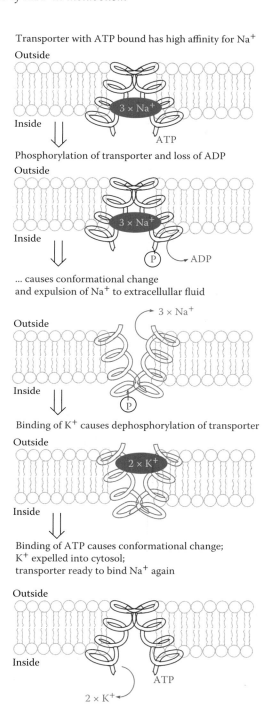

Figure 3.7 The role of ATP in active transport: P-type transporters that have to be phosphorylated to permit transport across the cell membrane (see also the animation on the CD).

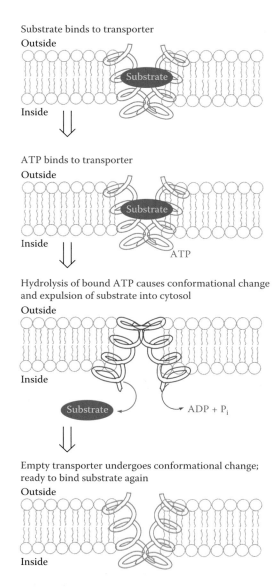

Figure 3.8 The role of ATP in active transport: ABC transporters that bind and hydrolyse ATP but are not phosphorylated (see also the animation on the CD).

The transporter with the ligand binds ATP. Hydrolysis of the bound ATP causes a conformational change in the protein so that the ligand is transported to the opposite face of the membrane, and expelled. Expulsion of the ligand causes the reverse conformational change; thus, the transporter is open at the opposite side of the membrane, ready to bind more ligand. The intestinal transport proteins that expel sterols into the lumen (Section 4.3.1.3) are ABC transporters, as is the chloride transport protein that is defective in cystic fibrosis. There is an animation to show the action of an ABC transporter on the CD.

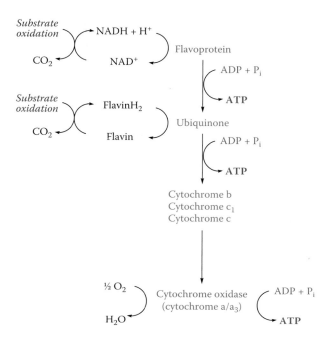

Figure 3.18 An overview of the mitochondrial electron transport chain.

occur with solubilised preparations from mitochondria, nor with open fragments of mitochondrial inner membrane. Under normal conditions, these three processes are linked, and none can occur without the others.

3.3.1.2   The mitochondrial electron transport chain

The mitochondrial electron transport chain is a series of enzymes and coenzymes in the crista membrane, each of which is reduced by the preceding coenzyme and in turn reduces the next, until finally, the protons and electrons that have entered the chain from either NADH or reduced flavin reduce oxygen to water. The sequence of the electron carriers (Figure 3.18) has been determined in two ways:

1. By consideration of their electrochemical redox potentials, which permits determination of which carrier is likely to reduce another and which is likely to be reduced. There is a steady fall in redox potential between the enzyme that oxidises NADH and that which reduces oxygen to water.
2. By incubation of mitochondria with substrates, in the absence of oxygen, when all of the carriers become reduced, then introducing a limited amount of oxygen, and following the sequence in which the carriers become oxidised, shown by changes in their absorption spectra.

Studies with inhibitors of specific electron carriers and with artificial substrates that oxidise or reduce one specific carrier permit the dissection of the electron transport chain into four complexes of electron carriers:

1. Complex I catalyses the oxidation of NADH and the reduction of ubiquinone and is associated with the phosphorylation of ADP to ATP.

2. Complex II catalyses the oxidation of reduced flavins and the reduction of ubiquinone. This complex is not associated with phosphorylation of ADP to ATP.
3. Complex III catalyses the oxidation of reduced ubiquinone and the reduction of cytochrome c and is associated with the phosphorylation of ADP to ATP.
4. Complex IV catalyses the oxidation of reduced cytochrome c and the reduction of oxygen to water, and is associated with the phosphorylation of ADP to ATP.

To understand how the transfer of electrons through the electron transport chain is linked to the phosphorylation of ADP to ATP, it is necessary to consider the chemistry of the various electron carriers. They can be classified into two groups, hydrogen carriers and electron carriers.

Hydrogen carriers (NAD, flavins, and ubiquinone) undergo reduction and oxidation reactions involving both protons and electrons. NAD undergoes a two-electron oxidation/reduction reaction (Figure 2.20), whilst the flavins (Figure 2.19) may undergo a two-electron or two single-electron reactions to form a half-reduced radical, then the fully reduced coenzyme. Ubiquinone (Figure 3.19) undergoes only two single-electron reactions to form a half-reduced radical, then the fully reduced coenzyme.

Electron carriers (the cytochromes and non-haem iron proteins, Figure 3.20) contain iron (and in the case of cytochrome oxidase also copper); they undergo oxidation and reduction by electron transfer alone. In the cytochromes, the iron is present in a haem molecule; in the non-haem iron proteins, the iron is bound to the protein through the sulphur atoms of the amino acid cysteine—these are sometimes called iron–sulphur proteins.

Three different types of haem occur in cytochromes:

1. Haem (protoporphyrin IX) is tightly but non-covalently bound to proteins, including cytochromes b and b_1 as well as enzymes such as catalase, and the oxygen transport proteins haemoglobin and myoglobin.
2. Haem C is covalently bound to protein in cytochromes c and c_1.
3. Haem A is anchored in the membrane by its hydrophobic side chain, in cytochromes a and a_3 (which together form cytochrome oxidase).

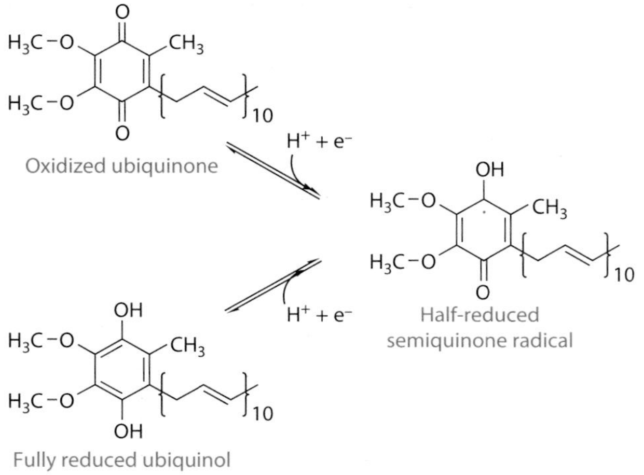

Figure 3.19 Oxidation and reduction of ubiquinone (coenzyme Q).

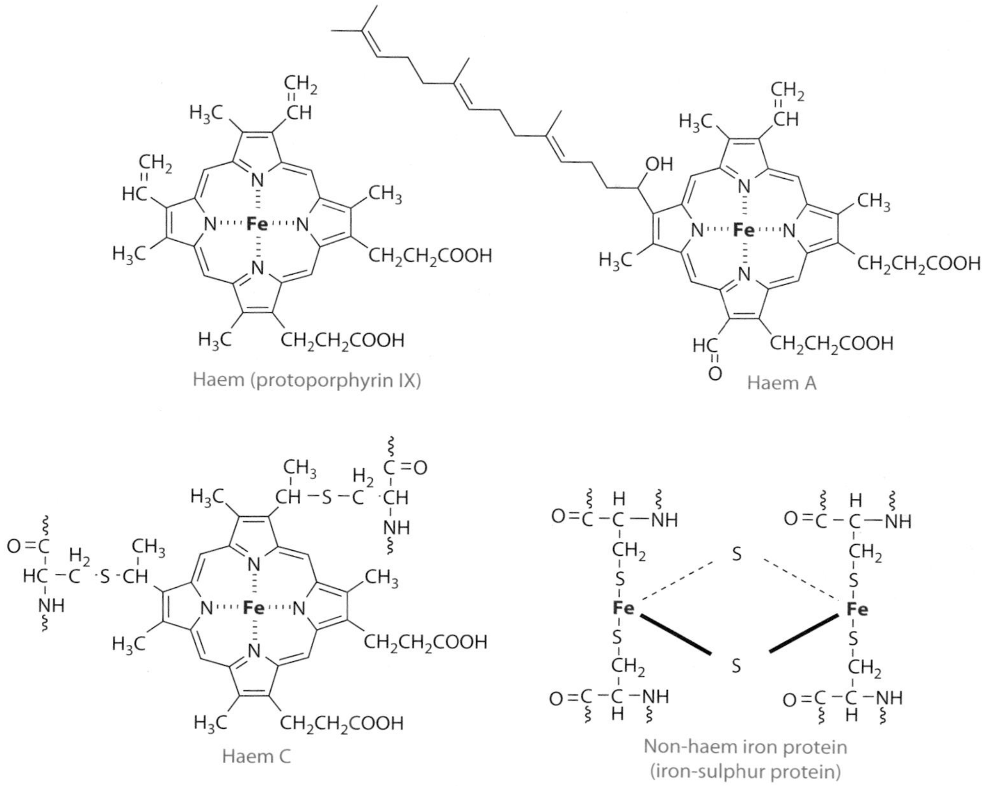

Figure 3.20 Iron-containing carriers of the electron transport chain: haem and non-haem iron proteins.

The hydrogen and electron carriers of the electron transport chain are arranged in sequence in the crista membrane (Figure 3.21). Some carriers are located entirely within the membrane, whilst others are at the inner or outer surface of the membrane.

There are two steps in which a hydrogen carrier reduces an electron carrier: the reaction between the flavin and non-haem iron protein in complex I and the reaction between ubiquinol and cytochrome b plus a non-haem iron protein in complex III. The reaction between non-haem iron protein and ubiquinone in complex I is the reverse—a hydrogen carrier is reduced by an electron carrier.

When a hydrogen carrier reduces an electron carrier, there is a proton that is not transferred onto the electron carrier but is extruded from the membrane into the crista space (Figure 3.22).

When an electron carrier reduces a hydrogen carrier, there is a need for a proton to accompany the electron that is transferred. This is acquired from the mitochondrial matrix, thus shifting the equilibrium between $H_2O \rightleftharpoons H^+ + OH^-$, resulting in an accumulation of hydroxyl ions in the matrix.

3.3.1.3   *Phosphorylation of ADP linked to electron transport*

The result of electron transport through the electron transport chain and the alternation between hydrogen carriers and electron carriers is a separation of protons and hydroxyl

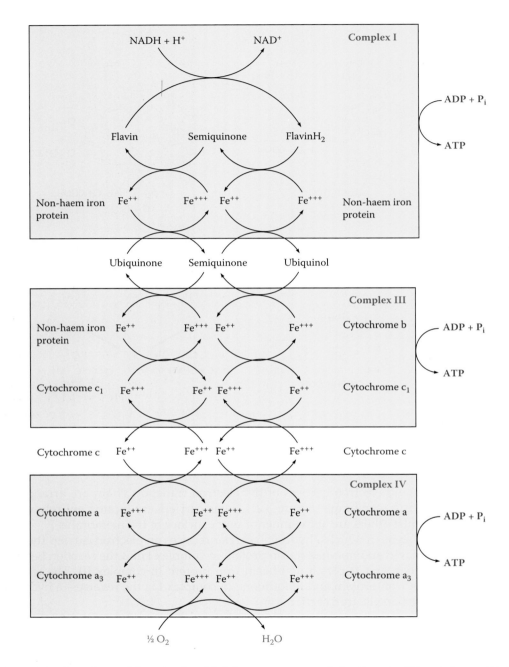

Figure 3.21 Complexes of the mitochondrial electron transport chain. Complex II is not shown; it is the reduction of ubiquinone by flavoproteins and is not associated with the phosphorylation of ADP to ATP.

ions across the crista membrane, with an accumulation of protons in the crista space, and an accumulation of hydroxyl ions in the matrix—i.e., creation of a pH gradient across the inner membrane. Overall, approximately 10 protons are expelled into the inter-membrane space when NADH is oxidised and 7 when reduced flavin is oxidised. These protons re-enter the mitochondrial matrix through a proton transport pore that forms the stalk of

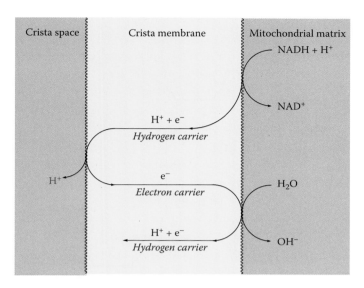

Figure 3.22 Hydrogen and electron carriers in the mitochondrial electron transport chain—generation of a transmembrane proton gradient.

ATP synthase (Figure 3.23), and the proton gradient provides the driving force for the highly endothermic phosphorylation of ADP to ATP (Figure 3.24).

ATP synthase acts as a molecular motor, driven by the flow of protons down the concentration gradient from the crista space into the matrix, through the transmembrane stalk of the primary particle. As protons flow through the stalk, they cause rotation of the core of the multi-enzyme complex that makes up ATP synthase.

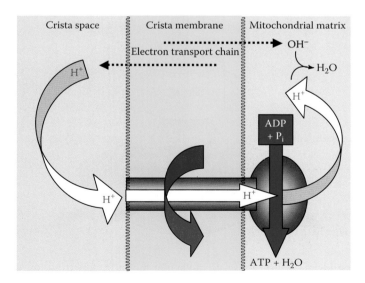

Figure 3.23 The re-entry of protons into the mitochondrial matrix through the stalk of ATP synthase. As protons travel through the stalk, they cause rotation of the central core of ATP synthase, which affects the conformation of the three active sites of the enzyme.

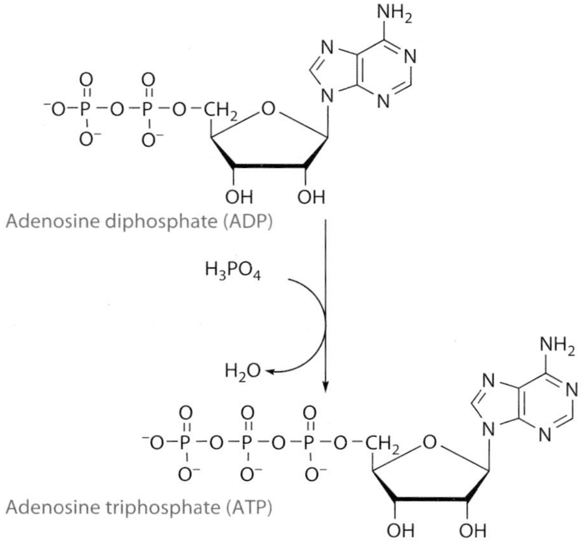

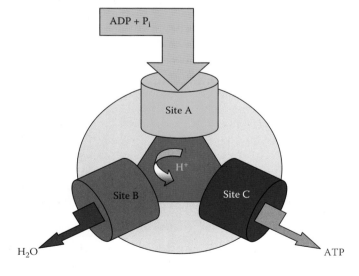

Figure 3.24 Condensation of ADP + phosphate → ATP.

There are three equivalent catalytic sites in ATP synthase, and each one-third turn of the central core causes a conformational change at each active site (Figure 3.25):

A. At one site, the conformational change permits binding of ADP and phosphate.
B. At the next site, the conformational change brings ADP and phosphate close enough together to undergo condensation and expel water.

Figure 3.25 Mitochondrial ATP synthase—a molecular motor. At any time, one site (shown here as site A) is binding ADP + P_i, the next (site B) is condensing ADP + P_i → ATP, and the third site (site C) is expelling ATP. The central core rotates in response to protons flowing through the transmembrane stalk of the enzyme, each site in turn undergoes a conformational change, site A becoming equivalent to B, B to C, and C to A.

C. At the third site, the conformational change causes expulsion of ATP from the site, leaving it free to accept ADP and phosphate at the next turn.

At any time, one site is binding ADP and phosphate, one is undergoing condensation, and the third is expelling ATP. If ADP is not available to bind at the empty site, then rotation cannot occur—and if rotation cannot occur, then protons cannot flow through the stalk from the crista space into the matrix.

3.3.1.4   The coupling of electron transport, oxidative phosphorylation, and fuel oxidation

The processes of oxidation of reduced coenzymes and phosphorylation of ADP → ATP are normally tightly coupled:

- ADP phosphorylation cannot occur unless there is a proton gradient across the crista membrane resulting from the oxidation of NADH or reduced flavins.
- If there is no ADP available, the oxidation of NADH and reduced flavins cannot occur because the protons cannot re-enter through the stalk of ATP synthase, and so the proton gradient becomes large enough to inhibit further transport of protons into the crista space. Indeed, experimentally, it is possible to force reverse electron transport and reduction of NAD^+ and flavins by creating a proton gradient across the crista membrane.

Metabolic fuels can only be oxidised when NAD^+ and oxidised flavoproteins are available. Therefore, if there is little or no ADP available in the mitochondria (i.e. it has all been phosphorylated to ATP), there will be an accumulation of reduced coenzymes, and hence a slowing of the rate of oxidation of metabolic fuels. This means that substrates are only oxidised when ADP is available and there is a need for formation of ATP. The availability of ADP is dependent on the utilisation of ATP is performing physical and chemical work (Figure 3.2). The rate of oxidation of metabolic fuels, and hence utilisation of oxygen, is controlled by energy expenditure in physical and chemical work.

3.3.1.5   Uncouplers

It is possible to uncouple electron transport and ADP phosphorylation by adding a weak acid such as dinitrophenol, which transports protons across the crista membrane. In the presence of such an uncoupler, the protons expelled during electron transport do not accumulate in the crista space but are transported into the mitochondrial matrix, bypassing the ATP synthase (Figure 3.26). This means that ADP is not phosphorylated to ATP, and the oxidation of NADH and reduced flavins can continue unimpeded until all the available oxygen (or substrate) has been consumed. Figure 3.27 shows the oxygen electrode trace in the presence of an uncoupler—there is rapid and more or less complete utilisation of oxygen, whether or not ADP has been added to the incubation.

The result of uncoupling electron transport from the phosphorylation of ADP is that a great deal of substrate is oxidised, with little production of ATP, although heat is produced. A moderate degree of uncoupling provides a physiological mechanism for non-shivering thermogenesis (heat production to maintain body temperature without performing physical work) by activating uncoupling proteins in mitochondria.

The first such uncoupling protein to be identified was in brown adipose tissue and was called thermogenin because of its role in thermogenesis. Brown adipose tissue is anatomically and functionally distinct from the white adipose tissue that is the main site of fat

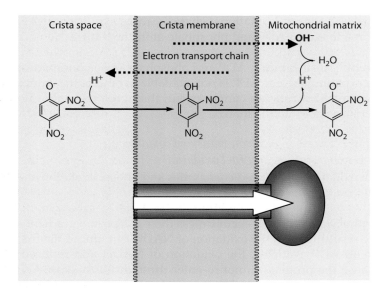

Figure 3.26 Uncoupling of electron transport and oxidative phosphorylation by a weak acid such as 2,4-dinitrophenol. The acid transports protons into the mitochondrial matrix, discharging the proton gradient before protons can enter through the transmembrane stalk of ATP synthase.

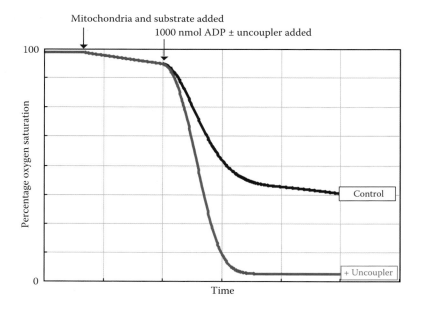

Figure 3.27 Oxygen consumption by mitochondria incubated with malate and ADP, with and without an uncoupler. In the presence of the uncoupler, there will be rapid and more or less complete consumption of oxygen whether or not ADP is present.

storage in the body. It has a red-brown colour because of the large number of mitochondria it contains. Brown adipose tissue is especially important in the maintenance of body temperature in infants, but it remains active in adults, although its importance compared with uncoupling proteins in muscle and other tissues is unclear. As discussed in Section 7.2.3, inter-organ abdominal adipose tissue, which is important in the development of insulin resistance and prediabetes (the metabolic syndrome), is metabolically more active than subcutaneous white adipose tissue and has probably developed from brown adipose tissue, whose original function was thermogenesis. In response to a high fat intake, it has differentiated into storage (white) adipose tissue.

In addition to maintenance of body temperature, uncoupling proteins are important in overall energy balance and maintenance of body weight. One of the actions of the hormone leptin secreted by (white) adipose tissue (Section 1.4.2) is to increase the expression of uncoupling proteins in muscle and adipose tissue, thus increasing energy expenditure and the utilisation of adipose tissue fat reserves.

3.3.1.6   Respiratory poisons

Much of our knowledge of the processes involved in electron transport and oxidative phosphorylation has come from studies using inhibitors. Figure 3.28 shows the oxygen electrode traces from mitochondria incubated with malate and an inhibitor of electron transport, with or without the addition of dinitrophenol as an uncoupler. When electron transport is inhibited, no oxygen can be consumed. Inhibitors of electron transport include

    a. Rotenone, the active ingredient of derris powder, an insecticide prepared from the roots of the leguminous plant *Lonchocarpus nicou*. It is an inhibitor of complex I (NADH → ubiquinone reduction). The same effect is seen in the presence of amytal

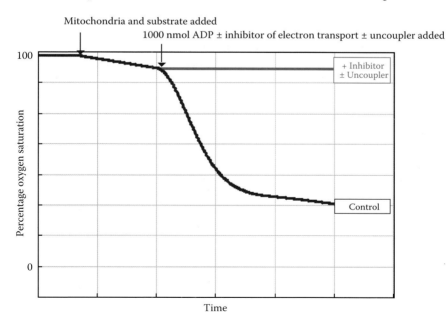

Figure 3.28 Oxygen consumption by mitochondria incubated with malate and ADP, plus an inhibitor of electron transport, with and without an uncoupler. When electron transport is inhibited, there can be no consumption of oxygen, even in the presence of an uncoupler.

(amobarbital), a barbiturate sedative drug, which again inhibits complex I. These two compounds inhibit oxidation of malate, which requires complex I, but not succinate, which reduces ubiquinone directly. The addition of the uncoupler has no effect on malate oxidation in the presence of these two inhibitors of electron transport but leads to uncontrolled oxidation of succinate.

b. Antimycin A, an antibiotic produced by *Streptomyces* spp., which is used as a fungicide against fungi that are parasitic on rice. It inhibits complex III (ubiquinone → cytochrome c reduction) and so inhibits the oxidation of both malate and succinate because both require complex III and the addition of the uncoupler has no effect.

c. Cyanide, azide, and carbon monoxide, all of which bind irreversibly to the iron of cytochrome a_3, and thus inhibit complex IV. Again, these compounds inhibit oxidation of both malate and succinate because both rely on cytochrome oxidase, and again, the addition of the uncoupler has no effect.

Figure 3.29 shows the oxygen electrode traces from mitochondria incubated with malate and an inhibitor of ATP synthesis, with or without the addition of dinitrophenol as an uncoupler. Oligomycin is a toxic, and therefore clinically useless, antibiotic produced by *Streptomyces* spp.; it inhibits the transport of protons across the stalk of ATP synthase. This results in inhibition of oxidation of both malate and succinate because if the protons cannot be transported back into the matrix, they will accumulate and inhibit further electron

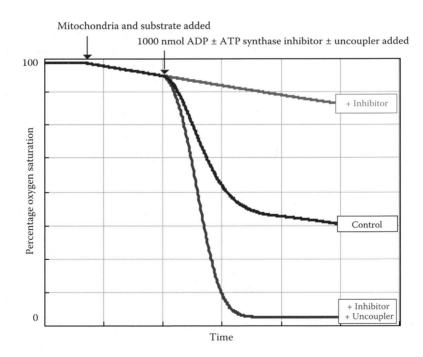

Figure 3.29 Oxygen consumption by mitochondria incubated with malate and ADP, plus an inhibitor of ATP synthesis such as oligomycin, with and without an uncoupler. Even when ATP synthesis is inhibited, addition of the uncoupler permits rapid and more or less complete utilisation of oxygen because electron transport is not inhibited.

transport. In this case, addition of the uncoupler permits re-entry of protons across the crista membrane and hence uncontrolled oxidation of substrates.

Two further compounds also inhibit ATP synthesis, not by inhibiting the ATP synthase, but by inhibiting the transport of ADP into, and ATP out of, the mitochondria:

1. Atractyloside is a toxic glycoside from the rhizomes of the Mediterranean thistle *Atractylis gummifera*; it competes with ADP for binding to the carrier protein at the outer face of the membrane and so prevents the entry of ADP into the matrix.
2. Bongkrekic acid is a toxic antibiotic formed by *Pseudomonas cocovenenans* growing on coconut; it is named after bongkrek, an Indonesian mould-fermented coconut product that becomes highly toxic when *Pseudomonas* outgrows the mould. It fixes the carrier protein at the inner face of the membrane so that ATP cannot be transported out, nor ADP in.

Both compounds thus inhibit ATP synthesis and therefore the oxidation of substrates. However, as with oligomycin (Figure 3.29), addition of an uncoupler permits rapid and complete utilisation of oxygen because electron transport can now continue uncontrolled by the availability of ADP.

Key points

- Endothermic reactions are coupled to the (exothermic) hydrolysis of ATP → ADP + phosphate. This may involve intermediate phosphorylation of either the enzyme or the substrate, or in some cases, adenylation of the substrate.
- Compounds that enter cells by passive or carrier-mediated diffusion may be accumulated to a higher concentration than in the extracellular fluid by binding to proteins or by phosphorylation at the expense of ATP (metabolic trapping).
- Active transport is the accumulation of a substance against a concentration gradient, linked to utilisation of ATP in one of three ways:
  - The carrier may be phosphorylated, leading to a conformational change.
  - The carrier may bind and hydrolyse ATP, but not be phosphorylated, again leading to a conformational change.
  - ATPase action in a membrane leads to formation of a proton gradient; protons re-enter the cell in exchange for Na^+ ions, which then re-enter the cell together with, or in exchange for, substrates and metabolites.
- Muscle contraction involves conformational changes in myosin due to the displacement of ADP by ATP, hydrolysis of ATP → ADP + phosphate and expulsion of phosphate from the active site of the protein.
- A relatively small amount of ATP is formed by substrate-level phosphorylation of ADP; most is formed in the mitochondria, linked to electron transport and the oxidation of educed coenzymes and reduction of oxygen to water.
- The oxidation of NADH yields approximately 2.5 mol of ATP and of reduced flavins 1.5.
- Transfer of electrons along the electron transport chain from reduced coenzymes to oxygen results in pumping of protons across the crista membrane and formation of a pH gradient across the membrane.

- Protons re-enter the mitochondrial matrix through a proton transport pore that forms the stalk of ATP synthase. This causes rotation of the central core of the enzyme and provides the driving force for the synthesis of ATP from ADP and phosphate.
- Electron transport and ATP synthesis are tightly coupled; thus, the oxidation of metabolic fuels and utilisation of oxygen are controlled by the availability of ADP and hence by the utilisation of ATP in physical and chemical work.
- Uncouplers permit uncontrolled oxidation of substrates (and hence generation of heat) by providing an alternative route for protons to re-enter the mitochondrial matrix, bypassing ATP synthase.

Further resources on the CD

The oxidative phosphorylation computer simulation in the virtual laboratory on the CD.

chapter four

Digestion and absorption

The major components of the diet are starches, sugars, fats, and proteins. These have to be hydrolysed to their constituent smaller molecules for absorption and metabolism. Starches and sugars are absorbed mainly as monosaccharides; fats are absorbed as free fatty acids and glycerol (plus a small amount of intact triacylglycerol); proteins are absorbed as their constituent amino acids and small peptides.

The fat-soluble vitamins (A, D, E, and K) are absorbed dissolved in dietary lipids; there are active transport systems (Section 3.2.2.3) in the small intestinal mucosa for the absorption of the water-soluble vitamins. The absorption of vitamin B_{12} (Section 4.5.2.1) requires a specific binding protein that is secreted in the gastric juice to bind to the mucosal transport system.

Minerals generally enter the intestinal mucosal cells by carrier-mediated diffusion and are accumulated intracellularly by binding to specific binding proteins (Section 3.2.2.1). They are then transferred into the bloodstream by active transport mechanisms (P-type transport proteins, Section 3.2.2.4) at the serosal side of the epithelial cells, usually onto plasma-binding proteins.

Objectives

After reading this chapter you should be able to

- Describe the major functions of each region of the gastrointestinal tract
- Describe and explain the classification of carbohydrates according to their chemical and nutritional properties; explain what is meant by glycaemic index
- Describe and explain the digestion and absorption of carbohydrates
- Describe and explain the classification of dietary lipids and the different types of fatty acid
- Describe and explain the digestion and absorption of lipids, the role of bile salts, and the formation of lipid micelles and chylomicrons
- Describe and explain the classification of amino acids according to their chemical and nutritional properties
- Describe the levels of protein structure and explain what is meant by denaturation
- Describe and explain the digestion and absorption of proteins
- Describe the absorption of vitamins and minerals, especially vitamin B_{12}, iron, and calcium

4.1   The gastrointestinal tract

The gastrointestinal tract is shown in Figure 4.1. The major functions of each region are as follows:

Mouth:

- Hydrolysis of a small amount of starch catalysed by amylase, secreted by the salivary glands
- Hydrolysis of a small amount of fat, catalysed by lingual lipase, secreted by the tongue
- Absorption of small amounts of vitamin C and a variety of non-nutrients (including nicotine)

Stomach:

- Denaturation of dietary proteins (Section 4.4.2.3) and the release of vitamin B_{12}, iron, and other minerals from protein binding, for which gastric acid is important
- Hydrolysis of protein catalysed by pepsin

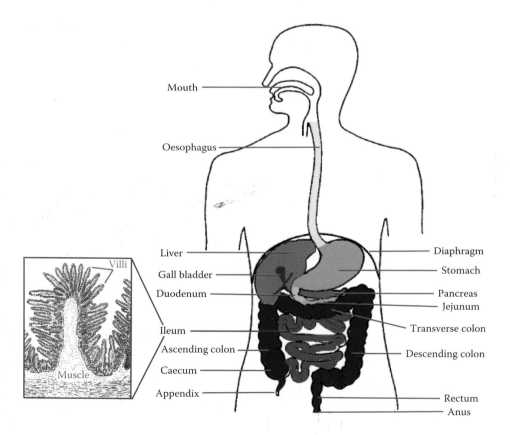

Figure 4.1 The gastrointestinal tract. The inset box shows the microscopic appearance of the small intestine and villi.

- Hydrolysis of fat catalysed by lipase
- Secretion of intrinsic factor for the absorption of vitamin B_{12}

Small intestine (duodenum, jejunum, and ileum):

- Hydrolysis of starch catalysed by amylase secreted by the pancreas
- Hydrolysis of disaccharides at the luminal surface of the intestinal mucosal cells
- Hydrolysis of fat catalysed by lipase, phospholipase, and esterase secreted by the pancreas
- Hydrolysis of protein catalysed by a variety of exopeptidases and endopeptidases (Section 4.4.3) secreted by the pancreas and small intestinal mucosa
- Hydrolysis of dipeptides and tripeptides within the brush border of the intestinal mucosal cells
- Absorption of the products of digestion, including minerals and vitamins
- Absorption of water (failure of water absorption, as in severe diarrhoea, can lead to dehydration)

Large intestine (caecum and colon):

- Bacterial metabolism of undigested carbohydrates, proteins, bile salts, and shed intestinal mucosal cells
- Absorption of some of the products of bacterial metabolism
- Absorption of water

Rectum:

- Storage of undigested gut contents prior to evacuation as faeces

Throughout the gastrointestinal tract, and especially in the small intestine, the surface area of the mucosa is considerably greater than would appear from its superficial appearance. As shown in the inset in Figure 4.1, the intestinal mucosa is folded into the lumen. The surface of these folds is covered with villi; finger-like projections into the lumen, some 0.5–1.5 mm long. There are some 20–40 villi/mm², giving a total absorptive surface area of some 300 m² in the small intestine.

Each villus has both blood capillaries, which drain into the hepatic portal vein, and a lacteal, which drains into the lymphatic system (Figure 4.2). Water-soluble products of digestion (carbohydrates and amino acids) are absorbed into the blood capillaries, and the liver has a major role in controlling the availability of the products of carbohydrate and protein digestion to other tissues in the body. Lipids are absorbed into the lacteals; the lymphatic system joins the bloodstream at the thoracic duct, and extrahepatic tissues are exposed to the products of lipid digestion uncontrolled by the liver, which functions to clear the remnants from the circulation (Section 5.6.2.1). In addition to absorptive cells in the intestinal mucosa, whose luminal surface area is considerably increased by the presence of a brush border, there are also mucus secreting goblet cells. The function of mucus is to protect the intestinal cells from attack by the digestive enzymes secreted into the lumen; its main constituent is the protein mucin, which is particularly rich in two amino acids (threonine and cysteine) and is resistant to enzymic hydrolysis. Indeed, a significant part of the requirement for a dietary intake of protein (Section 9.1.2) is to replace the amino acids lost in mucin, which is largely excreted unhydrolysed in the faeces.

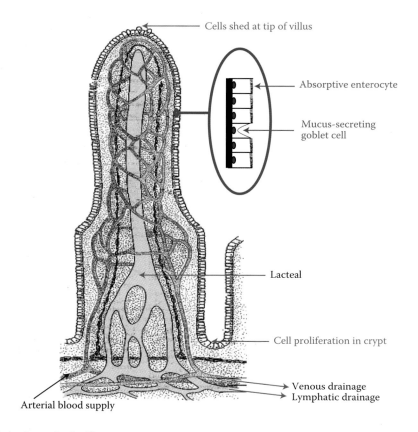

Figure 4.2 An intestinal villus.

There is rapid turnover of the cells of the intestinal mucosa; epithelial cells proliferate in the crypts, alongside the cells that secrete digestive enzymes and mucus, and migrate to the tip of the villus, where they are shed into the lumen. The average life of an intestinal mucosal epithelial cell is about 48 h. This rapid turnover of epithelial cells is important in controlling the absorption of iron, and possibly other minerals (Section 4.5.3.1).

4.2   Digestion and absorption of carbohydrates

Carbohydrates are compounds of carbon, hydrogen, and oxygen in the ratio $C_nH_{2n}O_n$. The basic unit of the carbohydrates is the sugar molecule or monosaccharide. Note that sugar is used here in a chemical sense and includes a variety of simple carbohydrates, which are collectively known as sugars. Ordinary table sugar (cane sugar or beet sugar) is correctly known as sucrose—it is a disaccharide (Section 4.2.1.4). It is only one of a number of different sugars found in the diet.

4.2.1   The classification of carbohydrates

Dietary carbohydrates can be considered in three main groups: sugars, oligosaccharides, and polysaccharides; the polysaccharides can be further subdivided into starches and non-starch polysaccharides (Figure 4.3).

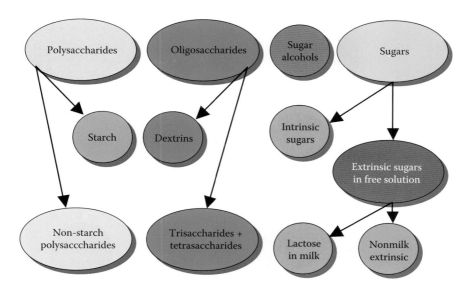

Figure 4.3 Nutritional classification of carbohydrates.

The simplest type of sugar is a monosaccharide—a single sugar unit (Section 4.2.1.2). Monosaccharides consist of between 3 and 7 carbon atoms (and the corresponding number of hydrogen and oxygen atoms). A few larger monosaccharides also occur, although they are not important in nutrition and metabolism.

Disaccharides (Section 4.2.1.4) are formed by condensation between two monosaccharides to form a glycoside bond. The reverse reaction, cleavage of the glycoside bond to release the individual monosaccharides, is a hydrolysis.

Oligosaccharides consist of three or four monosaccharide units (trisaccharides and tetrasaccharides), and occasionally more, linked by glycoside bonds. Most are not digested, but they are fermented by intestinal bacteria, yielding short-chain fatty acids that provide a metabolic fuel to intestinal mucosal cells, and may be protective against colorectal cancer (Section 6.3.3.2). The bacterial fermentation of oligosaccharides also makes a significant contribution to the production of intestinal gas.

Nutritionally, it is useful to consider sugars (both monosaccharides and disaccharides) in two groups:

1. Intrinsic sugars that are contained within plant cell walls in foods.
2. Sugars that are in free solution in foods, and therefore provide a substrate for oral bacteria, leading to the formation of dental plaque and caries. These are known as extrinsic sugars; it is considered desirable to reduce the consumption of extrinsic sugars (Section 6.3.3.1), both because of their role in dental decay and also because of the ease with which excessive amounts of sweet foods can be consumed, thus leading to obesity (Chapter 7).

A complication in the classification of sugars as intrinsic (which are considered desirable in the diet) and extrinsic (which are considered undesirable in the diet) is that lactose is in free solution in milk, and hence is an extrinsic sugar. However, lactose is not a cause of dental decay, and milk is an important source of calcium (Section 11.15.1), protein (Chapter 9), and vitamin B_2 (Section 11.7). It is not considered desirable to reduce intakes of milk, which

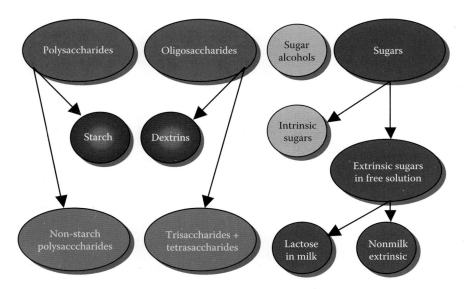

Figure 4.4 Classification of dietary carbohydrates by their glycaemic index. Blue shows glycaemic carbohydrates; red, non-glycaemic carbohydrates.

is the only significant source of lactose, and extrinsic sugars are further subdivided into milk sugar and non-milk extrinsic sugars.

Polysaccharides are polymers of many hundreds of monosaccharide units, again linked by glycoside bonds. The most important are starch and glycogen (Section 4.2.1.6), both of which are polymers of glucose. There are a number of other polysaccharides, composed of other monosaccharides, or of glucose units linked differently from the linkages in starch and glycogen. Collectively, these are known as non-starch polysaccharides. They are generally not digested, but they have important roles in nutrition (Section 4.2.1.7).

4.2.1.1   Glycaemic index

An alternative way of classifying carbohydrates is by the extent to which they increase the plasma concentration of glucose after consumption. The glycaemic index of a carbohydrate (or carbohydrate-containing food) is the increase in blood glucose after the test meal compared with that after consumption of an equivalent amount of glucose either as a solution of glucose or from a reference food such as white bread or boiled rice. A carbohydrate that is completely digested to yield glucose and/or galactose will have a glycaemic index of 1. As shown in Figure 4.4, sugar alcohols have a lower glycaemic index because they are only absorbed slowly and are only incompletely converted to glucose. Similarly, intrinsic sugars, within plant cell walls in foods, have a low glycaemic index because they are protected against digestion by the indigestible cellulose of the cell walls. Starch and dextrins have a variable glycaemic index, depending on their state of crystallisation, and non-starch polysaccharides, trisaccharides, and tetrasaccharides that are not digested at all have a glycaemic index of zero.

4.2.1.2   Monosaccharides

The classes of monosaccharides are named by the number of carbon atoms in the ring, using the Greek names for the numbers, with the ending *-ose* to show that they are sugars. The names of all sugars end in *-ose*:

- Three-carbon monosaccharides are trioses.
- Four-carbon monosaccharides are tetroses.
- Five-carbon monosaccharides are pentoses.
- Six-carbon monosaccharides are hexoses.
- Seven-carbon monosaccharides are heptoses.

In general, trioses, tetroses, and heptoses are important as intermediate compounds in the metabolism of pentoses and hexoses. Hexoses are the nutritionally important sugars.

The pentoses and hexoses can exist either as straight-chain compounds or can form heterocyclic rings (Figure 4.5). By convention, the ring of sugars is drawn with the bonds of one side thicker than the other. This is to show that the rings are planar and can be considered to lie at right angles to the plane of the page. The boldly drawn part of the molecule comes forward out of the paper, and the lightly drawn part goes behind the page. The hydroxyl groups lie above or below the plane of the ring, in the plane of the page. Each carbon has a hydrogen atom attached as well as a hydroxyl group; this is generally omitted when the structures are drawn as rings.

The nutritionally important hexoses are glucose, galactose, and fructose. Glucose and galactose differ from each other only in the arrangement of the hydroxyl group at carbon

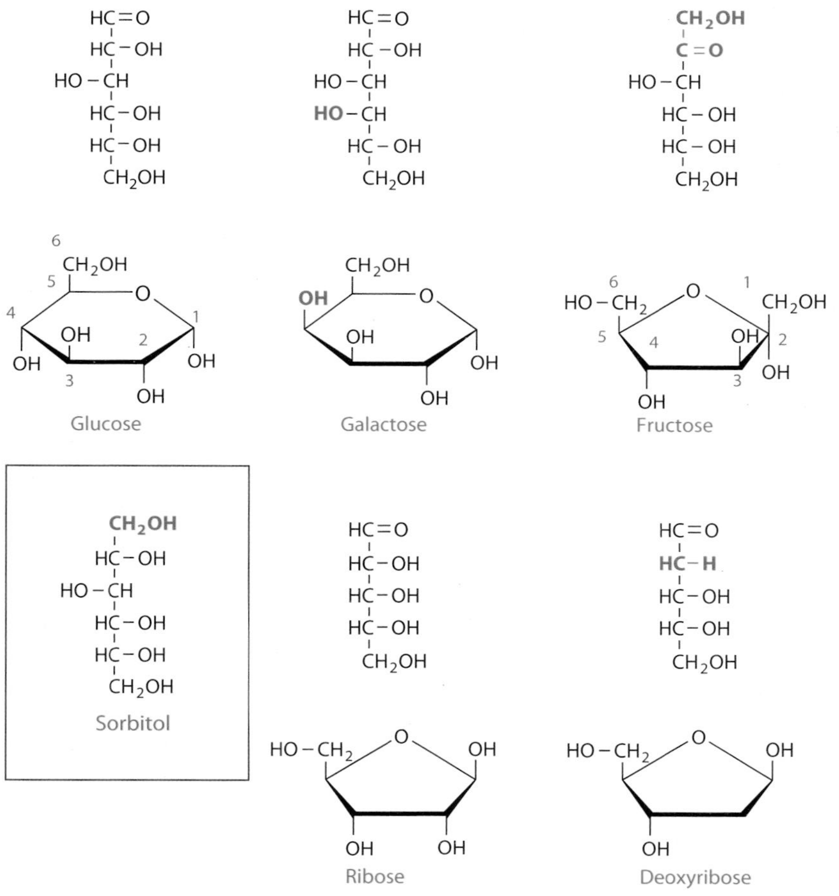

Figure 4.5 The nutritionally important monosaccharides.

4 above or below the plane of the ring. Fructose differs from glucose and galactose in that it has a C = O (keto) group at carbon 2, whilst the other two have an H – C = O (aldehyde) group at carbon 1.

There are two important pentose sugars, ribose and deoxyribose. Deoxyribose is unusual, in that it has lost one of its hydroxyl groups. The main role of ribose and deoxyribose is in the nucleotides (Figure 3.1) and the nucleic acids; RNA, in which the sugar is ribose (Section 9.2.2), and DNA, in which the sugar is deoxyribose (Section 9.2.1). Although pentoses do occur in the diet, they are also readily synthesised from glucose (Section 5.4.2).

4.2.1.3 *Sugar alcohols*

Sugar alcohols (or polyols) are formed by the reduction of the aldehyde group of a monosaccharide to a hydroxyl (–OH) group. Quantitatively, the most important is sorbitol, formed by the reduction of glucose (see Figure 4.5). It is poorly absorbed from the intestinal tract; thus, it has a lower glycaemic index than other carbohydrates. Because of this, it is widely used in preparation of foods suitable for use by diabetics because it tastes sweet and can replace sucrose and other sugars in food manufacture. Like sucrose, but unlike intense (artificial) sweeteners (Section 7.3.4.9), sorbitol adds bulk to manufactured foods and also provides a high osmolarity in foods such as jams, which prevents spoilage by the growth of bacteria, yeasts, and fungi. However, sorbitol is metabolised as a metabolic fuel, although because of its poor absorption, it has an energy yield approximately half that of glucose; thus, it is not suitable for the replacement of sugar in weight-reducing diets.

Sugar alcohols are poor substrates for metabolism by the plaque-forming bacteria that are associated with dental caries and are used in the manufacture of 'tooth-friendly' sweets and chewing gum. There is some evidence that xylitol, the sugar alcohol formed by reduction of the 5-carbon sugar xylose (an isomer of ribose), may have a positive effect in preventing dental caries.

4.2.1.4 *Disaccharides*

The major dietary disaccharides (Figure 4.6) are:

- Sucrose, cane, or beet sugar, which is glucosyl-fructose
- Lactose, the sugar of milk, which is galactosyl-glucose
- Maltose, the sugar originally isolated from malt and a product of starch digestion, which is glucosyl-glucose
- Isomaltose, a product of starch digestion, which is glucosyl-glucose linked 1 → 6
- Trehalose, found especially in mushrooms, but also as the blood sugar of some insects, which is glucosyl-glucoside

4.2.1.5 *Reducing and non-reducing sugars*

Chemically, the aldehyde group of glucose is a reducing agent. This provides a simple test for glucose in urine (Figure 4.7). Glucose reacts with copper (Cu^{2+}) ions in alkaline solution, reducing them to Cu^+ oxide, and itself being oxidised. The original solution of Cu^{2+} ions has a blue colour; the copper oxide forms a red-brown precipitate. This reaction is not specific for glucose. Other sugars with a free aldehyde group at carbon 1, including vitamin C (Section 11.14) and a number of pentose sugars that occur in foods, can undergo the same reaction, giving a false-positive result.

Whilst alkaline copper reagents are still sometimes used to measure urine glucose in monitoring diabetic control (Section 10.7), there is a more specific test using the enzyme glucose oxidase, which only measures glucose. Glucose oxidase catalyses the reduction of

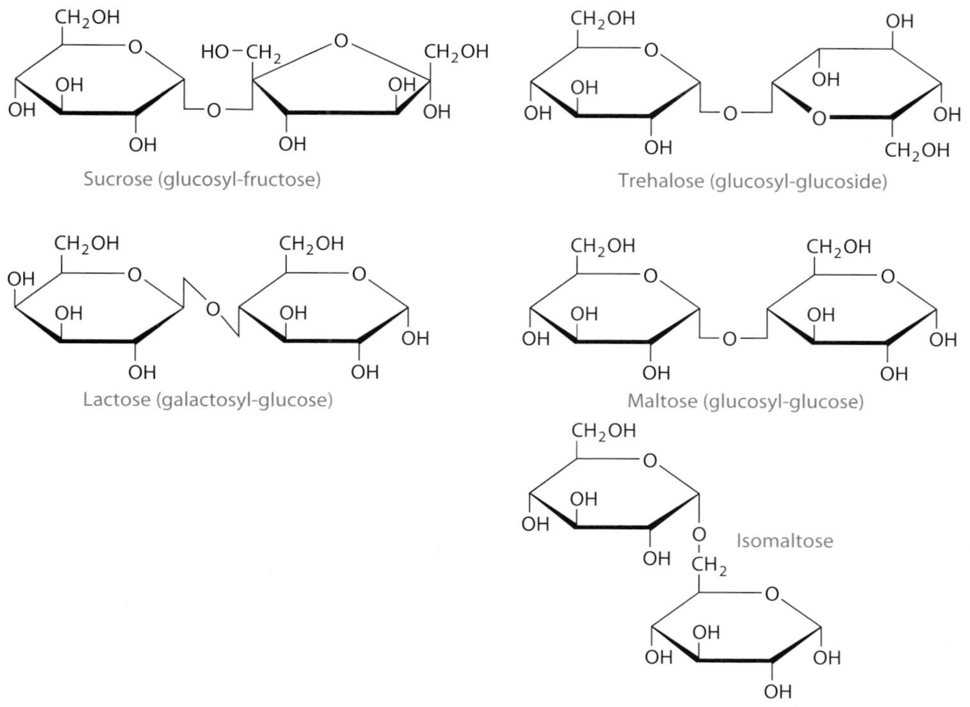

Figure 4.6 The nutritionally important disaccharides.

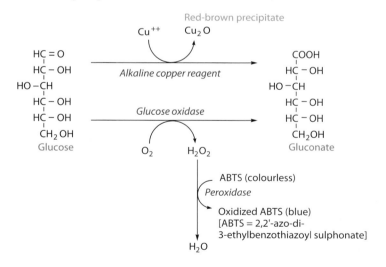

Figure 4.7 Measurement of glucose using alkaline copper reagents and glucose oxidase.

oxygen to hydrogen peroxide, which, in the presence of a second enzyme, catalase, can be reduced to water by oxidation of the colourless compound ABTS to yield a blue colour that can readily be measured. The glucose oxidase reaction can be fully quantitative when used in solution, or semi-quantitative when incorporated into 'dip sticks' that are commonly used to monitor glycaemic control in diabetes by estimating the concentration of glucose in urine.

Although the glucose oxidase test is specific for glucose, high concentrations of vitamin C (Section 11.14), as may occur in the urine of people taking supplements of the vitamin, can react with hydrogen peroxide before it oxidises the colourless precursor or can reduce the dyestuff back to its colourless form. This means that tests using glucose oxidase can yield a false-negative result in the presence of high concentrations of vitamin C.

The term *reducing sugars* reflects a chemical reaction of the sugars—the ability to reduce a suitable acceptor such as copper ions or ABTS. It has nothing to do with weight reduction and slimming, although some people erroneously believe that reducing sugars somehow help one to reduce excessive weight. This is not correct—the energy yield from reducing sugars and non-reducing sugars is exactly the same, and an excess of either will contribute to obesity.

4.2.1.6 *Polysaccharides: starches and glycogen*

Starch is a polymer of glucose, containing a large, but variable, number of glucose units. It is thus impossible to quote a relative molecular mass for starch or to discuss amounts of starch in terms of mol. It can, however, be hydrolysed to glucose, and the results expressed as mol of glucose.

The simplest type of starch is amylose, a straight chain of glucose molecules, with glycoside links between carbon 1 of one glucose unit and carbon 4 of the next. Amylopectin has a branched structure, where every 30th glucose molecule has glycoside links to three others instead of just two. The branch is formed by linkage between carbon 1 of one glucose unit and carbon 6 of the next (Figure 4.8).

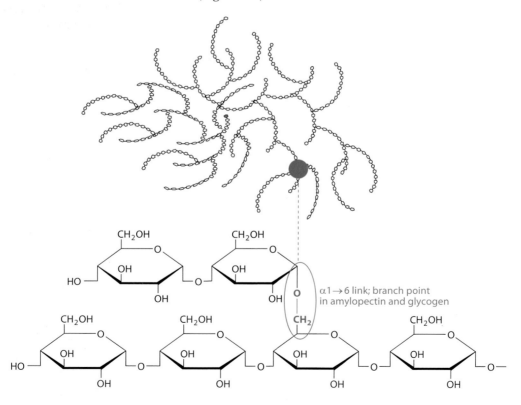

Figure 4.8 The branched structure of starch and glycogen.

Starches are the storage carbohydrates of plants, and relative amounts of amylose and amylopectin differ in starches from different sources, as indeed does the size of the overall starch molecule. On average, about 20%–25% of dietary starch is amylose, and the remaining 75%–80% is amylopectin. Uncooked starch is crystalline and highly resistant to digestion (and so has a very low glycaemic index). The process of cooking expands the starch granules, permitting a large amount of water to be trapped in the molecule and allowing access to digestive enzymes; thus, the glycaemic index may be as high as 1. However, as starchy foods stale, some of the starch recrystallises (the process of retrogradation), and the glycaemic index falls.

Glycogen is the storage carbohydrate of mammalian muscle and liver. It is synthesised from glucose in the fed state (Section 5.6.3), and its constituent glucose units are used as a metabolic fuel in the fasting state. Glycogen is a branched polymer, with a similar structure to amylopectin, but more highly branched, with a 1 → 6 bond about every 10th glucose unit. Because of its highly branched structure, glycogen traps a great deal of water in the cell; as glycogen stores are depleted during a period of fasting or reduced food intake, this water is released, leading to a considerable loss of body weight during the early stages of food restriction.

4.2.1.7   Non-starch polysaccharides (dietary fibre)

There are a number of other polysaccharides in foods. Collectively, they are known as non-starch polysaccharides and are the major components of dietary fibre. Non-starch polysaccharides are not digested by human enzymes, although all can be fermented to some extent by intestinal bacteria, and the products of bacterial fermentation may be absorbed and metabolised as metabolic fuels. The major non-starch polysaccharides (Figure 4.9) are

- Cellulose, a polymer of glucose in which the configuration of the glycoside bond between the glucose units is in the opposite configuration (β1→4) from that in starch (α1→4) and cannot be hydrolysed by human enzymes

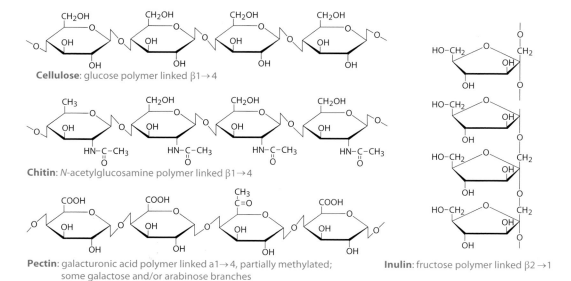

Cellulose: glucose polymer linked β1→4

Chitin: *N*-acetylglucosamine polymer linked β1→4

Pectin: galacturonic acid polymer linked α1→4, partially methylated; some galactose and/or arabinose branches

Inulin: fructose polymer linked β2→1

Figure 4.9 The major types of dietary non-starch polysaccharide.

- Hemicelluloses, branched polymers of pentose (5-carbon) and hexose (6-carbon) sugars.
- Inulin, a polymer of fructose, which is the storage carbohydrate of Jerusalem artichoke and some other root vegetables.
- Pectin, a complex polymer of a variety of monosaccharides, including some methylated sugars.
- Plant gums such as gum Arabic, gum tragacanth, acacia, carob, and guar gums—complex polymers of mixed monosaccharides.
- Mucilages such as alginates, agar, and carrageen; complex polymers of mixed monosaccharides found in seaweeds and other algae.

Cellulose, hemicelluloses, and inulin are insoluble non-starch polysaccharides, whilst pectin and plant gums and mucilages are soluble. The other major constituent of dietary fibre, lignin, is not a carbohydrate at all, but a complex polymer of a variety of aromatic alcohols.

Soluble non-starch polysaccharides increase the viscosity of the intestinal contents, and so slow the absorption of the products of digestion. This can be valuable in the treatment of diabetes mellitus (Section 10.7). A number of studies have shown that consuming a relatively large amount of soluble non-starch polysaccharides before a meal lowers the post-prandial increase in blood glucose, thus enhancing glycaemic control. Insoluble non-starch polysaccharides increase the bulk of the intestinal contents, thus aiding peristalsis; they may also adsorb the bile salts and potential carcinogens in the diet, thus reducing their absorption.

Both soluble and insoluble non-starch polysaccharides, as well as oligosaccharides and starch resistant to digestion (Section 4.2.2.1), are substrates for bacterial fermentation in the large intestine, yielding short-chain fatty acids (especially butyrate) that are absorbed and provide a significant metabolic fuel for intestinal enterocytes and may provide protection against the development of colorectal cancer. Provision of a substrate for bacterial fermentation in the form of oligosaccharides, resistant starch, and non-starch polysaccharides alters the composition of the intestinal flora, enhancing the growth of beneficial bacteria at the expense of potential pathogens. Carbohydrates that occur in, or are added to, foods for this purpose are known as prebiotics. Foods that contain the bacteria themselves (mainly *Lactobacillus* and *Bifidobacterium* spp.) are known as probiotics. One of the advantages of breast-feeding over infant formula is that human milk is rich in prebiotic oligosaccharides that enhance the infant's ability to develop a desirable intestinal bacterial flora.

4.2.2   Carbohydrate digestion and absorption

The digestion of carbohydrates is by hydrolysis to liberate small oligosaccharides, then free monosaccharides and disaccharides. The glycaemic index of a carbohydrate (Section 4.2.1.1) measures the extent and speed with which a carbohydrate is hydrolysed and the resultant monosaccharides are absorbed.

Glucose and galactose have a glycaemic index of 1, as do lactose, maltose, isomaltose, and trehalose, which give rise to these monosaccharides on hydrolysis. However, because plant cell walls are largely cellulose, which is not digested, intrinsic sugars in fruits and vegetables have a lower glycaemic index. Other monosaccharides (e.g. fructose) and the sugar alcohols are absorbed less rapidly (Section 4.2.2.3) and have a lower glycaemic index, as does sucrose, which yields glucose and fructose on hydrolysis. The glycaemic index of starch is variable and that of non-starch polysaccharides is zero.

Carbohydrates with a high glycaemic index lead to a greater secretion of insulin after a meal than do those with a lower glycaemic index; this results in increased synthesis of fatty acids and triacylglycerol (Section 5.6.1) and may therefore be a factor in the development of obesity (Chapter 7) and diabetes mellitus (Section 10.7).

4.2.2.1   Starch digestion

The enzymes that catalyse the hydrolysis of starch are amylases, which are secreted both in the saliva and the pancreatic juice. (Salivary amylase is sometimes known by its old name of ptyalin.) Both salivary and pancreatic amylases catalyse random hydrolysis of glycoside bonds, yielding initially dextrins and other oligosaccharides, then a mixture of glucose, maltose, and isomaltose (from the branch-points in amylopectin).

The digestion of starch begins when food is chewed, and continues for a time in the stomach. Hydrolysis of starch to sweet sugars in the mouth may be a factor in determining food and nutrient intake (Section 1.4.3.1).

The gastric juice is very acidic (about pH 1.5–2), and amylase is inactive at this pH; as the food bolus is mixed with gastric juice, starch digestion ceases. When the food leaves the stomach and enters the small intestine, it is neutralised by the alkaline pancreatic juice (pH 8.8) and bile (pH 8). Amylase secreted by the pancreas continues the digestion of starch begun by salivary amylase.

Starches can be classified as

1. Rapidly hydrolysed, with a glycaemic index near 1; these are more or less completely hydrolysed in the small intestine.
2. Slowly hydrolysed, with a glycaemic index significantly <1; a proportion remains in the gut lumen and is a substrate for bacterial fermentation in the colon.
3. Resistant to hydrolysis, with a glycaemic index near to zero; most remains in the gut lumen and is a substrate for bacterial fermentation in the colon. A proportion of the starch in foods is, like intrinsic sugars (Section 4.2.1), enclosed by plant cells walls, and is therefore protected against digestion.

Like non-starch polysaccharides, much of the resistant and slowly hydrolysed starch is fermented by bacteria in the colon, and a proportion of the products of bacterial metabolism, including short-chain fatty acids, may be absorbed and metabolised.

4.2.2.2   Digestion of disaccharides

The enzymes that catalyse the hydrolysis of disaccharides (the disaccharidases) are located on the luminal face of the brush border of the intestinal mucosal cells; the resultant monosaccharides are absorbed together with dietary monosaccharides and glucose arising from the digestion of starch (Section 4.2.2.1). There are four disaccharidases:

1. Maltase catalyses the hydrolysis of maltose to two molecules of glucose.
2. Lactase catalyses the hydrolysis of lactose to glucose and galactose.
3. Trehalase catalyses the hydrolysis of trehalose to two molecules of glucose.
4. Sucrase-isomaltase is a bifunctional enzyme that catalyses the hydrolysis of sucrose to glucose and fructose, and of isomaltose to two molecules of glucose.

Deficiency of the enzyme lactase is common. Indeed, it is mainly in people of north European origin that lactase persists after adolescence. In most other people, and in a number of Europeans, lactase is gradually lost through early adult life—the condition of alactasia. The persistence of lactase after adolescence in northern European and Indian subcontinent populations is a mutation in a gene adjacent to that for lactase. Different mutations are responsible for the persistence of lactase in African populations.

In the absence of lactase, lactose cannot be absorbed, but remains in the intestinal lumen, where it is a substrate for bacterial fermentation to lactate (Section 5.4.1.2). This results in a considerable increase in the osmolality of the intestinal contents, since 1 mol of lactose yields 4 mol of lactate and 4 mol of protons. In addition, bacterial fermentation produces carbon dioxide, methane, and hydrogen. For a person who is alactasic, the result of consuming a moderate amount of lactose is explosive watery diarrhoea with severe abdominal pain. Even the relatively small amounts of lactose in milk may upset people with a complete deficiency of lactase. Such people can normally tolerate yoghurt and other fermented milk products, since much of the lactose has been converted to lactic acid. Fortunately, for people who suffer from alactasia, milk is the only significant source of lactose in the diet; thus, it is relatively easy to avoid consuming it. Lactose is widely used in the manufacture of pharmaceuticals, but the small amounts consumed seem to be tolerated by most people who are alactasic.

Rarely, people may lack sucrase-isomaltase, maltase, and/or trehalase. This may either be a genetic lack of the enzyme or an acquired loss as a result of intestinal infection, when all four disaccharidases are lost. These people are intolerant of the sugar(s) that cannot be hydrolysed and suffer in the same way as alactasic subjects given lactose. It is relatively easy to avoid maltose and trehalose, since there are few sources in the diet. People who lack sucrase-isomaltase have a more serious problem, since as well as the obvious sugar in cakes, biscuits, and jams, many manufactured foods contain added sucrose.

Genetic lack of sucrase-isomaltase is very common amongst the Inuit of North America. In their traditional diet, this caused no problems, since they had no significant sources of sucrose or isomaltose. With the adoption of a more Western diet, sucrose-induced diarrhoea has become a significant cause of undernutrition amongst infants and children.

4.2.2.3   *The absorption of monosaccharides*

There are two separate mechanisms for the absorption of monosaccharides in the small intestine (Figure 4.10).

Glucose and galactose are absorbed by sodium-dependent active transport (Section 3.2.2.6). The sodium pump and the sodium/potassium ATPase, as well as sodium secreted in the alkaline pancreatic juice, create a sodium gradient across the membrane. The sodium ions then enter the cell together with glucose or galactose. These two monosaccharides are carried by the same transport protein and compete with each other for intestinal absorption.

Other monosaccharides are absorbed by carrier-mediated diffusion; there are at least three distinct carrier proteins, one for fructose, one for other monosaccharides, and one for sugar alcohols. Because they are not actively transported, fructose and sugar alcohols are only absorbed to a limited extent, and after a moderately high intake, a significant amount will avoid absorption and remain in the intestinal lumen, acting as a substrate for colon bacteria, and, like unabsorbed disaccharides in people with disaccharidase deficiency, causing abdominal pain and diarrhoea.

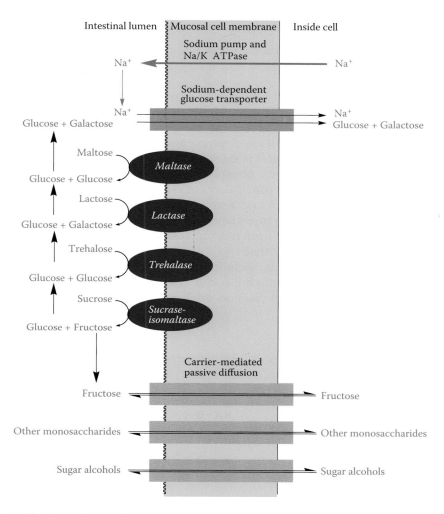

Figure 4.10 The hydrolysis of disaccharides and absorption of monosaccharides. Glucose and galactose are absorbed by Na⁺-dependent active transport, fructose, other monosaccharides and sugar alcohols by carrier-mediated passive diffusion.

4.3   Digestion and absorption of fats

The major fats in the diet are triacylglycerols and, to a lesser extent, phospholipids. Lipids are hydrophobic and have to be emulsified to very small droplets (micelles, Section 4.3.2) before they can be absorbed. This emulsification is achieved by hydrolysis of triacylglycerols to monoacyl and diacylglycerols and free fatty acids and also by the action of the bile salts (Section 4.3.2.1).

4.3.1   *The classification of dietary lipids*

Four groups of metabolically important compounds can be considered under the heading of lipids:

1. Triacylglycerols (sometimes also known as triglycerides), in which glycerol is esterified to three fatty acids (Figure 4.11). These are the oils and fats of the diet, which provide between 30% and 45% of average energy intake. The difference between oils and fats is that oils are liquid at room temperature, whereas fats are solid.
2. Phospholipids, in which glycerol is esterified to two fatty acids, with a hydrophilic group esterified to carbon 3 by a phosphate diester bond (Section 4.3.1.2 and Figure 4.12). Phospholipids are major constituents of cell membranes.
3. Steroids, including cholesterol and a variety of plant sterols and stanols (Section 4.3.1.3 and Figure 4.14) and extremely small amounts of steroid hormones. Chemically, these are completely different from triacylglycerols and phospholipids and are not a significant source of metabolic fuel.
4. A variety of other compounds, including vitamin A and carotenes (Section 11.2), vitamin D (Section 11.3), vitamin E (Section 11.4), and vitamin K (Section 11.5). They are absorbed in lipid micelles (Section 4.3.2), and their absorption depends on an adequate intake of fat.

4.3.1.1   *Fatty acids*

There are a number of different fatty acids, differing in both the length of the carbon chain and whether or not they have one or more double bonds (–CH = CH–) in the chain (Figure 4.11).

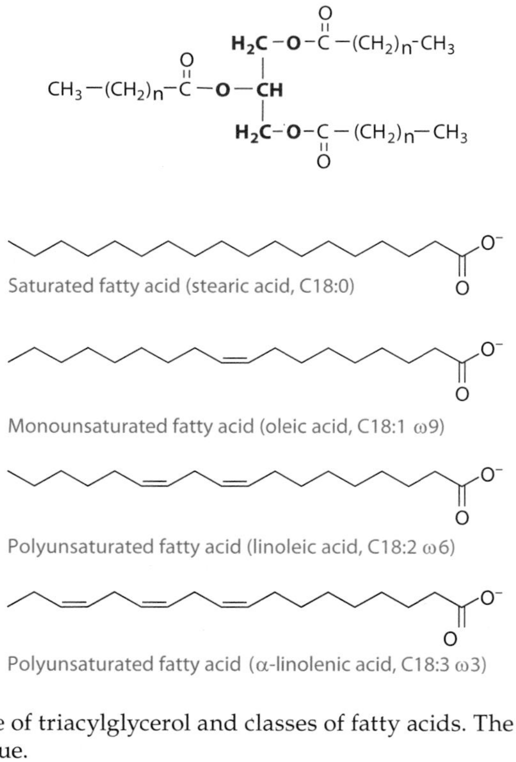

$$H_2C-O-\overset{\overset{O}{\|}}{C}-(CH_2)_n-CH_3$$
$$CH_3-(CH_2)_n-\overset{\overset{O}{\|}}{C}-O-CH$$
$$H_2C-O-\underset{\underset{O}{\|}}{C}-(CH_2)_n-CH_3$$

Saturated fatty acid (stearic acid, C18:0)

Monounsaturated fatty acid (oleic acid, C18:1 ω9)

Polyunsaturated fatty acid (linoleic acid, C18:2 ω6)

Polyunsaturated fatty acid (α-linolenic acid, C18:3 ω3)

Figure 4.11 The structure of triacylglycerol and classes of fatty acids. The glycerol moiety of a triacylglycerol is shown in blue.

4.4   Digestion and absorption of proteins

Proteins are polypeptides—polymers of amino acids, linked by peptide bonds. Unlike starch and glycogen, which are polymers of only a single type of monomer unit (glucose), proteins contain 21 different amino acids that are incorporated during synthesis (Section 9.2.3) as well as a number of others that are formed as a result of post-synthetic modification of precursor proteins. Since any individual polypeptide chain may contain 50–1000 amino acids, there is an almost infinite possible variety of proteins. There are some 30–40,000 different proteins and polypeptides in the human body; each has a specific sequence of amino acids.

Small proteins have a molecular mass of about $50–100 \times 10^3$, whilst some of the large complex proteins have a molecular mass of up to 10^4 or more. Large multi-enzyme complexes such as the fatty acid synthase complex (Section 5.6.1) have molecular masses of the order of 10^6 or more. Smaller polypeptides (containing between 3 and 50 amino acids) are important in the regulation of metabolism.

4.4.1   The amino acids

Chemically, the amino acids all have the same basic structure—an amino group ($-NH_3^+$) and a carboxylic acid group ($-COO^-$) attached to the same carbon atom (the α-carbon); what differs between the amino acids is the nature of the other group that is attached to the α-carbon. In the simplest amino acid, glycine, there are two hydrogen atoms, whilst in all other amino acids, there is one hydrogen atom and a side chain, varying in chemical complexity from the simple methyl group ($-CH_3$) of alanine to the aromatic ring structures of phenylalanine, tyrosine, and tryptophan.

Nine of the amino acids are dietary essentials that cannot be synthesised in the body (Section 9.1.3); these are marked by a star in Figure 4.19. The amino acids can be classified according to the chemical nature of the side chain; whether it is hydrophobic (on the left of Figure 4.19) or hydrophilic (on the right of Figure 4.19) and the nature of the group:

- Small hydrophobic amino acids: glycine, alanine, and proline
- Large hydrophobic amino acids: methionine and the branched-chain amino acids leucine, isoleucine, and valine
- Aromatic amino acids: phenylalanine, tyrosine, and tryptophan
- Neutral hydrophilic amino acids: serine, threonine, cysteine, and selenocysteine
- Acidic amino acids: glutamic and aspartic acids (the salts of these acids are glutamate and aspartate, respectively)
- Amides of the acidic amino acids: glutamine and asparagine
- Basic amino acids: lysine, arginine, and histidine

It is sometimes convenient to consider the two sulphur-containing amino acids, cysteine and methionine, together, since cysteine is synthesised in the body from methionine, and what is nutritionally important is the sum of [cysteine + methionine] (Section 9.1.3).

In addition to the three-letter abbreviations that are commonly used for the amino acids, there is a single-letter code for each (apart from selenocysteine) that is generally used for showing protein sequences.

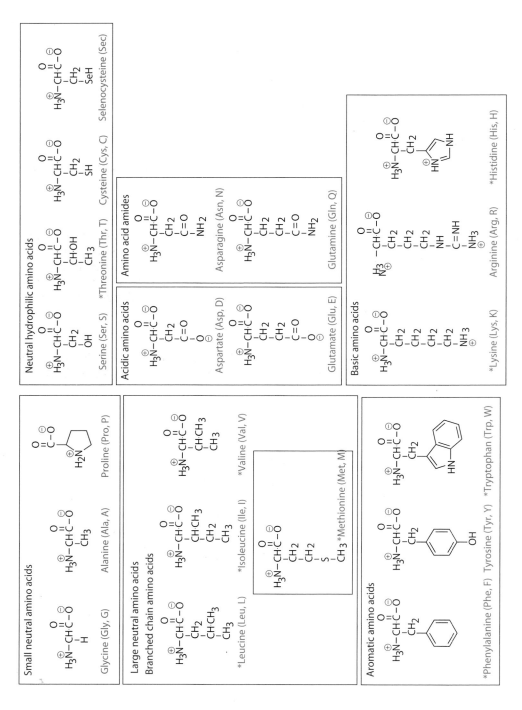

Figure 4.19 The amino acids, showing their three- and single-letter codes. *Starred amino acids are dietary essentials that cannot be synthesised in the body. There is no single-letter code for selenocysteine.

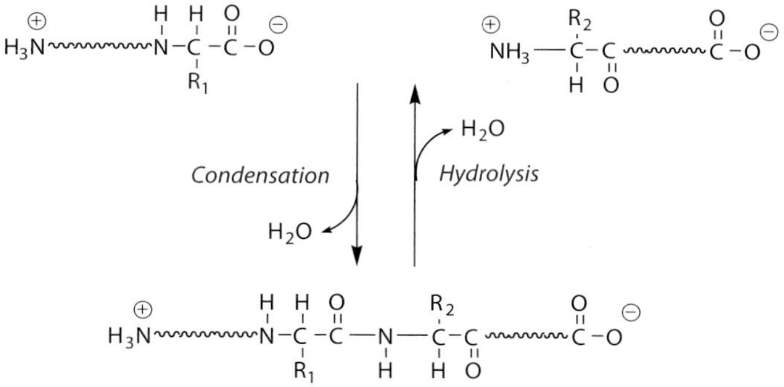

Figure 4.20 Condensation of amino acids to form a peptide bond and hydrolysis of a peptide bond.

4.4.2 Protein structure and denaturation of proteins

Proteins are composed of linear chains of amino acids, joined by condensation of the carboxyl group of one with the amino group of another, to form a peptide bond (Figure 4.20). The sequence of amino acids in a protein is its primary structure. It is different for each protein, although proteins that are closely related to each other often have very similar primary structures. The primary structure of a protein is determined by the gene containing the information for that protein (Section 9.2).

4.4.2.1 Secondary structure of proteins

Polypeptide chains fold up in a variety of ways, stabilised by hydrogen bonds between the oxygen of one peptide bond and the nitrogen of another (Figure 4.21). Interactions between

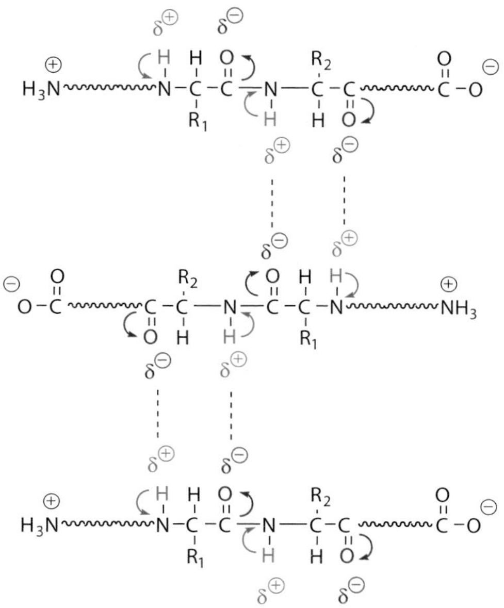

Figure 4.21 Hydrogen bonds in peptide chains.

the side chains of the amino acids determine which of the following patterns of secondary structure any given region of a protein adopts:

- α-helix, in which the peptide backbone of the protein adopts a spiral (helix) form. The hydrogen bonds are formed between peptide bonds that are near each other in the primary sequence.
- β-pleated sheet, in which regions of the polypeptide chain lie alongside one another, forming a 'corrugated' or pleated surface. The hydrogen bonds are between peptide bonds in different parts of the primary sequence and the regions of polypeptide chain forming a pleated sheet may run parallel or antiparallel.
- Hairpins and loops, in which small regions of the polypeptide chain form very tight bends.
- Random coil, in which there is no recognisable organised structure. Although this appears to be random, for any one protein, the shape of a random coil region will always be the same, although at the terminal regions many proteins have small regions that are not hydrogen bonded to other regions, and do indeed have a random secondary structure.

A protein may have several regions of α-helix, β-pleated sheet (with the peptide chains running parallel or anti-parallel), hairpins, and random coil, all in the same molecule.

4.4.2.2 Tertiary and quaternary structures of proteins

Having formed regions of secondary structure, the whole protein molecule then folds up into a compact shape. This is the third (tertiary) level of structure and is largely the result of interactions of the side chains of the amino acids with each other and with their environment. Proteins in an aqueous medium in the cell generally adopt a tertiary structure in which hydrophobic side chains are inside the molecule and can interact with each other, whilst hydrophilic side chains are exposed to interact with water. By contrast, proteins that are embedded in membranes (Figure 4.13) have a hydrophobic region on the outside to interact with the membrane lipids.

Two further interactions between amino acid side chains may be involved in tertiary structure, in this case forming covalent bonds between regions of the peptide chain (Figure 4.22):

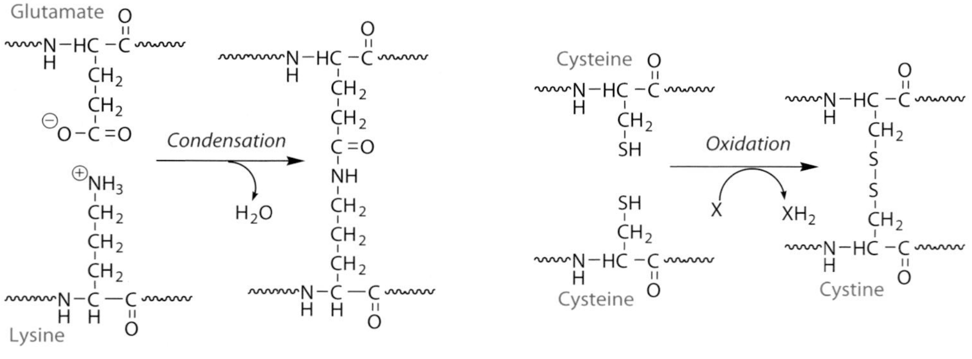

Figure 4.22 Covalent links between peptide chains—on the left, a side-chain peptide (an isopeptide bond) between the ε-amino group of lysine and the γ-carboxyl group of glutamate; on the right, a disulphide bridge formed by oxidation of two cysteine residues.

1. The ε-amino group on the side chain of lysine can form a peptide bond with the carboxyl group on the side chain of aspartate or glutamate. This is nutritionally important, since the side-chain peptide bond is not hydrolysed by digestive enzymes, and the lysine, which is an essential amino acid is not available for absorption (Section 9.1.3).
2. The sulfydryl (–SH) groups of two cysteine molecules may be oxidised, forming a disulfide bridge between two parts of the protein chain.

Some proteins consist of more than one polypeptide chain. The way in which the chains interact with each other, after each has formed its secondary and tertiary structures, is the quaternary structure of the protein. Interactions between the subunits of multi-subunit proteins, involving changes in quaternary structure and the conformation of the protein, are important in a number of regulatory enzymes (Section 10.2.1).

4.4.2.3   Denaturation of proteins

Because of their compact secondary and tertiary structures, most proteins are resistant to digestive enzymes—few bonds are accessible to the proteolytic enzymes that catalyse hydrolysis of peptide bonds. However, apart from covalent links formed by reaction between the side chains of lysine and aspartate or glutamate and disulfide bridges, the native structure of proteins is maintained by relatively weak non-covalent forces: ionic interactions, hydrogen bonding, and van der Waals forces.

The denaturation of a protein is loss of its compact secondary and tertiary structures, opening out the molecule so that it becomes insoluble (and in the case of an enzyme loses its catalytic activity, Section 2.3.2). Denatured proteins are susceptible to the action of digestive enzymes; thus, denaturation is an important precursor to protein digestion. The relatively weak bonds that maintain the native structure of proteins can be disrupted by heat and extremes of pH; thus, both cooking and gastric acid are important in protein digestion.

4.4.3   Protein digestion

Protein digestion occurs by hydrolysis of the peptide bonds between amino acids. There are two main classes of protein digestive enzymes (proteases), with different specificities for the amino acids forming the peptide bond to be hydrolysed (Table 4.2):

Table 4.2 Protein Digestive Enzymes

	Secreted by	Specificity
Endopeptidases		
Pepsin	Gastric mucosa	Adjacent to aromatic amino acid, leucine or methionine
Trypsin	Pancreas	Lysine or arginine esters
Chymotrypsin	Pancreas	Aromatic esters
Elastase	Pancreas	Neutral aliphatic esters
Enteropeptidase	Intestinal mucosa	Trypsinogen → trypsin
Exopeptidases		
Carboxypeptidases	Pancreas	Carboxy terminal amino acids
Aminopeptidases	Intestinal mucosa	Amino terminal amino acids
Tripeptidases	Mucosal brush border	Tripeptides
Dipeptidases	Mucosal brush border	Dipeptides

1. *Endopeptidases* cleave proteins by hydrolysing peptide bonds between specific amino acids throughout the molecule.
2. *Exopeptidases* remove amino acids one at a time from either the amino or carboxyl end of the molecule, again by the hydrolysis of the peptide bond.

The first enzymes to act on dietary proteins are the endopeptidases: pepsin in the gastric juice, and trypsin, chymotrypsin, and elastase in the small intestine. (The different specificities of trypsin, chymotrypsin, and elastase are discussed in Section 2.2.1.) The result of the combined action of the endopeptidases is that the large protein molecules are broken down into smaller polypeptides with a large number of amino and carboxy terminals for the exopeptidases to act on. There are two classes of exopeptidase:

1. *Carboxypeptidases*, secreted in the pancreatic juice, release amino acids from the free carboxyl terminal of peptides.
2. *Aminopeptidases*, secreted by the intestinal mucosal cells, release amino acids from the amino terminal of peptides.

Both aminopeptidases and carboxypeptidases continue to act until the final product is a dipeptide or tripeptide, which is hydrolysed by dipeptidases and tripeptidases inside the brush border of the mucosal cell.

4.4.3.1   Activation of zymogens of proteolytic enzymes

The proteases are secreted as inactive precursors (zymogens)—this is essential if they are not to digest themselves and tissue proteins before they are secreted. In each case, the active site of the enzyme is masked by a small region of the peptide chain that has to be removed for the enzyme to have activity. This is achieved by hydrolysis of a specific peptide bond in the precursor molecule, releasing the blocking peptide and revealing the active site of the enzyme.

Pepsin is secreted in the gastric juice as pepsinogen, which is activated by the action of gastric acid, and also by the action of already activated pepsin. In the small intestine, trypsinogen, the precursor of trypsin, is activated by the action of a specific enzyme, enteropeptidase (sometimes known by its obsolete name of enterokinase), which is secreted by the duodenal epithelial cells; trypsin can then activate chymotrypsinogen to chymotrypsin, pro-elastase to elastase, procarboxypeptidase to carboxypeptidase, and pro-aminopeptidase to aminopeptidase.

4.4.3.2   Absorption of the products of protein digestion

The end product of the action of endopeptidases and exopeptidases is a mixture of free amino acids, dipeptides and tripeptides, and oligopeptides.

Free amino acids are absorbed across the intestinal mucosa by sodium-dependent active transport (Section 3.2.2.6). There are a number of different amino acid transport systems, with specificity for the chemical nature of the side chain (large or small neutral, acidic or basic). Similar group-specific amino acid transporters occur in the renal tubules (for reabsorption of amino acids filtered at the glomerulus) and for uptake of amino acids into tissues. The various amino acids carried by any one transporter compete with each other for absorption and tissue uptake.

Dipeptides and tripeptides enter the brush border of the intestinal mucosal cells, where they are hydrolysed to free amino acids, which are then transported into the bloodstream. Patients with (rare) genetic defects of one or other of the amino acid transporters can still absorb dipeptides and tripeptides, thus having a (limited) dietary source of all of the amino acids.

Relatively large peptides can be absorbed intact, either by uptake into mucosal epithelial cells (the transcellular route) or by passing between epithelial cells (the paracellular route). These peptides may be large enough to stimulate antibody production; this is the basis of allergic reactions to foods. In infants, there is greater absorption of intact small proteins and oligopeptides than in adults. This permits the infant to gain passive immunity by absorbing immunoglobulins in breast milk. However, it also means that early exposure to foreign proteins can result in the development of a food allergy; cow's milk, egg, and peanut proteins are common food allergens.

4.5   The absorption of vitamins and minerals

In addition to compounds that enter the small intestine from the diet, a number of vitamins and other compounds are secreted in the bile, then reabsorbed from the small intestine—a process of enterohepatic circulation. For example, the total amount of cholesterol entering the gut is some fourfold to fivefold higher than the dietary intake; thus, inhibition of cholesterol absorption has a considerably greater effect than might be expected (Figure 4.15). Folate and vitamin B_{12} undergo similar enterohepatic circulation. In the case of vitamin B_{12}, this serves to remove degradation products and metabolites that have antivitamin activity, since the intestinal binding protein that is required for vitamin B_{12} absorption (intrinsic factor, Section 4.5.2.1) binds only biologically active vitamin B_{12} and none of its analogues.

4.5.1   Absorption of lipid-soluble vitamins and cholesterol

Absorption of the lipid soluble vitamins (A, D, E, and K) depends on an adequate total amount of fat in the diet because they are absorbed dissolved in the core of lipid micelles, then incorporated into chylomicrons together with re-esterified fatty acids (Section 4.3.2.2). Vitamins D and E, and carotenes, are absorbed passively, by diffusion. Vitamin A enters enterocytes by carrier-mediated transport, followed by esterification to permit accumulation; when the carrier is saturated, there is also passive uptake of the vitamin. Vitamin K is transported into enterocytes by an ATP-dependent transporter. Cholesterol enters enterocytes by carrier-mediated transport.

4.5.2   Absorption of water-soluble vitamins

The absorption of water-soluble vitamins requires a transport protein at the luminal surface of the mucosal cell; this may involve active or passive transport and may be followed by metabolic trapping (Section 3.2.2.2) to permit accumulation. In some cases, active transport is also involved in the efflux of the vitamin from the enterocyte into the bloodstream.

Thiamin (vitamin B_1, Section 11.6.1) enters the enterocyte by active transport via a proton pumping ATPase. Some is phosphorylated intracellularly, and there is Na^+-dependent active transport into the bloodstream. The active transport of thiamin out of the enterocyte into the bloodstream is inhibited by alcohol, which, together with a poor diet, explains the relatively common occurrence of thiamin deficiency in alcoholics and heavy drinkers.

Riboflavin (vitamin B_2, Section 11.7.1) enters the enterocyte by Na^+-dependent active transport, followed by metabolic trapping as riboflavin monophosphate. The niacin vitamers nicotinic acid and nicotinamide (Section 11.8) enter the enterocyte by Na^+-dependent active transport.

Vitamin B_6 (Section 11.9.1) enters the enterocyte by carrier-mediated passive transport, followed by metabolic trapping as pyridoxal phosphate. However, much is dephosphorylated by alkaline phosphatase at the serosal surface of the cell; thus, it is mainly pyridoxal rather than pyridoxal phosphate that enters the bloodstream.

Dietary folate (Section 11.11) is a mixture of derivatives with different lengths of a poly-γ-glutamyl side chain. In the intestinal lumen the side chain is removed by conjugase (a zinc-dependent enzyme), and folate monoglutamate enters the enterocyte by carrier-mediated passive uptake, followed by reduction and methylation; thus, what enters the bloodstream is mainly methyl-tetrahydrofolate.

Despite their very different structures, biotin (Section 11.12) and pantothenic acid (Section 11.13) enter the enterocyte using the same Na^+-dependent active transport protein.

Vitamin C (Section 11.14.1) enters the enterocyte by Na^+-dependent active transport. This transport protein is found elsewhere in the gastrointestinal tract, and a modest amount of vitamin C can be absorbed in the mouth.

4.5.2.1   *Absorption of vitamin B_{12}*

Very small amounts of vitamin B_{12} (Section 11.10) can be absorbed by passive diffusion across the intestinal mucosa, but under normal conditions this is insignificant, accounting for less than 1% of a large oral dose; the major route of vitamin B_{12} absorption is by way of attachment to a specific binding protein in the intestinal lumen. This binding protein is 'intrinsic factor', so-called because in the early studies of pernicious anaemia (Section 11.10.2), it was found that two curative factors were involved—an extrinsic or dietary factor, which we now know to be vitamin B_{12}, and an intrinsic or endogenously produced factor. Intrinsic factor is a small glycoprotein secreted by the parietal cells of the gastric mucosa, which also secrete hydrochloric acid.

Both gastric acid and pepsin have a role in vitamin B_{12} absorption, serving to release the vitamin from the proteins it is bound to in foods. Atrophic gastritis is a relatively common problem of advancing age; in the early stages, there is impaired acid secretion, but more or less normal secretion of intrinsic factor. This can result in vitamin B_{12} depletion due to failure to release the vitamin from dietary proteins, but the absorption of free vitamin B_{12} (as in nutritional supplements) is unaffected. Inhibition of gastric acid secretion to treat gastric ulcers and hiatus hernia will also impair the release of vitamin B_{12} from dietary proteins, but there is no evidence that even prolonged use of the proton pump inhibiting drugs results in vitamin B_{12} deficiency.

In the stomach, vitamin B_{12} binds to cobalophilin, a binding protein secreted in the saliva. Cobalophilin is hydrolysed in the duodenum, releasing the vitamin B_{12} for binding to intrinsic factor. Pancreatic insufficiency can therefore be a factor in the development of vitamin B_{12} deficiency, since failure to hydrolyse cobalophilin will result in the excretion of cobalophilin-bound vitamin B_{12} rather than transfer to intrinsic factor. Intrinsic factor only binds biologically active vitamin B_{12} and not analogues that have no biological activity. Considerably more intrinsic factor is normally secreted than is needed for the binding and absorption of dietary vitamin B_{12}, which requires only about 1% of the total intrinsic factor available.

Vitamin B_{12} is absorbed from the distal third of the ileum by receptor-mediated endocytosis. There are intrinsic factor–vitamin B_{12} binding sites on the brush border of the mucosal cells in this region; free intrinsic factor does not interact with these receptors. The absorption of vitamin B_{12} is limited by the number of binding sites in the ileal mucosa; thus, not more than about 1–1.5 μg of a single oral dose of the vitamin is absorbed.

Within the mucosal cell, the vitamin is released by lysosomal proteolysis of intrinsic factor and is bound to transcobalamin II, a binding protein synthesised in the enterocytes and stored in vesicles destined for export from the cell. In plasma, vitamin B_{12} circulates bound to transcobalamin I, which is required for tissue uptake of the vitamin, and transcobalamin II, which seems to be a storage form of the vitamin.

There is a considerable enterohepatic circulation of vitamin B_{12}. Vitamin B_{12} and its metabolites (some of which are biologically inactive) are transferred from peripheral tissues to the liver bound to transcobalamin III. They are then secreted into the bile, bound to cobalophilins; 3–8 µg of vitamin B_{12} may be secreted in the bile each day, about the same as the average dietary intake. Like dietary vitamin B_{12} bound to salivary cobalophilin, the biliary cobalophilins are hydrolysed in the duodenum, and the vitamin binds to intrinsic factor, thus permitting reabsorption in the ileum. Whilst cobalophilins and transcorrin III have low specificity and will bind a variety of vitamin B_{12} analogues, intrinsic factor binds only cobalamins, and so only the biologically active vitamin will be reabsorbed to any significant extent.

4.5.3   Absorption of minerals

Mineral ions require a transport protein at the luminal surface of the mucosal cell and are accumulated inside the mucosal cell by binding to intracellular proteins. Transfer from mucosal cells into the bloodstream is usually by ATP-dependent active transport (Section 3.2.2.3), commonly onto a plasma-binding protein. Genetic defects of the intracellular binding proteins or the active transport systems at the basal membrane of the mucosal cell can result in deficiency despite an apparently adequate intake of the mineral.

The absorption of calcium is dependent on vitamin D (Section 11.3.3). Synthesis of calbindin, the intracellular binding protein that is required for accumulation of calcium, requires the nuclear action of vitamin D; thus, when vitamin D deficient animals are repleted with the vitamin, there is a significant time lag before calcium absorption increases. The calcium transport protein only migrates from intracellular vesicles to the cell surface, to permit uptake of calcium, in response to rapid (cell surface receptor mediated) actions of vitamin D.

The absorption of many minerals is affected by other compounds present in the intestinal lumen. Reducing compounds can enhance the absorption of iron (Section 4.5.3.1), and chelating compounds enhance the absorption of other minerals. For example, zinc absorption is dependent on the secretion by the pancreas of a zinc-binding ligand (tentatively identified as the tryptophan metabolite picolinic acid). Failure to synthesise and secrete this zinc binding ligand, as a result of a genetic disease, leads to the condition of acrodermatitis enteropathica—functional zinc deficiency despite an apparently adequate intake.

Diets based on unleavened wheat bread contain a relatively large amount of phytic acid (inositol hexaphosphate), which can bind calcium, iron, and zinc to form insoluble complexes that are not absorbed. Zinc deficiency, leading to delayed puberty, is relatively common in tropical countries where there is a considerable loss of zinc in sweat and the diet is based on unleavened wheat breads. Leavened breads do not impair zinc absorption. Phytases in yeast catalyse dephosphorylation of phytate to products that do not chelate minerals. Polyphenols (flavonoids, Section 6.7.2.3), especially tannic acid in tea, can also chelate iron and other minerals, reducing their absorption. Large amounts of free fatty acids in the gut lumen (associated with defects of fat absorption) can impair the absorption of calcium and magnesium by forming insoluble soaps. Oxalic acid (as found in rhubarb and some other foods) can also impair absorption of calcium and magnesium by forming insoluble oxalate salts in the intestinal lumen.

4.5.3.1 Iron absorption

Only about 10%–15% of total dietary iron is absorbed, depending on the state of body iron reserves, and as little as 1%–5% of the inorganic iron in plant foods. Haem iron in meat is better absorbed by a separate transport system (Figure 4.23).

Inorganic iron is absorbed only in the Fe^{2+} (reduced) form. This means that a variety of reducing agents present in the intestinal lumen together with dietary iron will enhance its absorption. The most effective such compound is vitamin C (Section 11.14). Whilst intakes of 40–100 mg of vitamin C/day are more than adequate to meet requirements, an intake of 25–50 mg per meal is sometimes recommended to enhance iron absorption. For this reason, it is, or should be, common practice to prescribe vitamin C supplements together with iron supplements to treat iron deficiency anaemia (Sections 11.15.2.3 and 11.16) or recommend that the iron tablets are taken together with a fruit juice. Alcohol, fructose, and a number of organic acids also enhance iron absorption.

Inorganic iron enters the mucosal cells by a proton-linked active transport mechanism, the divalent metal ion transporter. There is a separate transporter for the uptake of haem. Haem iron is released as Fe^{2+} by the action of haem oxygenase. Iron can only leave the mucosal cell via the transport protein ferroportin, and only if there is free apo-transferrin in the bloodstream to oxidise it to Fe^{3+} and bind it. When all or most of the transferrin in the bloodstream has iron bound, no more iron can leave the mucosal cells. The activity of ferroportin (and possibly also that of the divalent metal transporter) is down-regulated by hepcidin, a peptide secreted by the liver. In response to anaemia, hypoxia or haemorrhage, hepcidin secretion is reduced, and the activity of ferroportin increases; thus, more iron can enter the bloodstream from the mucosal cells. Iron in the mucosal cell that is not transported out by ferroportin is oxidised to Fe^{3+} and bound to ferritin. It is then lost into the intestinal lumen when the cells are shed at the tip of the villus.

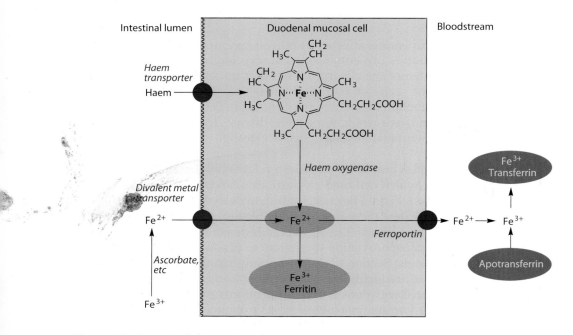

Figure 4.23 Intestinal absorption of iron.

This mucosal barrier to the absorption of iron has a protective function. There is no pathway for excretion of iron from the body, although there are obligatory losses in shed skin and intestinal cells. The body's iron reserves are controlled by regulation of intestinal absorption. About 10% of the population are genetically susceptible to iron overload (haemochromatosis). This is a serious condition, with deposition of inappropriately large amounts of iron in haemosiderin in tissues, and the accumulation of free iron ions, which generate tissue-damaging oxygen radicals (Section 6.5). The consequences of haemochromatosis include enlargement of the liver, diabetes mellitus as a result of radical damage to pancreatic β-islet cells (because of the skin pigmentation associated with haemochromatosis, the condition is sometimes called bronze diabetes), painful inflammation of joints, heart disease, and depletion of vitamin C, leading to scurvy (Section 11.14.3).

By contrast, at least 10% of women have higher losses of iron in menstrual blood loss than can readily be replaced from the diet, and iron-deficiency anaemia, or very low tissue reserves of iron, are common amongst women of child-bearing age. In men, the ratio of storage iron (in ferritin and haemosiderin) to the functional pool of iron (in haemoglobin, myoglobin, transferrin, cytochromes, and enzymes) ranges between 0.17 and 0.52; in women of child-bearing age, this ratio ranges between 0 and 0.16. One of the reasons why women are less at risk of atherosclerosis than are men may be because of their lower iron reserves. This raises the interesting problem of whether or not it is desirable to recommend high intakes of iron for women of child-bearing age to increase their iron reserves to the same level as seen in men. This would prevent the development of iron deficiency but might also put them at risk of iron overload and increased risk of atherosclerosis.

Key points

- Carbohydrates provide the main source of metabolic fuel. They can be classified into three main groups: sugars (monosaccharides and disaccharides), oligosaccharides, and polysaccharides. Starch is the nutritionally important polysaccharide; a variety of non-starch polysaccharides occur in foods, but are not digested, although they provide a substrate for intestinal bacterial fermentation.
- Dietary carbohydrates can be classified according to their glycaemic index—the extent to which they raise blood glucose compared with an equivalent amount of glucose or a reference carbohydrate.
- Starch digestion begins with the action of amylase secreted in saliva, then continues with pancreatic amylase, yielding a mixture of glucose, maltose, and isomaltose. The extent and rate of starch digestion, and hence its glycaemic index, depend on the degree of crystallisation of the starch.
- Dietary disaccharides are hydrolysed by disaccharidases on the luminal face of the brush border of the intestinal mucosa. Glucose and galactose are absorbed by Na$^+$-linked active transport, other sugars and sugar alcohols are absorbed by facilitated (passive) diffusion.
- Disaccharides that cannot be hydrolysed because of lack of the relevant disaccharidase, and unabsorbed monosaccharides and sugar alcohols provide substrates for bacterial fermentation, leading to osmotic diarrhoea and intestinal pain.
- Triacylglycerols contain saturated or unsaturated fatty acids esterified to glycerol; the amount of saturated, monounsaturated, and polyunsaturated fatty acids in the diet has significant health effects. *Trans*-isomers of unsaturated fatty acids have adverse health effects.

- Triacylglycerols are hydrolysed by lipase secreted by the tongue, in gastric juice and by the pancreas, leading to liberation of free fatty acids and 2-monoacylglycerol; the latter is hydrolysed by pancreatic and intracellular esterases.
- The bile salts are required to complete the emulsification of dietary lipids to micelles that are small enough to be absorbed into intestinal mucosal cells.
- Within the mucosal cell, fatty acids are re-esterified to triacylglycerol and packaged with proteins to form chylomicrons, which enter the lymphatic system. Peripheral tissues take up fatty acids from chylomicrons by the action of extracellular lipoprotein lipase; the liver clears chylomicron remnants.
- Proteins are polymers of amino acids; 21 amino acids are involved in protein synthesis, and others are formed by postsynthetic modification of proteins. Nine of the amino acids are dietary essentials that cannot be synthesised in the body.
- Protein digestion involves denaturation of dietary proteins by heat and the action of gastric acid, followed by the action of endopeptidases that cleave the proteins into smaller peptides, then of exopeptidases that sequentially remove amino and carboxy terminal amino acids.
- Free amino acids are absorbed by Na^+-linked active transport; dipeptides and tripeptides are absorbed by a separate mechanism and are hydrolysed inside the mucosal cell. Significant amounts of relatively large peptides can be absorbed intact; this may result in allergic reactions to foods.
- Absorption of the lipid-soluble vitamins requires an adequate amount of dietary fat.
- Water-soluble vitamins are absorbed in various ways, generally involving active transport into or out of the mucosal cell, sometimes with metabolic trapping to achieve intracellular accumulation.
- Vitamin B_{12} absorption requires gastric acid to release the vitamin from binding to dietary proteins, and specific binding proteins secreted in saliva and by the gastric mucosa. There is considerable enterohepatic cycling of vitamin B_{12}.
- The absorption of minerals generally involves active transport into and out of the mucosal cell as well as intracellular protein binding. A variety of non-nutrient compounds present in foods (especially phytate and polyphenols) can impair the absorption of minerals.
- The absorption of iron is limited and controlled by the state of body iron reserves.

Additional resources on the CD

The peptide sequence computer simulation program in the virtual laboratory on the CD.

chapter five

Energy nutrition
The metabolism of carbohydrates and fats

If the intake of metabolic fuels is equivalent to energy expenditure, there is a state of energy balance. Overall, there will be equal periods of fed state metabolism (during which nutrient reserves are accumulated as liver and muscle glycogen, adipose tissue triacylglycerols, and labile protein stores), and fasting state metabolism, during which these reserves are utilised. Averaged out over several days, there will be no change in body weight or body composition.

By contrast, if the intake of metabolic fuels is greater than is required to meet energy expenditure, the body will spend more time in the fed state than the fasting state; there will be more accumulation of nutrient reserves than utilisation. The result of this is an increase in adipose tissue stores. If continued for long enough, this will result in overweight or obesity, with potentially serious health consequences (Chapter 7).

The opposite state of affairs is when the intake of metabolic fuels is lower than is required to meet energy expenditure. Now the body has to mobilise its nutrient reserves and overall spends more time in the fasting state than in the fed state. The result of this is undernutrition, starvation, and eventually death (Chapter 8).

Objectives

After reading this chapter, you should be able to

- Define the terms used in energy metabolism and explain how energy expenditure is measured.
- Describe the sources of metabolic fuels in the fed and fasting states.
- Describe and explain the relationship among energy intake, energy expenditure, and body weight.
- Describe the pathway of glycolysis and explain how anaerobic glycolysis under conditions of maximum exertion leads to oxygen debt.
- Describe the pentose phosphate pathway, and explain its importance in tissues synthesising fatty acids, and how deficiency of glucose 6-phosphate dehydrogenase results in haemolytic crisis.
- Describe the metabolic fates of pyruvate arising from glycolysis.
- Describe the citric acid cycle and explain how it acts both as a central energy-yielding pathway and also for interconversion of metabolites.
- Explain the importance of carnitine in fatty acid uptake into mitochondria and describe the β-oxidation of fatty acids.
- Describe the formation and utilisation of ketone bodies and explain their importance in fasting and starvation.
- Describe the synthesis of fatty acids and triacylglycerol as a major energy reserve in the body.

- Describe the roles of plasma lipoproteins in transport of lipids around the body.
- Describe the synthesis and utilisation of glycogen and the pathways for gluconeo-genesis in the fasting state.

5.1 Estimation of energy expenditure

Energy expenditure can be determined directly, by measuring heat output from the body. This requires a thermally insulated chamber in which the temperature can be controlled to maintain the subject's comfort and in which it is possible to measure the amount of heat produced—for example, by the increase in temperature of the water used to cool the chamber. Calorimeters of this sort are relatively small; thus, it is only possible for measurements of direct heat production to be made for subjects performing a limited range of tasks, and only for a relatively short time. Most estimates of energy expenditure are based on indirect measurements—either measurement of oxygen consumption and carbon dioxide production (indirect calorimetry, Section 5.1.1) or indirect estimation of carbon dioxide production by use of dual isotopically labelled water (Section 5.1.2). From the results of a number of studies in which energy expenditure in different activities has been measured, it is possible to calculate total energy expenditure from the time spent in each type of activity (Section 5.1.3).

5.1.1 Indirect calorimetry and the respiratory quotient

Energy expenditure can be determined from the rate of consumption of oxygen. This is known as indirect calorimetry, since there is no direct measurement of the heat produced. There is an output or expenditure of approximately 20 kJ for each litre of oxygen consumed, regardless of whether the fuel being metabolised is carbohydrate, fat, or protein (Table 5.1). Measurement of oxygen consumption is quite simple using a spirometer. Such instruments are portable; thus, people can carry on more or less normal activities for several hours at a time, whilst their oxygen consumption is being measured.

Measurement of both oxygen consumption and carbon dioxide production at the same time provides information on the mixture of metabolic fuels being metabolised. In the metabolism of carbohydrates, the same amount of carbon dioxide is produced as oxygen is consumed—i.e., the ratio of carbon dioxide produced/oxygen consumed (the respiratory quotient, RQ) = 1.0. This is because the overall reaction is $C_6H_{12}O_6 + 6 O_2 \rightarrow 6 CO_2 + 6 H_2O$.

Proportionally more oxygen is required for the oxidation of fat. The major process involved is the oxidation of $-CH_2-$ units: $-CH_2 + 1\frac{1}{2} O_2 \rightarrow CO_2 + H_2O$. Allowing for the fact that, in triacylglycerols, there are also the glycerol and three carboxyl groups to be considered, overall for the oxidation of fat the RQ = 0.7.

Table 5.1 Oxygen Consumption and Carbon Dioxide Production
in the Oxidation of Metabolic Fuels

	Energy yield (kJ/g)	Oxygen consumed (L/g)	Carbon dioxide produced (L/g)	Respiratory quotient (CO_2/O_2)	Energy/oxygen consumption (kJ/L oxygen)
Carbohydrate	16	0.829	0.829	1.0	
Protein	17	0.966	0.782	0.809	~20
Fat	37	2.016	1.427	0.707	

The oxidation of the mixture of amino acids arising from proteins gives RQ = 0.8. The amount of protein being oxidised can be determined separately, by measuring the excretion of urea, the end product of amino acid metabolism (Section 9.3.1.4).

Measurement of the respiratory quotient and urinary excretion of urea thus permits calculation of the relative amounts of fat, carbohydrate, and protein being metabolised. In the fasting state (Section 5.3.2), when a relatively large amount of fat is being used as a fuel, the RQ is around 0.8–0.85; after a meal, when there is more carbohydrate available to be metabolised (Section 5.3.1), the RQ increases to about 0.9–1.0. If there is a significant amount of lipid being synthesised from carbohydrate (Section 5.6.1), then the respiratory quotient may increase above 1.0.

5.1.2 Long-term measurement of energy expenditure— the dual isotopically labelled water method

Measurement of oxygen consumption only permits measurement of energy expenditure over a period of a few hours. An alternative technique permits estimation of total energy expenditure over a period of 2–3 weeks by giving a dose of dual isotopically labelled water, $^2H_2^{18}O$, and determining the rate of loss of the isotopes from body water.

The deuterium (^2H) is lost from the body only in water. However, the labelled oxygen (^{18}O) can be lost in either water or carbon dioxide because of the rapid equilibrium between carbon dioxide and bicarbonate: $H_2O + CO_2 \rightleftharpoons H^+ + HCO_3^-$. This means that the rate of loss of ^{18}O is faster than that of ^2H (Figure 5.1). The difference between the rate of loss of the two isotopes from body water (plasma, saliva, or urine) thus reflects the total amount of carbon dioxide that has been produced:

$$CO_2 \text{ production} = (0.5 \times \text{total body water}) \times (k_O - k_H)$$

where k_O is the rate constant for loss of label from ^{18}O and k_H is the rate constant for loss of label from ^2H.

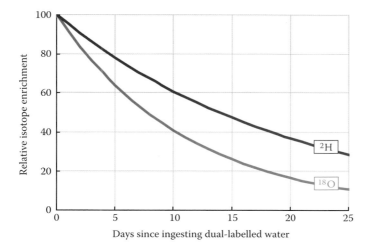

Figure 5.1 The estimation of energy expenditure using dual isotopically labelled water ($^2H_2^{18}O$).

Estimating the average respiratory quotient over the period from the proportions of fat, carbohydrate, and protein in the diet and allowing for any changes in body fat permits calculation of the total amount of oxygen that has been consumed and hence the total energy expenditure over a period of 2–3 weeks. This technique thus provides a non-invasive way of estimating energy expenditure over several days in normal activities.

5.1.3   Calculation of energy expenditure

Key terms in energy metabolism are defined in Table 5.2. Energy expenditure depends on

- The requirement for maintenance of normal body structure, function, and metabolic integrity—the basal metabolic rate (Section 5.1.3.1).
- The energy required for work and physical activity (Section 5.1.3.2).
- The energy cost of synthesising reserves of fat and glycogen and the increase in protein synthesis in the fed state (Section 5.1.3.3).

5.1.3.1   Basal metabolic rate

Basal metabolic rate (BMR) is the energy expenditure by the body when at rest, but not asleep, under controlled conditions of thermal neutrality and about 12 h after the last meal. It is the energy requirement for the maintenance of metabolic integrity, nerve and muscle tone, circulation, and respiration (see Figure 1.2 for the contribution of different organs to resting energy expenditure). It is important that the subject is awake, since some people show an increased metabolic rate (and hence increased heat output) when they are asleep, whilst others have a reduced metabolic rate and a slight fall in body temperature. Where the measurement of metabolic rate has been made under less strictly controlled conditions, the result is more correctly called the resting metabolic rate.

Table 5.2 Definitions in Energy Metabolism

BMR	Basal metabolic rate	Energy expenditure in the post-absorptive state; measured under standardised conditions of thermal neutrality (environmental temperature 26°C–30°C), awake but completely at rest
RMR	Resting metabolic rate	Energy expenditure at rest, not measured under strictly standardised conditions
PAR	Physical activity ratio	The energy cost of physical activity expressed as multiple of BMR
MET	Metabolic equivalent of the task	The energy cost of physical activity expressed as multiple of BMR
IEI	Integrated energy index	Energy cost of an activity over a period of time, including time spent pausing or resting, expressed as the average (integrated) value over the time, as a multiple of BMR
PAL	Physical activity level	Sum of PAR or IEI × hours spent in each activity/24 h, expressed as multiple of BMR
DIT	Diet-induced thermogenesis	Increased energy expenditure after a meal
TEE	Total energy expenditure	(PAL × BMR) + DIT

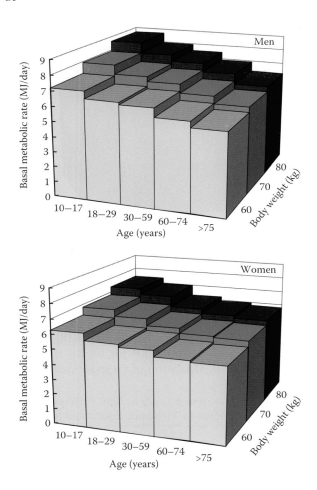

Figure 5.2 The effects of age and gender on basal metabolic rate.

BMR depends on body weight, age, and gender (Figure 5.2):

- Body weight affects BMR because there is a greater amount of metabolically active tissue in a larger body. Although adipose tissue contains 80% by weight triacylglycerol, it is still metabolically active.
- The decrease in BMR with increasing age is due to changes in body composition. With increasing age, even if body weight remains constant, there is loss of muscle and replacement by adipose tissue, which is metabolically less active, since 80% of the weight of adipose tissue consists of reserves of triacylglycerol.
- Women have a significantly lower BMR than men of the same weight because the proportion of body weight that is adipose tissue reserves in lean women is higher than in men (Figure 5.3).

5.1.3.2   *Energy costs of physical activity*

The most useful way of expressing the energy cost of physical activities is as a multiple of BMR. Two equivalent terms are used to describe this: physical activity ratio (PAR) and metabolic equivalent of the task (MET). The PAR (or MET) for an activity is the ratio of

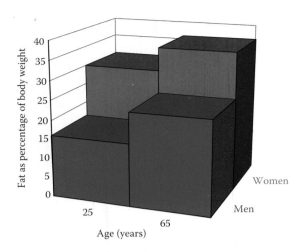

Figure 5.3 Body fat as a percentage of weight with age and gender.

the energy expended whilst performing the activity/that expended at rest (= BMR). Very gentle, sedentary activities use only about 1.1–1.2 × BMR. By contrast, vigorous exertion, such as climbing stairs or walking uphill, may use 6–8 × BMR.

Using data such as those in Table 5.3 and allowing for the time spent during each type of activity through the day permits calculation of an individual's PAL. This is the sum of

Table 5.3 Energy Expenditure in Different Types of Activity Expressed as Multiple of BMR (Physical Activity Ratio or Metabolic Equivalent of the Task)

PAR (or MET)	
1.0–1.4	Lying, standing, or sitting at rest, e.g., watching TV, reading, writing, eating, playing cards and board games
1.5–1.8	*Sitting:* sewing, knitting, playing piano, driving
	Standing: preparing vegetables, washing dishes, ironing, general office, and laboratory work
1.9–2.4	*Standing:* mixed household chores, cooking, playing snooker or bowls
2.5–3.3	*Standing:* dressing, undressing, showering, making beds, vacuum cleaning
	Walking: 3–4 km/h, playing cricket
	Occupational: tailoring, shoemaking, electrical and machine tool industry, painting, and decorating
3.4–4.4	*Standing:* mopping floors, gardening, cleaning windows, table tennis, sailing
	Walking: 4–6 km/h, playing golf
	Occupational: motor vehicle repairs, carpentry and joinery, chemical industry, bricklaying
4.5–5.9	*Standing:* polishing furniture, chopping wood, heavy gardening, volley ball
	Walking: 6–7 km/h
	Exercise: dancing, moderate swimming, gentle cycling, slow jogging
	Occupational: labouring, hoeing, road construction, digging and shovelling, felling trees
6.0–7.9	*Walking:* uphill with load or cross-country, climbing stairs
	Exercise: jogging, cycling, energetic swimming, skiing, tennis, football

Table 5.4 Classification of Types of Occupational Work by Physical Activity Ratio

Work intensity	PAR (or MET)[a]	
Light	1.7	Professional, clerical, and technical workers, administrative and managerial staff, sales representatives, housewives
Moderate	2.2–2.7	Sales staff, domestic service, students, transport workers, joiners, roofing workers
Moderately heavy	2.3–3.0	Machine operators, labourers, agricultural workers, bricklaying, masonry
Heavy	2.8–3.8	Labourers, agricultural workers, bricklaying, masonry where there is little or no mechanisation

Note: Figures show the average PAR through an 8-h working day, excluding leisure activities.

[a] Where a range of PAR (or MET) is shown, the lower figure is for women and the higher for men.

the PAR of each activity performed × hours spent in that activity/24. A desirable level of physical activity, in terms of cardiovascular and respiratory health, is a PAL of 1.7.

Table 5.4 shows the classification of different types of occupational work by PAR. This is the average PAR during the 8-h working day and makes no allowance for leisure activities. From these figures, it might seem that there would be no problem in achieving the desirable PAL of 1.7. However, in Britain, the average PAL is only 1.4, and the desirable level of 1.7 is achieved by only 22% of men and 13% of women.

The energy cost of physical activity is obviously affected by body weight because more energy is required to move a heavier body. Figure 5.4 shows the effects of body weight on BMR and total energy expenditure at different levels of physical activity. Table 5.5 shows

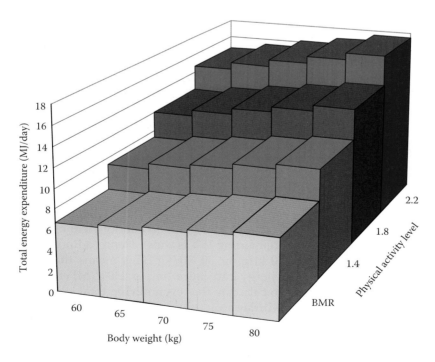

Figure 5.4 The effects of body weight and physical activity on total energy expenditure.

Table 5.5 Average Requirements for Energy, Based on Desirable
Body Weight (BMI = 20–25) and for Adults Assuming PAL = 1.4

Age (years)	Males (MJ/day)	Females (MJ/day)
1–3	5.2	4.9
4–6	7.2	6.5
7–10	8.2	7.3
11–14	9.3	7.9
15–18	11.5	8.8
Adults	10.6	8.0

average energy requirements at different ages, assuming a desirable and constant body weight (BMI 20–25, see Section 7.1.1), and for adults, the average PAL of 1.4 × BMR.

5.1.3.3   Diet-induced thermogenesis

There is a considerable increase in metabolic rate after a meal. A small part of this is the energy cost of secreting digestive enzymes and the energy cost of active transport of the products of digestion (Section 3.2.2). The major part is the energy cost of synthesising reserves of glycogen (Section 5.6.3) and triacylglycerol (Section 5.6.1.2) as well as the increased protein synthesis that occurs in the fed state (Section 9.2.3.3). For an adult in nitrogen balance (Section 9.1), an amount of amino acids equivalent to the dietary intake of protein will be catabolised each day. The metabolism of these amino acids includes a number of steps that are thermogenic and metabolically inefficient, in that ATP is both consumed and produced, leading to heat production without ATP formation. The pathway of glycolysis (Section 5.4.1) similarly involves inefficient thermogenesis; 2 mol of ATP are consumed and 4 mol are produced in the anaerobic metabolism of glucose to pyruvate.

The cost of synthesising glycogen from glucose is about 5% of the ingested energy, whilst the cost of synthesising triacylglycerol from glucose is about 20% of the ingested energy. Depending on the relative amounts of fat, carbohydrate, and protein in the diet and the amounts of triacylglycerol and glycogen being synthesised, diet-induced thermogenesis may account for 10% or more of the total energy yield of a meal.

5.2   Energy balance and changes in body weight

When energy intake is greater than expenditure (positive energy balance), there is increased storage of surplus metabolic fuel, largely as triacylglycerol in adipose tissue; similarly, if energy intake is inadequate to meet expenditure (negative energy balance), adipose tissue triacylglycerol reserves are utilised.

Adipose tissue contains 80% triacylglycerol (with an energy yield of 37 kJ/g) and 5% protein (energy yield 17 kJ/g)—the remaining 15% is water. Hence, adipose tissue reserves are equivalent to approximately 30 kJ/g, or 30 MJ/kg. This means that the theoretical change in body weight is 33 g/MJ energy imbalance/day, or 230 g/MJ energy imbalance/week. On this basis, it is possible to calculate that even during total starvation, a person with an energy expenditure of 10 MJ/day would lose only 330 g body weight per day or 2.3 kg/week.

This calculation suggests that there will be a constant change of body weight with a constant excessive or deficient energy intake, but this is not observed in practice. The rate of weight gain in positive energy balance is not as great as would be predicted and

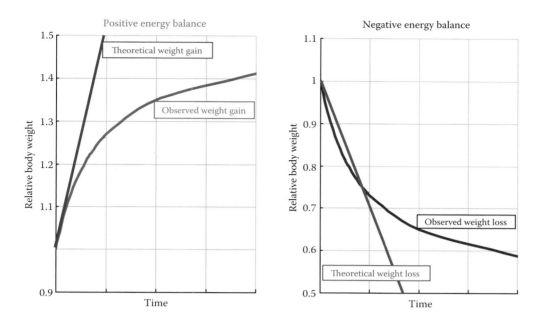

Figure 5.5 Predicted and observed changes in body weight with energy imbalance.

gradually slows down, so that after a time, the subject regains energy balance, albeit with a higher body weight (Figure 5.5). Similarly, in negative energy balance, weight is not lost at a constant rate; the rate of loss slows down, and (assuming that the energy deficit is not too severe) levels off, and the subject regains energy balance, at a lower body weight.

A number of factors contribute to this adaptation to changing energy balance:

- As more food is eaten, there is an increased energy cost of digestion and absorption.
- When intake is in excess of requirements, a greater proportion is used for synthesis of adipose tissue triacylglycerol reserves; thus, there is more diet-induced thermogenesis. Conversely, in negative energy balance, there is less synthesis of adipose tissue reserves and so less diet-induced thermogenesis.
- The rate of protein turnover increases with greater energy intake (Section 9.2.3.3) and decreases with lower energy intake.
- Although adipose tissue is less metabolically active than muscle, 5% of its weight is metabolically active, and therefore, the BMR increases as body weight rises and decreases as it falls.
- The energy cost of physical activity is markedly affected by body weight; thus, even with a constant level of physical activity, total energy expenditure will increase with increasing body weight (Figure 5.4). There is some evidence that people with habitually low energy intakes are more efficient in their movements and so have a lower energy cost of activity.

Figure 5.5 shows that in the early stages of negative energy balance, the rate of weight loss may be greater than the theoretical rate calculated from the energy yield of adipose tissue. This is because of the loss of relatively large amounts of water associated with liver and muscle glycogen reserves (Section 4.2.1.6), which are considerably depleted during energy restriction.

5.3   Metabolic fuels in the fed and fasting states

Energy expenditure is relatively constant throughout the day, but food intake normally occurs in two or three meals. There is therefore a need to ensure that there is a constant supply of metabolic fuel, regardless of the variation in intake. See Section 10.5 for a more detailed discussion of the hormonal control of metabolism in the fed and fasting states.

5.3.1   The fed state

During the 3–4 h after a meal, there is an ample supply of metabolic fuel entering the circulation from the gut (Figure 5.6). Glucose from carbohydrate digestion (Section 4.2.2) and amino acids from protein digestion (Section 4.4.3) are absorbed into the portal circulation, and to a considerable extent, the liver controls the amounts that enter the peripheral circulation. After a meal, the concentration of glucose in the hepatic portal vein may be as high as 20 mmol/L, but that entering the peripheral circulation does not normally increase above 8–9 mmol/L. By contrast, the products of fat digestion are absorbed into the lymphatic system as chylomicrons (Sections 4.3.2.2 and 5.6.2.1) and are available to peripheral tissues first; the liver acts to clear chylomicron remnants. Much of the triacylglycerol in chylomicrons goes directly to adipose tissue for storage; when there is a plentiful supply of glucose, it is the main metabolic fuel for most tissues.

  The increased concentration of glucose and amino acids in the portal blood stimulates the β-cells of the pancreas to secrete insulin, and suppresses the secretion of glucagon by the α-cells of the pancreas. In response to insulin, there is

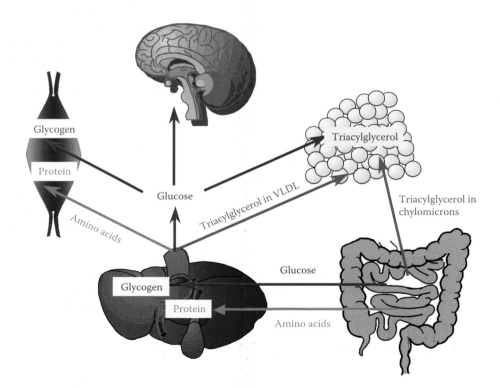

Figure 5.6 An overview of metabolism in the fed state.

- Increased uptake of glucose into muscle and adipose tissue, as a result of migration to the cell surface of glucose transporters that are in intracellular vesicles in the fasting state.
- Increased synthesis of glycogen (Section 5.6.3) from glucose in both liver and muscle, as a result of increased availability of glucose and activation of glycogen synthetase.
- Increased synthesis of fatty acids in adipose tissue (Section 5.6.1) by activation of acetyl CoA carboxylase and inhibition of fatty acid release by inactivation of hormone-sensitive lipase.
- Increased uptake of fatty acids from chylomicrons and very-low-density lipoprotein (VLDL) (Sections 5.6.2.1 and 5.6.2.2) by increasing the synthesis of lipoprotein lipase and stimulating its migration into blood capillaries.
- Increased amino acid uptake into tissues and stimulation of protein synthesis.

In the liver, glucose uptake is by carrier-mediated diffusion and metabolic trapping as glucose 6-phosphate (Section 3.2.2.2) and is independent of insulin. The uptake of glucose into the liver increases very significantly as the concentration of glucose in the portal vein increases, and the liver has a major role in controlling the amount of glucose that reaches peripheral tissues after a meal. There are two isoenzymes that catalyse the formation of glucose 6-phosphate in liver:

1. Hexokinase has a K_m of approximately 0.15 mmol/L and is saturated, therefore acting at its V_{max}, under all conditions. It acts mainly to ensure an adequate uptake of glucose into the liver to meet the demands for liver metabolism.
2. Glucokinase has a K_m of approximately 20 mmol/L and will have very low activity in the fasting state, when the concentration of glucose in the portal blood is between 3 and 5 mmol/L. However, after a meal the portal concentration of glucose may well reach 20 mmol/L or higher, and under these conditions, glucokinase has significant activity, and there is increased formation of glucose 6-phosphate. Most of this will be used for synthesis of glycogen (Section 5.6.3), although some will also be used for synthesis of fatty acids that will be exported in VLDL (Section 5.6.2.2).

5.3.2 The fasting state

In the fasting or the post-absorptive state (beginning about 4–5 h after a meal, when the products of digestion have been absorbed) metabolic fuels enter the circulation from the reserves of glycogen, triacylglycerol, and protein laid down in the fed state (Figure 5.7).

As the concentration of glucose and amino acids in the portal blood decreases, the secretion of insulin by the β-cells of the pancreas decreases and the secretion of glucagon by the α-cells increases. In response to glucagon, there is

- Increased breakdown of liver glycogen to glucose 1-phosphate, to release glucose into the circulation (muscle glycogen cannot be used directly as a source of free glucose).
- Increased synthesis of glucose from amino acids in liver and kidney (gluconeogenesis, Section 5.7).

At the same time, in response to the reduced secretion of insulin, there is

- Decreased uptake of glucose into muscle and adipose tissue because the glucose transporter is internalised in the absence of insulin.

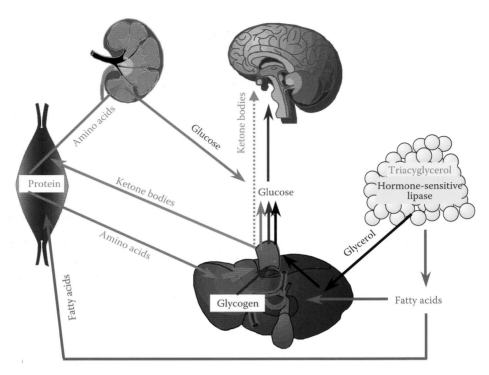

Figure 5.7 An overview of metabolism in the fasting state.

- Decreased protein synthesis; the amino acids arising from protein catabolism (Section 9.1.1.1) are available for gluconeogenesis (Sections 5.7 and 9.3.2).
- Release of non-esterified fatty acids from adipose tissue, as a result of relief of the inhibition of hormone-sensitive lipase.

The metabolic imperative in the fasting state is that the brain is largely dependent on glucose as its metabolic fuel, and red blood cells (which lack mitochondria) and the renal medulla can only utilise glucose. Therefore, those tissues that can utilise other fuels do so to spare glucose for the brain, red blood cells, and renal medulla. Any metabolites that can be used for gluconeogenesis will be used to supplement the relatively small amount of glucose that is available from glycogen reserves—the total liver and muscle glycogen reserves would only meet requirements for 12–18 h. The main substrates for gluconeogenesis are amino acids (Sections 5.7 and 9.3.2) and the glycerol arising from hydrolysis of triacylglycerol. Fatty acids can never be substrates for gluconeogenesis.

Muscle and other tissues can utilise fatty acids as a metabolic fuel but only to a limited extent and not enough to meet their energy requirements completely. By contrast, the liver has a greater capacity for the oxidation of fatty acids than is required to meet its own energy needs. Therefore, in the fasting state the liver synthesises ketone bodies (acetoacetate and β-hydroxybutyrate, Section 5.5.3), which it exports to other tissues for use as a metabolic fuel.

The result of these metabolic changes is shown in Figure 5.8. The plasma concentration of glucose falls somewhat but is maintained through fasting into starvation, as a result of gluconeogenesis. The concentration of non-esterified fatty acids in plasma increases in fasting, but does not increase any further in starvation, whilst the concentration of ketone bodies increases continually through fasting into starvation. After about 2–3 weeks of starvation, the plasma

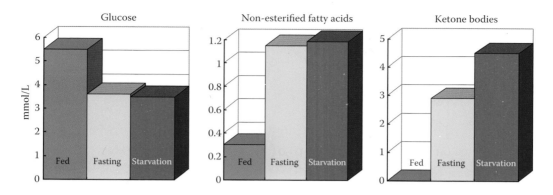

Figure 5.8 Plasma concentrations of metabolic fuels in the fed and fasting states and in starvation.

concentration of ketone bodies is high enough for them to be a significant fuel for the brain, providing about 20% of its energy requirement. This means that in prolonged starvation there is a decrease in the amount of tissue protein that needs to be catabolised for gluconeogenesis.

5.4   Energy-yielding metabolism

5.4.1   Glycolysis—the (anaerobic) metabolism of glucose

Overall, the pathway of glycolysis is cleavage of the 6-carbon glucose molecule into two 3-carbon units. The key steps in the pathway are

- Two phosphorylation reactions to form fructose-bisphosphate, at the expense of 2 mol of ATP
- Cleavage of fructose-bisphosphate to yield two molecules of triose (3-carbon sugar) phosphate
- Two steps in which phosphate is transferred from a substrate onto ADP, forming ATP (and hence a yield of 4 mol of ATP per mole of glucose metabolised)
- One step in which NAD$^+$ is reduced to NADH (equivalent to 2.5 mol ATP per mol of triose phosphate metabolised, or 5 mol ATP/mol of glucose metabolised when the NADH is re-oxidised in the mitochondrial electron transport chain (Section 3.3.1))
- Formation of 2 mol of pyruvate per mol of glucose metabolised

The immediate substrate for glycolysis is glucose 6-phosphate (Figure 5.9), which may arise by:

- Phosphorylation of glucose, catalysed by hexokinase (and also by glucokinase in the liver in the fed state) at the expense of ATP.
- Phosphorolysis of glycogen in liver and muscle to yield glucose 1-phosphate, catalysed by glycogen phosphorylase, using inorganic phosphate. Glucose 1-phosphate is readily isomerised to glucose 6-phosphate.

The pathway of glycolysis is shown in Figure 5.10. Although the aim of glucose oxidation is to phosphorylate ADP → ATP, the pathway involves two steps in which ATP is used, one to form glucose 6-phosphate when glucose is the substrate and the other to form fructose bisphosphate. In other words, there is a modest cost of ATP to initiate the metabolism

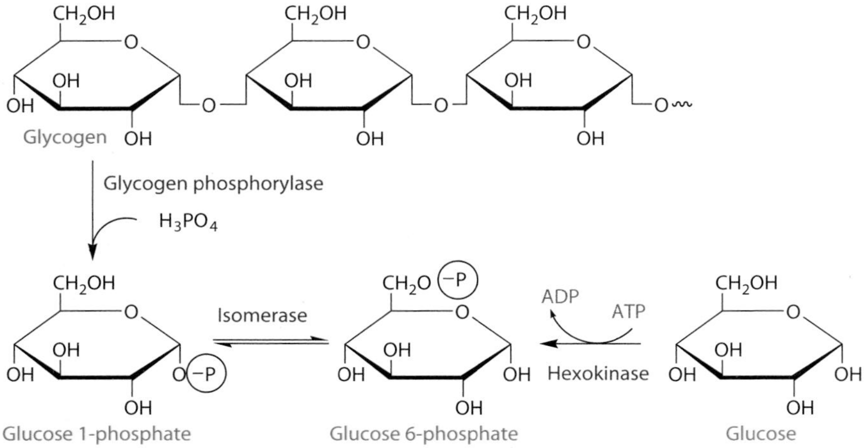

Figure 5.9 Sources of glucose 6-phosphate for glycolysis.

of glucose. When glycogen is the source of glucose 6-phosphate there is a cost of only 1 mol of ATP for glycolysis, but there is a cost of 2 mol of ATP equivalents for each mol of glucose added in glycogen synthesis (Section 5.6.3).

The formation of fructose bisphosphate, catalysed by phosphofructokinase, is an important step for the regulation of glucose metabolism (Section 10.2.2). Once it has been formed, fructose bisphosphate is cleaved to yield two interconvertible three-carbon compounds. The metabolism of these three-carbon sugars is linked to both the reduction of NAD^+ to NADH and direct (substrate-level) phosphorylation of ADP → ATP (Section 3.3). The result is the formation of 2 mol of pyruvate from each mol of glucose.

Glycolysis thus requires the utilisation of 2 mol of ATP (giving ADP) per mol of glucose metabolised and yields 4 mol of ATP by substrate-level phosphorylation and 2 mol of NADH (formed from NAD^+), equivalent to a further 5 mol of ATP when oxidised in the electron transport chain (Section 3.3.1). There is thus a net yield of 7 mol of ADP + phosphate → ATP from the oxidation of 1 mol of glucose to 2 mol of pyruvate.

The reverse of glycolysis is important as a means of glucose synthesis—the process of gluconeogenesis (Section 5.7). Most of the reactions of glycolysis are readily reversible, but at three points (the reactions catalysed by hexokinase, phosphofructokinase, and pyruvate kinase) there are separate enzymes involved in glycolysis and gluconeogenesis.

For two of these reactions, hexokinase and phosphofructokinase, the equilibrium is in the direction of glycolysis because of the utilisation of ATP in the reaction and the high ratio of ATP/ADP in the cell. The reactions of phosphofructokinase and hexokinase are reversed in gluconeogenesis by hydrolysis of fructose bisphosphate → fructose 6-phosphate + phosphate (catalysed by fructose bisphosphatase) and of glucose 6-phosphate → glucose + phosphate (catalysed by glucose 6-phosphatase).

The equilibrium of pyruvate kinase is also strongly in the direction of glycolysis because the immediate product of the reaction is enolpyruvate, which is chemically unstable, and undergoes a non-enzymic reaction to yield pyruvate.* This means that little of the product is available to undergo the reverse reaction in the direction of gluconeogenesis. The conversion of pyruvate to phosphoenolpyruvate for gluconeogenesis is discussed in Section 5.7.

* See Figure 5.36.

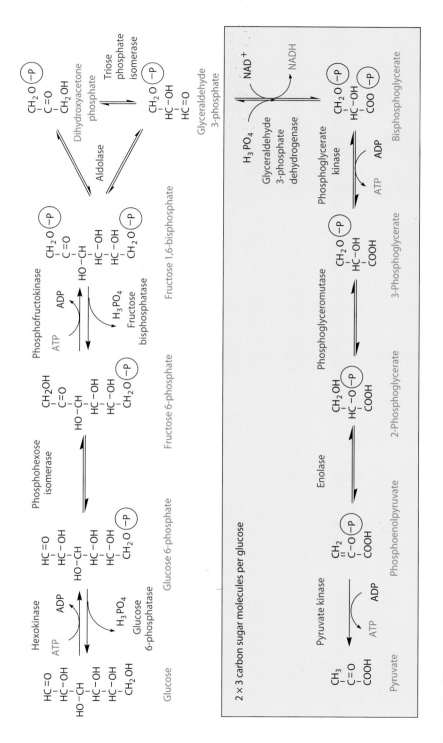

Figure 5.10 Glycolysis.

The glycolytic pathway also provides a route for the metabolism of fructose, galactose (which undergoes phosphorylation to galactose 1-phosphate and isomerisation to glucose 1-phosphate), and glycerol. Some fructose is phosphorylated directly to fructose 6-phosphate by hexokinase, but most is phosphorylated to fructose 1-phosphate by a specific enzyme, fructokinase. Fructose 1-phosphate is then cleaved to yield dihydroxyacetone phosphate and glyceraldehyde; the glyceraldehyde can be phosphorylated to glyceraldehyde 3-phosphate by triose kinase. This means that fructose enters glycolysis after the main regulatory step catalysed by phosphofructokinase (Section 10.2.2), and its utilisation is not controlled by the need for ATP formation. There is excessive formation of acetyl CoA, which is used for fatty acid synthesis; a high intake of fructose may be a significant factor in the development of obesity (Section 7.3).

Glycerol arising from the hydrolysis of triacylglycerols can be phosphorylated and oxidised to dihydroxyacetone phosphate. In triacylglycerol synthesis (Section 5.6.1.2), most glycerol phosphate is formed from dihydroxyacetone phosphate.

5.4.1.1   *Transfer of NADH formed during glycolysis into the mitochondria*

The mitochondrial inner membrane is impermeable to NAD, and therefore, the NADH produced in the cytosol in glycolysis cannot enter the mitochondria for re-oxidation. To transfer the reducing equivalents from cytosolic NADH into the mitochondria, two substrate shuttles are used.

The malate-aspartate shuttle (Figure 5.11) involves reduction of oxaloacetate in the cytosol to malate (with the oxidation of cytosolic NADH to NAD⁺). Malate enters the mitochondria and is reduced back to oxaloacetate, with the reduction of intra-mitochondrial NAD⁺ to NADH. Oxaloacetate cannot cross the mitochondrial inner membrane but undergoes transamination to aspartate (Section 9.3.1.2), with glutamate acting as amino donor, yielding α-ketoglutarate. α-Ketoglutarate then leaves the mitochondria using an antiporter that transports malate inward. Aspartate leaves the mitochondria in exchange for glutamate entering; in the cytosol, the reverse transamination reaction occurs, forming oxaloacetate (for reduction to malate) from aspartate, and glutamate (for transport back into the mitochondria) from α-ketoglutarate.

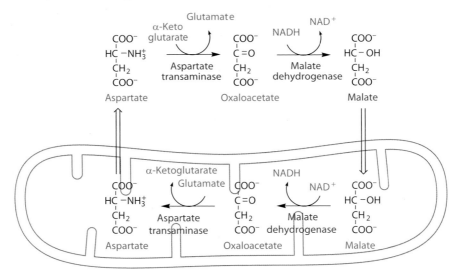

Figure 5.11 The malate-aspartate shuttle for transfer of reducing equivalents from the cytosol into the mitochondrion.

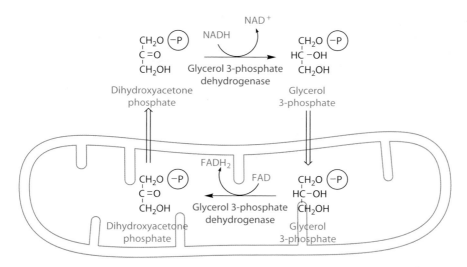

Figure 5.12 The glycerophosphate shuttle for transfer of reducing equivalents from the cytosol into the mitochondrion.

The glycerophosphate shuttle (Figure 5.12) involves reduction of dihydroxyacetone phosphate to glycerol 3-phosphate in the cytosol (with oxidation of NADH to NAD$^+$) and oxidation of glycerol 3-phosphate to dihydroxyacetone phosphate inside the mitochondrion. Dihydroxyacetone phosphate and glycerol 3-phosphate are transported in opposite directions by an antiporter in the mitochondrial membrane.

The cytosolic glycerol 3-phosphate dehydrogenase uses NADH to reduce dihydroxyacetone phosphate to glycerol 3-phosphate, but the mitochondrial enzyme uses FAD to reduce glycerol 3-phosphate to dihydroxyacetone phosphate. This means that when this shuttle is used, there is a yield of 1.5 mol of ATP rather than the 2.5 mol of ATP that would be expected from re-oxidation of NADH.

The malate–aspartate shuttle (Figure 5.11) is sensitive to the relative amounts of NADH and NAD$^+$ in the cytosol and mitochondria and cannot operate if the mitochondrial NADH/NAD$^+$ ratio is higher than that in the cytosol. However, the glycerophosphate shuttle does not use NAD$^+$ in the mitochondrion (Figure 5.12) and so can operate even when the mitochondrial NADH/NAD$^+$ ratio is higher than that in the cytosol.

The glycerophosphate shuttle is important in muscle where there is a very high rate of glycolysis (especially insect flight muscle); the malate–aspartate shuttle is especially important in heart and liver.

5.4.1.2   *The reduction of pyruvate to lactate: anaerobic glycolysis*

Under conditions of maximum exertion, for example, in sprinting, the rate at which oxygen can be transported into the muscle is not great enough to allow for the reoxidation of all the NADH formed in glycolysis. To maintain the oxidation of glucose and the net yield of 2 mol of ATP per mol of glucose oxidised (or 3 mol of ATP if the source is muscle glycogen), NADH is oxidised to NAD$^+$ by the reduction of pyruvate to lactate, catalysed by lactate dehydrogenase (Figure 5.13). In red blood cells, which lack mitochondria, formation of lactate is the only way to re-oxidise NADH.

The resultant lactate is exported from the muscle and red blood cells and taken up by the liver, where it is used for the resynthesis of glucose. As shown on the right of Figure

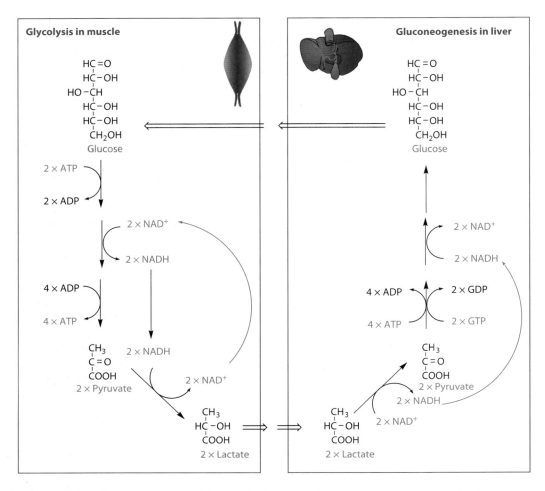

Figure 5.13 The Cori cycle—anaerobic glycolysis in muscle and gluconeogenesis in the liver.

5.13, synthesis of glucose from lactate is an ATP (and GTP) requiring process. The oxygen debt after strenuous physical activity is due to an increased rate of energy-yielding metabolism to provide the ATP and GTP that are required for gluconeogenesis from lactate. Although most of the lactate will be used for gluconeogenesis, a proportion will undergo oxidation to pyruvate and onward through the citric acid cycle (Sections 5.4.3 and 5.4.4) to provide the ATP and GTP needed.

Lactate may also be taken up by tissues such as the heart, where oxygen availability is not a limiting factor. Here it is oxidised to pyruvate, and the resultant NADH is oxidised in the mitochondrial electron transport chain, yielding 2.5 mol of ATP. The pyruvate is then a substrate for complete oxidation through the citric acid cycle. The isoenzyme of lactate dehydrogenase in heart muscle acts preferentially in the direction of lactate oxidation to pyruvate, whilst the skeletal muscle isoenzyme acts preferentially in the direction of pyruvate reduction to lactate.

Many tumours have a low capacity for oxidative metabolism and anaerobically metabolise glucose to lactate, which is exported to the liver for gluconeogenesis. This cycling of glucose between anaerobic glycolysis in the tumour and gluconeogenesis in the liver may account for much of the increased metabolism and consequent weight loss (cachexia) that is seen in patients with advanced cancer (Section 8.4.1).

Anaerobic glycolysis is the main pathway in microorganisms that are capable of living in the absence of oxygen. Here there are two possible fates for the pyruvate formed from glucose, both of which involve the oxidation of NADH to NAD⁺:

1. Reduction to lactate, as occurs in human muscle. This is the pathway in lactic acid bacteria, which are responsible for both the fermentation of lactose in milk for manufacture of yoghurt and cheese and also the gastrointestinal discomfort after consumption of lactose in people who lack intestinal lactase (Section 4.2.2.2).
2. Decarboxylation and reduction to ethanol. This is the pathway of fermentation in yeast, which is exploited to produce alcoholic beverages. Human gastrointestinal bacteria normally produce lactate rather than ethanol, although there have been reports of people with a high intestinal population of yeasts that produce significant amounts of ethanol after consumption of resistant starch.

5.4.2   *The pentose phosphate pathway—an alternative to glycolysis*

There is an alternative pathway for the conversion of glucose 6-phosphate to fructose 6-phosphate, the pentose phosphate pathway (sometimes known as the hexose monophosphate shunt; Figure 5.14).

Overall, the pentose phosphate pathway produces 2 mol of fructose 6-phosphate, 1 mol of glyceraldehyde 3-phosphate, and 3 mol of carbon dioxide from 3 mol of glucose 6-phosphate, linked to the reduction of 6 mol of NADP⁺ to NADPH. The sequence of reactions is as follows:

- 3 mol of glucose are oxidised to yield 3 mol of the 5-carbon sugar ribulose 5-phosphate + 3 mol of carbon dioxide.
- 2 mol of ribulose 5-phosphate are isomerised to yield 2 mol of xylulose 5-phosphate.
- 1 mol of ribulose 5-phosphate is isomerised to ribose 5-phosphate.
- 1 mol of xylulose 5-phosphate reacts with the ribose 5-phosphate, yielding (ultimately) fructose-6-phosphate and erythrose 4-phosphate.
- The other mol of xylulose-5-phosphate reacts with the erythrose 4-phosphate, yielding fructose 6-phosphate and glyceraldehyde 3-phosphate.

This is the pathway for the synthesis of ribose for nucleotide synthesis; more importantly, it is the source of half the NADPH required for fatty acid synthesis (Section 5.6.1). Tissues that synthesise large amounts of fatty acids have a high activity of the pentose phosphate pathway. It is also important in the respiratory burst of macrophages that are activated in response to infection (Section 6.5.2.2).

5.4.2.1   *The pentose phosphate pathway in red blood cells—favism*

The pentose phosphate pathway is also important in the red blood cell, where NADPH is required to maintain an adequate pool of reduced glutathione, which is used to reduce hydrogen peroxide.

The tripeptide glutathione (γ-glutamyl-cysteinyl-glycine, Figure 5.15) is the reducing agent for glutathione peroxidase, which reduces H_2O_2 to H_2O and O_2. (Glutathione peroxidase is a selenium-dependent enzyme, Section 11.15.2.5; this explains the antioxidant role of selenium, Section 6.5.3.2.)

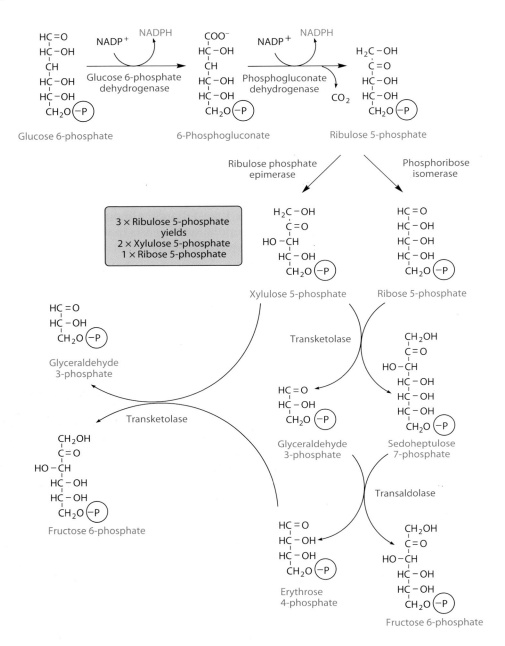

Figure 5.14 The pentose phosphate pathway (also known as the hexose monophosphate shunt).

Oxidised glutathione (GSSG) is reduced back to active GSH by glutathione reductase, which uses NADPH as the reducing agent. Glutathione reductase is a flavin-dependent enzyme, and its activity, or its activation after incubation with FAD, can be used as an index of vitamin B_2 status (Sections 2.7.3 and 11.7).

Partial or total lack of glucose 6-phosphate dehydrogenase (and hence impaired activity of the pentose phosphate pathway) is the cause of favism, an acute haemolytic anaemia

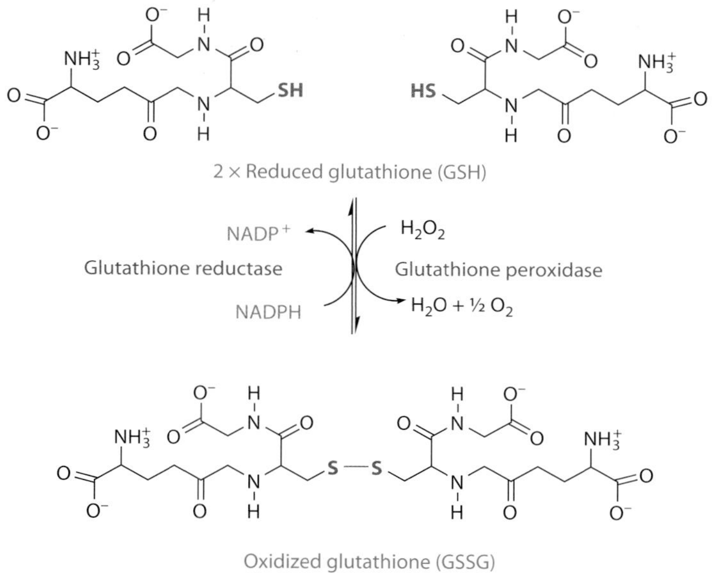

Figure 5.15 The reactions of glutathione peroxidase and glutathione reductase.

with fever and haemoglobinuria, precipitated in genetically susceptible people by the consumption of broad beans (fava beans, *Vicia faba*) and a variety of drugs, all of which, like the toxins in fava beans, undergo redox cycling and produce hydrogen peroxide. Infection can also precipitate an attack because of the increased production of oxygen radicals as part of the macrophage respiratory burst (Section 6.5.2.2).

Because of the low activity of glucose 6-phosphate dehydrogenase in affected people, there is a lack of NADPH in red blood cells, and hence an impaired ability to remove hydrogen peroxide, which causes oxidative damage to the cell membrane lipids, leading to haemolysis. Other tissues are unaffected because there are mitochondrial enzymes that can provide a supply of NADPH; red blood cells have no mitochondria.

Favism is one of the commonest genetic defects, affecting some 200 million people. It is an X-linked condition, and female carriers are resistant to malaria, an advantage that explains why defects in the gene are so widespread. A large number of variant forms of the glucose 6-phosphate dehydrogenase gene are known, some of which do not affect the activity of the enzyme significantly. There are two main types of favism:

1. A moderately severe form, in which there is between 10% and 50% of the normal activity of glucose 6-phosphate dehydrogenase in red blood cells. The abnormal enzyme is unstable; older red blood cells have low activity, but younger cells have nearly normal activity. This means that the haemolytic crisis is self-limiting, as only older red blood cells are lysed. This is the form of favism found amongst people of Afro-Caribbean descent. Crises are rarely precipitated by consumption of fava beans.
2. A severe form, in which there is less than 10% of normal activity of glucose 6-phosphate dehydrogenase in red blood cells. Here the problem is that the enzyme has either low catalytic activity (a low V_{max}) or an abnormally high K_m for NADP$^+$. In

extremely severe cases, haemolytic crises can occur without the stress of toxin or infection. This is the form of favism found amongst people of Mediterranean descent.

5.4.3   The metabolism of pyruvate

Pyruvate arising from glycolysis (or from amino acids, Section 9.3.2) can be metabolised in four different ways, depending on the metabolic state of the body:

1. Reduction to lactate (Section 5.4.1.2)
2. As a substrate for gluconeogenesis (Section 5.7)
3. Oxidation to acetyl CoA, which is then used for fatty acid synthesis (Section 5.6.1)
4. Oxidation to acetyl CoA, followed by complete oxidation to carbon dioxide and water (Sections 5.4.3.1 and 5.4.4)

5.4.3.1   The oxidation of pyruvate to acetyl CoA

The first step in the complete oxidation of pyruvate is a multistep reaction in which carbon dioxide is lost, and the resulting two-carbon compound is oxidised to acetate. The oxidation involves the reduction of NAD^+ to NADH. Since 2 mol of pyruvate are formed from each mol of glucose, this step represents the formation of 2 mol of NADH, equivalent to 5 mol of ATP for each mol of glucose metabolised. The acetate is released from the enzyme esterified to coenzyme A, as acetyl CoA (Figure 5.16). Coenzyme A (see Figure 5.23) is derived from the vitamin pantothenic acid (Section 11.13).

The decarboxylation and oxidation of pyruvate to form acetyl CoA requires the coenzyme thiamin diphosphate, which is formed from vitamin B_1 (Section 11.6.2). In thiamin deficiency, this reaction is impaired, and deficient subjects are unable to metabolise glucose normally. Especially after a test dose of glucose, or moderate exercise, they develop high

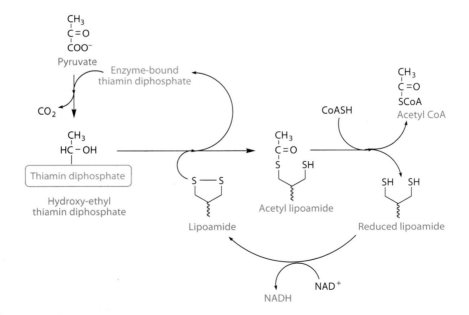

Figure 5.16 The reaction of the pyruvate dehydrogenase multi-enzyme complex.

blood concentrations of pyruvate and lactate. In some cases this may be severe enough to result in life-threatening acidosis.

5.4.4 Oxidation of acetyl CoA—the citric acid cycle

The acetate of acetyl CoA undergoes a stepwise oxidation to carbon dioxide and water in a cyclic pathway, the citric acid cycle (Figures 5.17 and 5.18). This pathway is sometimes known as the Krebs' cycle, after its discoverer, Sir Hans Krebs, and sometimes as the tricarboxylic acid cycle, because citric acid has three carboxylic acid groups. For each mol of acetyl CoA oxidised in this pathway, there is a yield of

1. 3 mol of NAD^+ reduced to NADH, equivalent to 7.5 mol of ATP
2. $1 \times$ flavoprotein reduced, leading to reduction of ubiquinone (Section 3.3.1.2), equivalent to 1.5 mol of ADP
3. 1 mol of ADP phosphorylated to ATP, or in liver and some other tissues, 1 mol of GDP phosphorylated to GTP

This is a total of 10 mol of ATP for each mole of acetyl CoA oxidised; since 2 mol of acetyl CoA are formed from each mole of glucose, this cycle yields 20 mol of ATP for each mol of glucose oxidised.

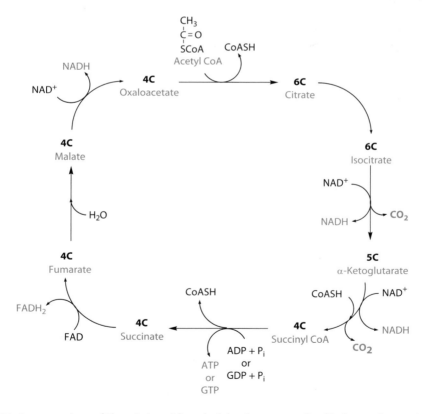

Figure 5.17 An overview of the citric acid cycle (also known as the Krebs cycle or tricarboxylic acid cycle).

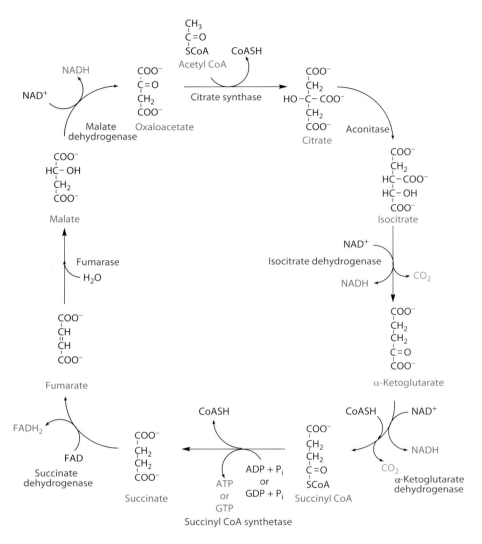

Figure 5.18 The citric acid cycle (also known as the Krebs cycle or tricarboxylic acid cycle). The reaction of succinyl CoA synthetase is linked to phosphorylation of ADP → ATP in most tissues, but also to GDP → GTP, in tissues that perform gluconeogenesis.

Although it appears complex at first sight, the citric acid cycle is a simple pathway. A four-carbon compound, oxaloacetate, reacts with acetyl CoA to form a six-carbon compound, citric acid. The cycle is then a series of reactions in which two carbon atoms are lost as carbon dioxide, followed by a series of oxidation and other reactions, eventually reforming oxaloacetate. The CoA of acetyl CoA is released and is available for further formation of acetyl CoA from pyruvate.

The citric acid cycle also catalyses the oxidation of acetyl CoA arising from other sources:

- β-oxidation of fatty acids (Section 5.5.2)
- metabolism of ketone bodies (Section 5.5.3)

- alcohol (Figure 2.21)
- those amino acids that give rise to acetyl CoA or acetoacetate (Figure 5.20 and Section 9.3.2)

Although oxaloacetate is the precursor for gluconeogenesis (Section 5.7), fatty acids and other compounds that give rise to acetyl CoA or acetoacetate cannot be used for net synthesis of glucose. As can be seen from Figure 5.18, although two carbons are added to the cycle by acetyl CoA, two carbons are lost as carbon dioxide in each turn of the cycle. Therefore, when acetyl CoA is the substrate there is no increase in the pool of citric acid cycle intermediates, and therefore oxaloacetate cannot be withdrawn for gluconeogenesis.

α-Ketoglutarate dehydrogenase catalyses a reaction similar to that of pyruvate dehydrogenase—oxidative decarboxylation and formation of an acyl CoA derivative. Like pyruvate dehydrogenase, it is a thiamin diphosphate dependent enzyme, and the reaction sequence is the same as that shown in Figure 5.16. However, thiamin deficiency does not have a significant effect on the citric acid cycle because α-ketoglutarate can undergo transamination to yield glutamate, which is decarboxylated to γ-aminobutyric acid (GABA, Figure 5.19). In turn, GABA can undergo onward metabolism to yield succinate. This pathway, the GABA shunt, thus provides an alternative to α-ketoglutarate dehydrogenase, and in thiamin deficiency, there is increased turnover of GABA, permitting normal oxidation of acetyl CoA and formation of ATP.

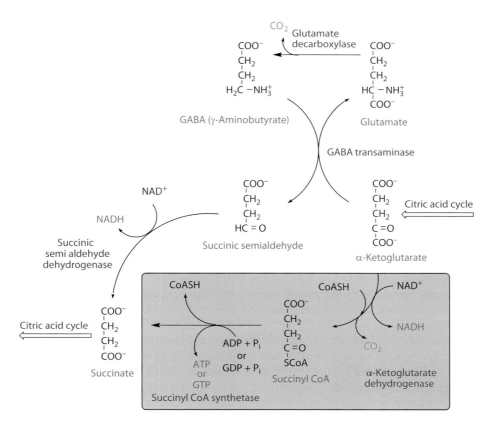

Figure 5.19 The GABA shunt—an alternative to α-ketoglutarate dehydrogenase in the citric acid cycle.

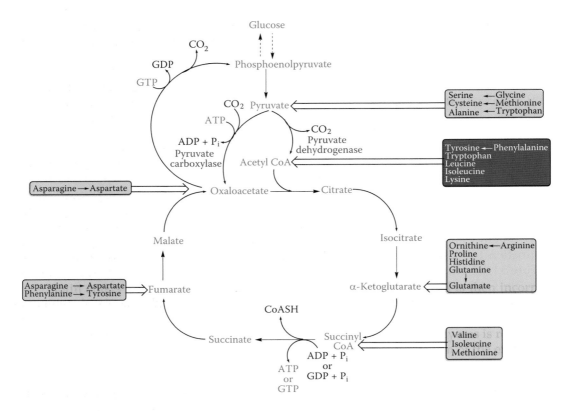

Figure 5.20 The entry of amino acid carbon skeletons into the citric acid cycle. Amino acids that give rise to pyruvate or intermediates of the cycle (in yellow boxes) provide a net increase in oxaloacetate and are therefore substrates for gluconeogenesis. Amino acids that give rise to acetyl CoA do not provide any increase in oxaloacetate and therefore cannot be substrates for gluconeogenesis—they are ketogenic.

The sequence of reactions between succinate and oxaloacetate is chemically the same as that involved in the β-oxidation of fatty acids (Section 5.5.2):

- Oxidation to yield a carbon-carbon double bond. Although this reaction is shown in Figure 5.18 as being linked to reduction of FAD, the coenzyme is tightly enzyme bound, and succinate dehydrogenase reacts directly with ubiquinone in the electron transport chain (Section 3.3.1.2).
- Addition of water across the carbon–carbon double bond, to yield a hydroxyl group.
- Oxidation of the hydroxyl group, linked to reduction of NAD^+, to yield an oxo-group.

5.4.4.1 *The citric acid cycle as pathway for metabolic interconversion*

In addition to its role in oxidation of acetyl CoA, the citric acid cycle provides the link between carbohydrate, fat, and amino acid metabolism. Many of the intermediates can be used for the synthesis of other compounds:

- α-Ketoglutarate and oxaloacetate can give rise to the amino acids glutamate and aspartate, respectively (Section 9.3.1.2).

- Oxaloacetate is the precursor for glucose synthesis in the fasting state (Section 5.7).
- Citrate is the source of acetyl CoA for fatty acid synthesis in the cytosol in the fed state (Section 5.6.1).

The toxicity of ammonia (Section 9.3.1.3) is due to the activity of glutamate dehydrogenase, which forms glutamate by reaction of α-ketoglutarate with ammonium; this depletes the citric acid cycle pool of intermediates, leading to impaired activity of the cycle and reduced formation of ATP.

If oxaloacetate is removed from the cycle for glucose synthesis (Section 5.7), it must be replaced, since if there is not enough oxaloacetate available to form citrate, the rate of acetyl CoA metabolism, and hence the rate of formation of ATP, will slow down. A variety of amino acids give rise to citric cycle intermediates, thus providing a net increase in oxaloacetate and permitting its removal for gluconeogenesis. In addition, the reaction of pyruvate carboxylase (Figure 5.20) is a source of oxaloacetate to maintain citric acid cycle activity.

There is a further control over the removal of oxaloacetate for gluconeogenesis. The decarboxylation and phosphorylation of oxaloacetate to form phosphoenolpyruvate uses GTP as the phosphate donor (Figure 5.20). In gluconeogenic tissues such as liver and kidney, the major mitochondrial source of GTP is the reaction of succinyl CoA synthetase. If so much oxaloacetate is withdrawn that the rate of cycle activity falls, there is not enough GTP to permit further removal. In tissues such as brain and heart, which do not carry out gluconeogenesis, there is a different isoenzyme of succinyl CoA synthetase, linked to phosphorylation of ADP rather than GDP.

5.4.4.2   Complete oxidation of 4- and 5-carbon compounds

Although the citric acid cycle is generally regarded as a pathway for the oxidation of 4- and 5-carbon compounds such as fumarate, oxaloacetate, α-ketoglutarate, and succinate arising from amino acids (Figure 5.20), it does not, alone, permit complete oxidation of these compounds. Four-carbon intermediates are not overall consumed in the cycle, since oxaloacetate is reformed. Addition of 4- and 5-carbon intermediates will increase the rate of cycle activity (subject to control by the requirement for ATP) only until the pool of intermediates is saturated.

Complete oxidation of 4- and 5-carbon intermediates requires removal of oxaloacetate from the cycle and conversion to pyruvate (Figure 5.20). This pyruvate may either undergo decarboxylation to acetyl CoA (Figure 5.16), which can be oxidised in the cycle or may be used as a substrate for gluconeogenesis.

Oxidation of 4- and 5-carbon citric acid cycle intermediates thus involves a greater metabolic activity than oxidation of acetyl CoA. This has been exploited as a means of overcoming the hypothermia that occurs in patients recovering from anaesthesia by giving an intravenous infusion of the amino acid glutamate. This provides α-ketoglutarate, which will largely be used for gluconeogenesis, and hence causes an increase in metabolic activity, and increased heat production.

5.5   The metabolism of fats

There are two sources of fatty acids available to tissues (Figure 5.21). In the fed state, chylomicrons assembled in the small intestine (Sections 4.3.2.2 and 5.6.2.1) and VLDL exported from the liver (Section 5.6.2.2) bind to lipoprotein lipase at the luminal surface of capillary epithelium. This enzyme catalyses hydrolysis of triacylglycerols to glycerol and non-esterified fatty acids. Most of the fatty acid released enters cells and is metabolised (or in

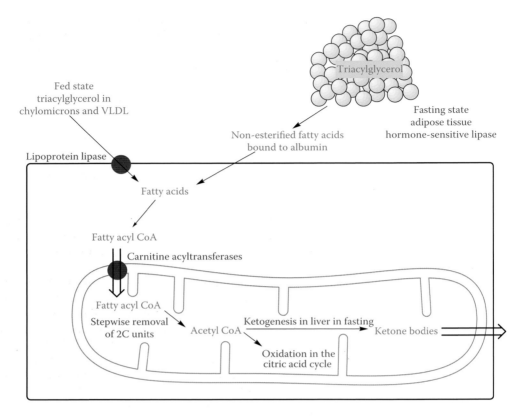

Figure 5.21 An overview of fatty acid metabolism.

adipose tissue, re-esterified to form triacylglycerol), but some remains in the bloodstream and is taken up by the liver, re-esterified and exported in VLDL; as discussed in Section 5.6.1.2, this is an ATP-expensive process.

In the fasting state, hormone-sensitive lipase in adipose tissue is activated in response to falling insulin secretion or the secretion of adrenaline and catalyses the hydrolysis of triacylglycerol, releasing non-esterified fatty acids into the bloodstream, where they bind to albumin and are transported to tissues. The binding of non-esterified fatty acids to albumin is important for two reasons:

1. Non-esterified fatty acids acts as detergents (soap consists of the salts of fatty acids). Because they have a hydrophobic tail, they can dissolve in cell membranes, leaving the carboxylic acid group exposed to the aqueous medium. This results in the lysis of cell membranes.
2. Fatty acids form insoluble salts with calcium ions. If this occurred in the circulation then there would be a loss of ionised calcium (Section 11.15.1.1) and blockage of blood capillaries by the insoluble calcium salts.

Increased activity of hormone-sensitive lipase in response to compounds secreted by some tumours leads to cycling of fatty acids between adipose tissue and liver and is a factor in the hypermetabolism seen in patients with cancer cachexia (Section 8.4.1).

The glycerol released by hormone-sensitive lipase or lipoprotein lipase is mainly taken up by the liver, where it may be used either as a metabolic fuel or for gluconeogenesis. The fatty acids are oxidised in the mitochondria by the β-oxidation pathway, in which two carbon atoms at a time are removed from the fatty acid chain as acetyl CoA. This acetyl CoA then enters the citric acid cycle, together with that arising from the metabolism of pyruvate.

5.5.1   *Carnitine and the transport of fatty acids into the mitochondrion*

As fatty acids enter the cell, they are esterified with coenzyme A to form acyl CoA. This protects membranes against the lytic action of free fatty acids. However, acyl CoA cannot cross the mitochondrial membranes to enter the matrix, where the enzymes for β-oxidation are located.

On the outer face of the outer mitochondrial membrane, the fatty acid is transferred from CoA onto carnitine, forming acylcarnitine, a reaction catalysed by carnitine acyl-transferase 1. Acylcarnitine enters the inter-membrane space through an acylcarnitine transporter (Figures 5.22 and 5.23).

Acylcarnitine can cross only the mitochondrial membranes using a counter-transport system that transports acylcarnitine inward in exchange for free carnitine being transported out. Once inside the mitochondrial inner membrane, the acyl group is transferred onto CoA, a reaction catalysed by carnitine acyltransferase 2. The resultant acyl CoA is a substrate for β-oxidation. This counter-transport system provides regulation of the uptake of fatty acids into the mitochondrion for oxidation. As long as there is free CoA available in the mitochondrial matrix, fatty acids can be taken up, and the carnitine returned to the outer membrane for uptake of more fatty acids. However, if most of the CoA in the mitochondrion is acylated, then there is no need for further fatty uptake, and indeed, it is not possible.

This carnitine shuttle also serves to prevent mitochondrial uptake and oxidation of fatty acids synthesised in the cytosol in the fed state. Malonyl CoA (the precursor for fatty acid synthesis, Section 5.6.1) is a potent inhibitor of carnitine acyltransferase I in the outer mitochondrial membrane.

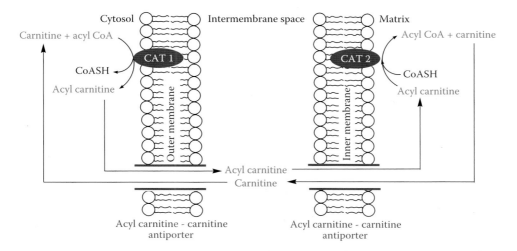

Figure 5.22 The role of carnitine in the transport of fatty acids into the mitochondrion (CAT = carnitine acyltransferase).

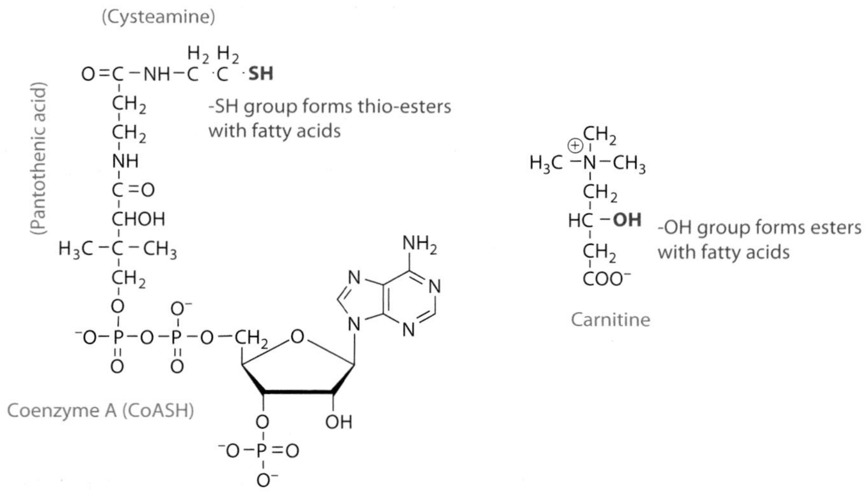

Figure 5.23 The structures of coenzyme A (CoA) and carnitine. Free coenzyme A is usually shown as CoASH to show that it has a free sulphydryl group.

Tissues such as muscle that oxidise fatty acids, but do not synthesise them, also have acetyl CoA carboxylase, and produce malonyl CoA. This controls the activity of carnitine acyltransferase I, and thus controls the mitochondrial uptake and β-oxidation of fatty acids. Tissues also have malonyl CoA decarboxylase, which acts to remove malonyl CoA and so reduce the inhibition of carnitine acyltransferase I. The two enzymes are regulated in opposite directions in response to

1. Insulin, which stimulates fatty acid synthesis and reduces β-oxidation.
2. Glucagon, which reduces fatty acid synthesis and increases β-oxidation.

Fatty acids are the major fuel for red muscle fibres, the main type involved in moderate exercise (Section 10.6). Children who lack one or the other of the enzymes for carnitine synthesis, and are therefore reliant on a dietary intake, have poor exercise tolerance because they have an impaired ability to transport fatty acids into the mitochondria for β-oxidation. Provision of supplements of carnitine to the affected children overcomes the problem. Extrapolation from this rare clinical condition has led to the use of carnitine as a so-called ergogenic aid to improve athletic performance. A number of studies have shown that relatively large supplements of carnitine increase the muscle content of carnitine to only a small extent, and most studies have shown no significant effect on athletic performance or endurance. This is not surprising—carnitine is readily synthesised from the amino acids lysine and methionine, and there is no evidence that any dietary intake is required.

5.5.2   The β-oxidation of fatty acids

Once it has entered the mitochondria, fatty acyl CoA undergoes a series of four reactions, resulting in the cleavage of the molecule to yield acetyl CoA and a new fatty acyl CoA that is two carbons shorter than the initial substrate (Figure 5.24). This shorter fatty acyl CoA is a substrate for the same sequence of reactions, which is repeated until the final result is

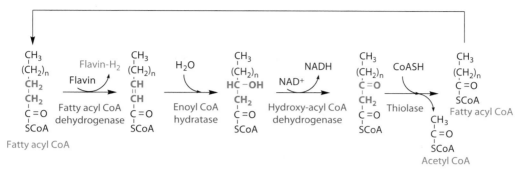

Figure 5.24 The β-oxidation of fatty acids.

cleavage to yield two molecules of acetyl CoA. This is the pathway of β-oxidation, so called because it is the β-carbon of the fatty acid that undergoes oxidation.

The reactions of β-oxidation are chemically the same as those in the conversion of succinate to oxaloacetate in the citric acid cycle (Figure 5.18):

- Removal of two hydrogens from the fatty acid, to form a carbon-carbon double bond—an oxidation reaction that linked to the reduction of flavin; thus, for each double bond formed in this way, there is a yield of 1.5 mol of ATP
- Hydration of the newly formed double bond to form hydroxyl group
- Oxidation of the hydroxyl group to an oxo group, linked to reduction of NAD^+, equivalent to 2.5 mol of ATP
- Cleavage of the oxo-acyl CoA by coenzyme A, to form acetyl CoA and the shorter fatty acyl CoA, which undergoes the same sequence of reactions

There are three separate sets of enzymes catalysing these four reactions, with specificity for long-, medium-, and short-chain fatty acyl CoA derivatives. Each set of enzymes is arranged as a membrane-bound array (a metabolon), and the product of one is passed directly to the active site of the next. The result of this is that whilst short- and medium-chain fatty acyl CoA can be detected in the mitochondrial matrix, as they pass from one array of enzymes to the next, none of the intermediates of the reaction sequence can be detected—they remain enzyme-bound.

The acetyl CoA formed by β-oxidation then enters the citric acid cycle (Figure 5.18). Almost all of the metabolically important fatty acids have an even number of carbon atoms; thus, the final cycle of β-oxidation is the conversion of a four-carbon fatty acyl CoA (butyryl CoA) to two molecules of acetyl CoA. Rare odd-carbon fatty acids yield propionyl CoA as the final product; this is carboxylated to succinyl CoA, which is an intermediate of the citric acid cycle. Because it increases the pool of 4-carbon intermediates in the cycle, propionyl CoA provides a net source of carbon for gluconeogenesis, whilst acetyl CoA does not.

5.5.3   Ketone bodies

Most tissues, and especially muscle, have a limited capacity for fatty acid oxidation, and in the fasting state cannot meet their energy requirements from fatty acid oxidation alone. By contrast, the liver is capable of forming considerably more acetyl CoA from fatty acids than is required for its own metabolism. It takes up fatty acids from the circulation and oxidises them to acetyl CoA, then synthesises and exports the four-carbon ketone bodies formed from acetyl CoA to other tissues (especially heart and skeletal muscle) for use as a metabolic fuel.

Acetoacetyl CoA is formed by reaction between two molecules of acetyl CoA (Figure 5.25). This is essentially the reverse of the final reaction of fatty acid β-oxidation (Figure 5.24). Acetoacetyl CoA then reacts with a further molecule of acetyl CoA to form hydroxy-methylglutaryl CoA, which is cleaved to acetyl CoA and acetoacetate.

Acetoacetate is chemically unstable and undergoes a non-enzymic reaction to yield acetone, which is only poorly metabolised. Most of it is excreted in the urine and in exhaled air—a waste of valuable metabolic fuel reserves in the fasting state. To avoid this, much of the acetoacetate is reduced to β-hydroxybutyrate before being released from the liver.

The first step in the utilisation of β-hydroxybutyrate and acetoacetate in extrahepatic tissues is oxidation of β-hydroxybutyrate to acetoacetate, yielding NADH (Figure 5.26). The synthesis of β-hydroxybutyrate in the liver can thus be regarded not only as a way of preventing loss of metabolic fuel as acetone, but also effectively as a means of exporting NADH (and therefore effectively ATP) to extrahepatic tissues. The liver synthesises and exports ketone bodies but does not oxidise them.

The utilisation of acetoacetate is controlled by the activity of the citric acid cycle. The reaction of acetoacetate succinyl CoA transferase provides an alternative to the reaction of succinyl CoA synthase (Figure 5.18), and there will only be an adequate supply of succinyl CoA to permit conversion of acetoacetate to acetoacetyl CoA as long as the rate of citric acid cycle activity is adequate. This means that even in the fasting state there may be a need for some metabolism of glucose or amino acids to provide pyruvate that can be carboxylated to oxaloacetate to maintain citric acid cycle activity.

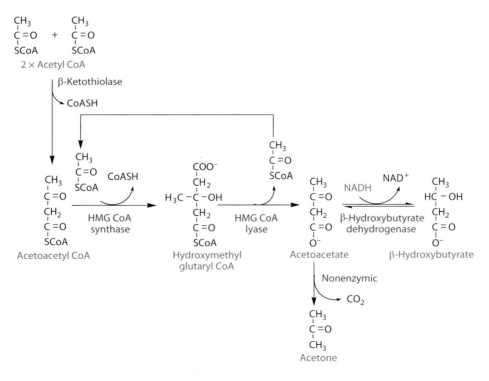

Figure 5.25 The synthesis of ketone bodies in the liver.

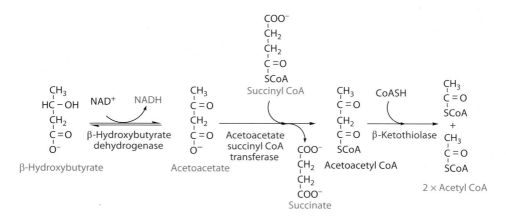

Figure 5.26 The utilisation of ketone bodies in extrahepatic tissues.

Acetoacetate, β-hydroxybutyrate, and acetone are collectively known as the ketone bodies, and the occurrence of increased concentrations of these three compounds in the bloodstream is known as ketosis. Although acetone and acetoacetate are chemically ketones, having a –C = O grouping, β-hydroxybutyrate is not chemically a ketone. It is classified with the other two because of its metabolic relationship. Actetoacetate and β-hydroxybutyrate are also acids, and will lower blood pH, potentially leading to metabolic acidosis. See Section 10.7 for a discussion of the problems of ketoacidosis in diabetes mellitus.

5.6   Tissue reserves of metabolic fuels

In the fed state, as well as providing for immediate energy needs, substrates are converted into storage compounds for use in the fasting state. There are two main stores of metabolic fuels:

1. Triacylglycerols in adipose tissue
2. Glycogen in liver and muscle

In addition, there is an increase in the synthesis of proteins after a meal, as a result of the increased availability of amino acids and metabolic fuel to provide the ATP and GTP needed for protein synthesis (Section 9.2.3.3) and stimulation of protein synthesis by insulin. The amino acid leucine also acts to stimulate protein synthesis, separately from the effect of generally increased availability of amino acids.

In the fasting state, which is the normal state between meals, these reserves are mobilised and used. Glycogen is a source of glucose, whilst adipose tissue provides both fatty acids and glycerol from triacylglycerol. The rate of protein synthesis is slower than that of protein catabolism, so that there is an increased supply of amino acids for gluconeogenesis.

5.6.1   Synthesis of fatty acids and triacylglycerols

Fatty acids are synthesised by the successive addition of two-carbon units from acetyl CoA, followed by reduction. Like β-oxidation, fatty acid synthesis is a spiral sequence of reactions. Unlike β-oxidation, which occurs in the mitochondrial matrix, fatty acid synthesis occurs in the cytosol. The enzymes required for fatty acid synthesis form a large multi-enzyme complex (Figure 5.27), and the growing fatty acid chain is carried from one catalytic site to the next by a flexible acyl carrier protein. The functional group of the acyl carrier protein is the same as that of CoA, derived from the vitamin pantothenic acid and cysteamine (Figure 5.23). Only the final 16-carbon fatty acid, and none of the intermediates, is released.

The only source of acetyl CoA is in the mitochondrial matrix, and acetyl CoA cannot cross the inner mitochondrial membrane. For fatty acid synthesis, citrate is formed inside the mitochondria by reaction between acetyl CoA and oxaloacetate (Figure 5.28) and is then transported into the cytosol, where it is cleaved to acetyl CoA and oxaloacetate. The acetyl CoA is used for fatty acid synthesis, whilst the oxaloacetate (indirectly) returns to the mitochondria to maintain citric acid cycle activity.

Fatty acid synthesis can only occur when there is citrate available in excess of the requirement for citric acid cycle activity for energy-yielding metabolism. Citrate is passed directly from the active site of citrate synthase to that of aconitase. It is only when isocitrate dehydrogenase is saturated, and hence aconitase is inhibited by its product, that citrate is released from the active site of citrate synthase into free solution, to be available for transport out of the mitochondria.

Oxaloacetate cannot re-enter the mitochondrion directly. It is reduced to malate, which then undergoes oxidative decarboxylation to pyruvate, linked to the reduction of $NADP^+$

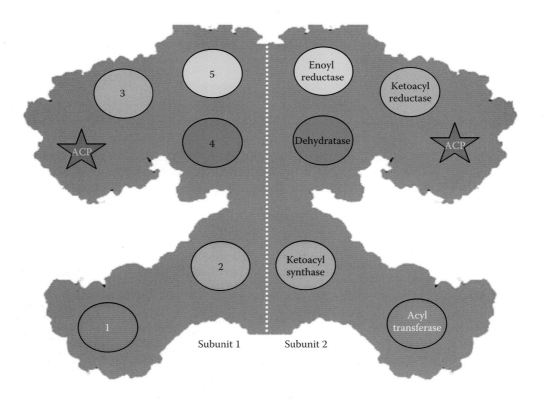

Figure 5.27 The fatty acid synthetase multi-enzyme complex.

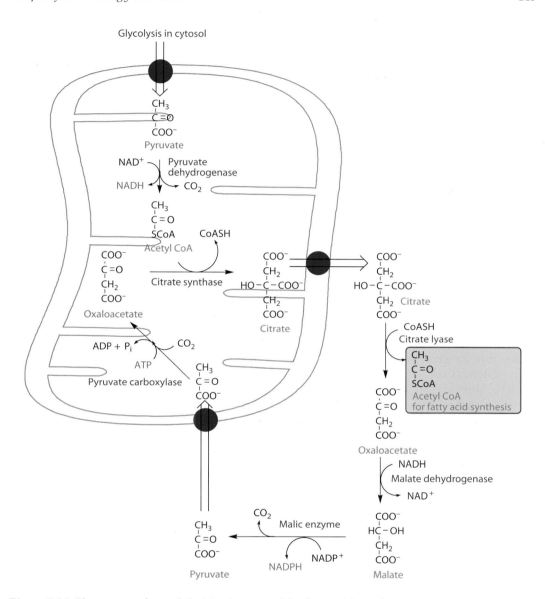

Figure 5.28 The source of acetyl CoA in the cytosol for fatty acid synthesis.

to NADPH. Pyruvate enters the mitochondrion, and is carboxylated to oxaloacetate in a reaction catalysed by pyruvate carboxylase.

The first reaction in the synthesis of fatty acids is carboxylation of acetyl CoA to malonyl CoA (Figure 5.29). This is a biotin-dependent reaction (Section 11.12.2). The activity of acetyl CoA carboxylase is regulated in response to insulin and glucagon. Malonyl CoA is not only the substrate for fatty acid synthesis, but also a potent inhibitor of carnitine acyltransferase, thus inhibiting the uptake of fatty acids into the mitochondrion for β-oxidation (Section 5.5.1).

The malonyl group is transferred onto an acyl carrier protein (ACP), and then reacts with the growing fatty acid chain, bound to the acyl carrier protein of the fatty acid synthase complex. The carbon dioxide that was added to form malonyl CoA is lost in this reaction.

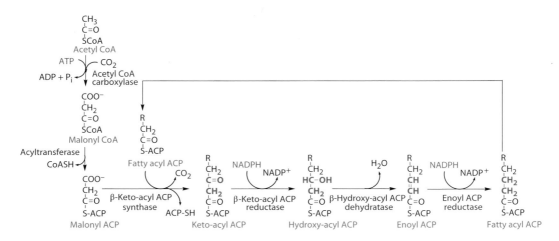

Figure 5.29 The synthesis of fatty acids.

For the first cycle of reactions, the central acyl carrier protein carries an acetyl group, and the product of reaction with malonyl CoA is acetoacetyl-ACP. In subsequent reaction cycles, it is the growing fatty acid chain that occupies the ACP, and the product of reaction with malonyl CoA is a keto-acyl-ACP.

The keto-acyl-ACP is then reduced to yield a hydroxyl group. In turn, this is dehydrated to yield a carbon–carbon double bond, which is reduced to yield a saturated fatty acid chain. Thus, the sequence of reactions is the reverse of that in β-oxidation (Section 5.5.2). For both reduction reactions in fatty acid synthesis, NADPH is the hydrogen donor. The source of half of this NADPH is the pentose phosphate pathway (Section 5.4.2), and of the remainder the oxidation of malate (arising from oxaloacetate) to pyruvate, catalysed by the malic enzyme (Figure 5.28).

The end product of cytosolic fatty acid synthesis in liver and adipose tissue is palmitate (C16:0); longer chain fatty acids (up to C24), and unsaturated fatty acids, are synthesised from palmitate in the endoplasmic reticulum and mitochondria. In the lactating mammary gland, fatty acid synthesis stops at myristate (C14:0) and the mammary gland does not synthesise longer chain or unsaturated fatty acids. The polyunsaturated fatty acids in milk are derived from synthesis in the liver, and, more importantly, the maternal diet.

5.6.1.1 *Unsaturated fatty acids*

Although fatty acid synthesis involves the formation of an unsaturated intermediate, the next step, reduction to the saturated fatty acid derivative, is an obligatory part of the reaction sequence and cannot be omitted. The product of the fatty acid synthase multi-enzyme complex is always saturated. Some unsaturated fatty acids can be synthesised from saturated fatty acids, by dehydrogenation to yield a carbon–carbon double bond.

Mammalian tissues have a cytochrome-dependent Δ^9-desaturase, which can introduce a carbon–carbon double bond between carbons 9 and 10 of the fatty acid (counting from the carboxyl group). As shown in Figure 5.30, this will yield oleic acid (C18:1 ω9) from stearic acid (C18:0). Other mammalian desaturases permit insertion of double bonds between Δ^{9-10} and the carboxyl group, but not between Δ^{9-10} and the methyl group (see Table 4.1).

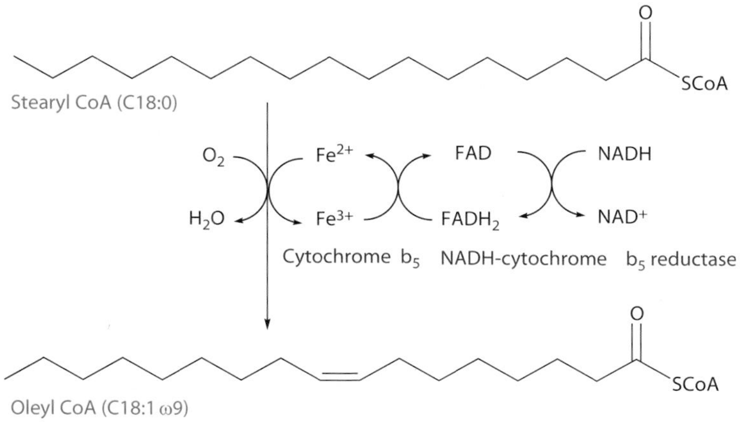

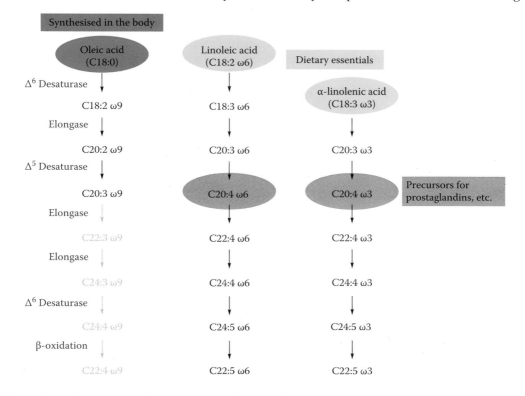

Figure 5.30 The reaction of fatty acid Δ^9 desaturase.

This means that fatty acids with double bonds between Δ^{9-10} and the methyl group must be provided in the diet. Linoleic acid (C18:2 ω6) is $\Delta^{9-10,12-13}$ and α-linolenic acid (C18:3 ω3) is $\Delta^{9-10,12-13,15-15}$. Both of these are dietary essentials and undergo chain elongation and further desaturation (between Δ^{9-10} and the carboxyl group) to yield the precursors of the eicosanoids.

As shown in Figure 5.31, the same series of enzymes catalyses elongation and desaturation of the ω3 and ω6 families of fatty acids and they compete with each other. Although

Figure 5.31 Elongation and desaturation of fatty acids.

it is considered desirable to increase intakes of polyunsaturated fatty acids (Section 6.3.2.1), there is some concern that an imbalance between intakes of ω6 polyunsaturated fatty acids (which come mainly from vegetable oils) and the ω3 series (which come mainly from fish oils) may lead to an imbalance in the synthesis of the two groups of eicosanoids synthesised from the polyunsaturated fatty acids.

5.6.1.2   Synthesis of triacylglycerol

The storage lipids in adipose tissue are triacylglycerols: glycerol esterified with three molecules of fatty acids. The three fatty acids in a triacylglycerol molecule are not always the same, and the fatty acid at carbon 2 is usually unsaturated. Triacylglycerol is synthesised in the small intestinal mucosa, liver, adipose tissue, lactating mammary gland, and skeletal muscle.

In adipose tissue, triacylglycerol is synthesised from the dietary fatty acids absorbed in lipid micelles that have been re-esterified and packaged into chylomicrons (Sections 4.3.2.2 and 5.6.2.1) and fatty acids from triacylglycerol in VLDL (Section 5.6.2.2). Adipose tissue can also synthesise fatty acids *de novo*. The triacylglycerol in VLDL comes from chylomicron remnants that have been taken up by the liver, *de novo* synthesis of fatty acids in the liver and from non-esterified fatty acids that have been released from adipose tissue and not taken up by muscle. Skeletal muscle also synthesises triacylglycerol for storage between muscle fibres. In this case all of the fatty acid comes from chylomicrons, VLDL, and plasma non-esterified fatty acids; muscle is not capable of *de novo* fatty acid synthesis.

The substrates for triacylglycerol synthesis are fatty acyl CoA esters (formed by reaction between fatty acids and coenzyme A, linked to the conversion of ATP → AMP + pyrophosphate), and glycerol phosphate (Figure 5.32). The main source of glycerol phosphate is by reduction of dihydroxy-acetone phosphate (an intermediate in glycolysis, Figure 5.10); the liver, but not adipose tissue, can also utilise glycerol directly.

Two fatty acids are esterified to the free hydroxyl groups of glycerol phosphate, by transfer from fatty acyl CoA, forming monoacylglycerol phosphate and then diacylglycerol phosphate (or phosphatidate). Diacylglycerol phosphate is then hydrolysed to diacylglycerol and phosphate before reaction with the third molecule of fatty acyl CoA to yield triacylglycerol. (The diacylglycerol phosphate can also be used for the synthesis of phospholipids, Section 4.3.1.2.)

Triacylglycerol synthesis incurs a considerable ATP cost; if the fatty acids are being synthesised from glucose then overall some 20% of the energy yield of the carbohydrate is expended in synthesising triacylglycerol reserves. The energy cost is lower if dietary fatty acids are being esterified to form triacylglycerols, but there is a cost of 2 mol of ATP (1 mol of ATP hydrolysed to AMP + pyrophosphate) for each mol of fatty acyl CoA formed. This explains the high energy cost of futile cycling of fatty acids that are released from adipose tissue and not taken up into adipose tissue, but re-esterified to triacylglycerol in the liver.

The enzymes for phosphatidate synthesis, acyl CoA synthetase, glycerol 3-phosphate acyltransferase, and monoacylglycerol acyltransferase, are on both the outer mitochondrial membrane and also the endoplasmic reticulum membrane. Diacylglycerol acyltransferase is only on the endoplasmic reticulum; it may use either diacylglycerol phosphate synthesised in the endoplasmic reticulum or that synthesised in mitochondria. Triacylglycerol synthesised on the endoplasmic reticulum membrane may then either enter lipid droplets in the cytosol, or, in the liver and intestinal mucosa, the lumen of the endoplasmic reticulum for assembly into lipoproteins—chylomicrons in the intestinal mucosa (Sections 4.3.2.2 and 5.6.2.1) and VLDL in the liver (Section 5.6.2.2).

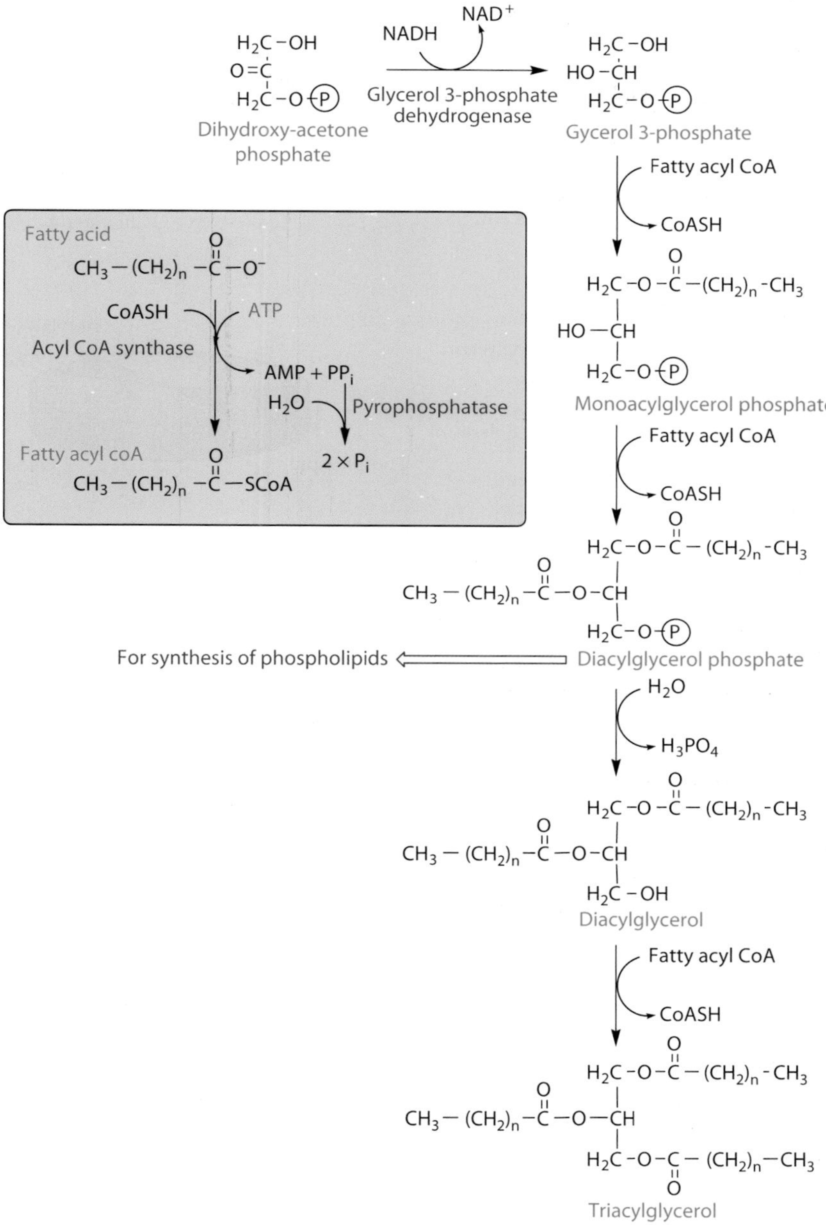

Figure 5.32 Esterification of fatty acids to form triacylglycerol.

5.6.2   *Plasma lipoproteins*

Triacylglycerol, cholesterol, and cholesterol esters as well as lipid-soluble vitamins are transported in plasma complexed with proteins; there are five classes of lipoproteins,

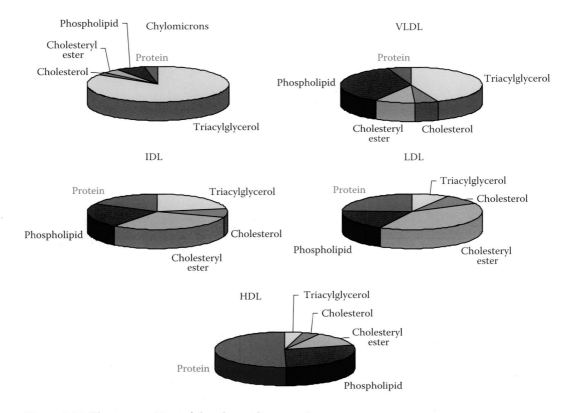

Figure 5.33 The composition of the plasma lipoproteins.

classified by their density, which in turn reflects their relative content of lipid and protein (Figure 5.33):

1. Chylomicrons, the least dense of the plasma lipoproteins are formed in the intestinal mucosa and circulate as a source of triacylglycerol in the fed state.
2. VLDLs are assembled in the liver and circulate as a source of cholesterol and triacylglycerol for extrahepatic tissues mainly in the fed state.
3. Intermediate-density lipoproteins (IDL) are formed in the circulation by removal of triacylglycerol from VLDL.
4. Low-density lipoproteins (LDL) are formed in the circulation by transfer of cholesterol from HDL onto IDL.
5. High-density lipoproteins (HDLs) are synthesised in the liver and small intestine as apoproteins, and acquire lipids (and especially cholesterol) from tissues for transport back to the liver, either directly or by transfer to IDL, forming LDL.

5.6.2.1   Chylomicrons

Newly absorbed fatty acids are re-esterified to form triacylglycerol in the intestinal mucosal cells, then assembled into chylomicrons (Section 4.3.2.2), which enter the lacteal of the villus (Figure 4.2), then the lymphatic system; they enter the bloodstream (the subclavian vein) at the thoracic duct. Chylomicrons begin to appear in the bloodstream about 60 min after a fatty meal, and have normally been cleared within 6–8 h by the action of lipoprotein lipase at the luminal surface of capillary blood vessels. The lipid-depleted chylomicron

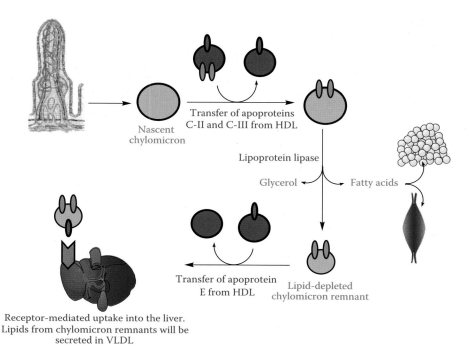

Figure 5.34 The life cycle of chylomicrons.

remnants are cleared by the liver by receptor-mediated endocytosis, followed by hydroly-sis of the proteins and residual lipids.

As shown in Figure 5.34, chylomicrons acquire three additional proteins from HDL after release into the bloodstream:

1. Apoprotein C-II activates lipoprotein lipase at the cell surface, permitting hydrolysis of chylomicron triacylglycerol to liberate fatty acids that are mainly taken up into adipose tissue and muscle cells.
2. Apoprotein C-III activates cholesterol esterase, permitting cells to take up cholesterol from chylomicron cholesteryl esters.
3. Apoprotein E is transferred onto lipid-depleted chylomicron remnants; it binds to hepatic receptors for receptor-mediated uptake of chylomicron remnants.

5.6.2.2   *Very-low-density lipoproteins, intermediate-density lipoprotein, and low-density lipoproteins*

As shown in Figure 5.35, VLDL is assembled in the liver, and contains both newly syn-thesised triacylglycerol, cholesterol, cholesteryl esters, and phospholipids, and also lipids from chylomicron remnants. These lipids are taken up by peripheral tissues that have cell surface lipoprotein lipase, phospholipase, and cholesterol esterase.

As the VLDL particles are progressively depleted of lipids, they transfer apoproteins C-I and C-II to HDL, becoming IDL. IDL takes up cholesteryl esters from HDL, becoming LDL.

LDL is cleared from the circulation by receptor-mediated uptake in the liver. Both the receptor and the LDL are internalised; the LDL is hydrolysed in lysosomes by proteases and lipases, and the receptor is recycled back to the cell surface.

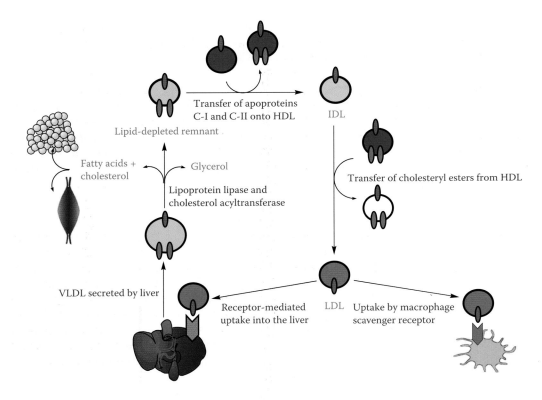

Figure 5.35 The life cycle of VLDL, IDL, and LDL.

Free (unesterified) cholesterol represses synthesis of the LDL receptor; thus, when there is an adequate amount of cholesterol in the liver, less LDL will be cleared. The hypo-cholesterolemic statin drugs both inhibit cholesterol synthesis and also increase clearance of LDL because there is now less repression of receptor synthesis.

Elevated LDL cholesterol is one of the major factors in the development of atherosclerosis and ischaemic heart disease. Two factors are involved in elevated LDL cholesterol:

1. Increased synthesis and secretion of VLDL. This in turn will be a consequence of a high fat intake, since there is more lipid from chylomicron remnants to be exported from the liver in VLDL.
2. Decreased clearance of LDL by receptor-mediated uptake. This may be due to
   i. Down-regulation of LDL receptor synthesis by free cholesterol in cells. Monosaturated and polyunsaturated fatty acids are good substrates for cholesterol esterification in cells, whilst saturated fatty acids are not. When saturated fatty acid levels are relatively high, less cholesterol is esterified; thus, the intracellular concentration rises, repressing the synthesis of LDL receptor (see also Section 6.3.2.1).
   ii. Poor affinity of some genetic variants of apoprotein E for the LDL receptor. This is the basis of some of the genetic susceptibility to atherosclerosis.
   iii. Genetic defects of the LDL receptor, in some cases of familial hyperlipidaemia.
   iv. Chemical modification of apoprotein E in the circulation, thus reducing its affinity for the hepatic receptors. Commonly, this is secondary to oxidative damage to

unsaturated fatty acids in LDL, hence the role of antioxidants in reducing the risk of atherosclerosis (Section 6.5.3). High levels of homocysteine (Section 6.6) can also lead to modification of apoprotein E.

LDL that is not cleared by the liver is taken up by macrophage scavenger receptors; unlike hepatic uptake, this is an unregulated process, and macrophages can take up an almost unlimited amount of lipid from LDL. Lipid-engorged macrophages (foam cells) infiltrate blood vessel endothelium, especially when there is already some degree of endothelial damage, then undergo necrosis to form fatty streaks which eventually develop into atherosclerotic plaque. Unesterified cholesterol and plant sterols are especially cytotoxic to macrophages.

5.6.2.3 High-density lipoproteins

Peripheral tissues take up more cholesterol from VLDL and LDL than they require and export the surplus onto HDL for return to the liver for excretion or catabolism. As shown in Figure 5.36, HDL is secreted from the liver as a lipid-poor protein and takes up cholesterol from tissues by the action of lecithin cholesterol acyltransferase at the lipoprotein surface.

Much of the cholesterol in HDL is transferred to LDL (and some into chylomicron remnants), for receptor-mediated uptake into the liver. However, cholesterol-rich HDL can also bind to a liver receptor, which has esterase activity, permitting uptake of cholesterol into the liver. The apoprotein is not internalised, as occurs with chylomicron remnants and LDL, but is released back into the circulation when most of the lipid has been removed.

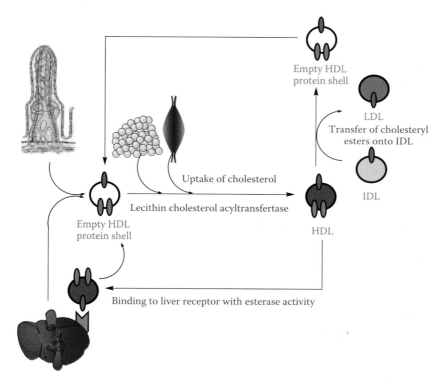

Figure 5.36 The life cycle of HDL.

5.6.3   Glycogen

In the fed state, glycogen is synthesised from glucose in both liver and muscle. The reaction is a step-wise addition of glucose units onto the glycogen that is already present (Figure 5.37).

Glycogen synthesis involves the intermediate formation of UDP-glucose (uridine diphosphate glucose) by reaction between glucose 1-phosphate and UTP (uridine triphosphate). As each glucose unit is added to the growing glycogen chain, UDP is released and must be rephosphorylated to UTP by reaction with ATP. There is thus a significant cost of ATP in the synthesis of glycogen: 2 mol of ATP are converted to ADP + phosphate for each glucose unit added, and overall the energy cost of glycogen synthesis may account for 5% of the energy yield of the carbohydrate stored.

Glycogen synthetase forms only the α1→4 links that form the straight chains of glycogen. The branch points are introduced by the transfer of a chain of 6–10 glucose units from carbon 4 to carbon 6 of the glucose unit at the branch point.

The branched structure of glycogen means that it traps a considerable amount of water within the molecule. In the early stages of food restriction there is depletion of muscle and liver glycogen, with the release and excretion of this trapped water. This leads to an initial rate of weight loss that is very much greater than can be accounted for by catabolism of

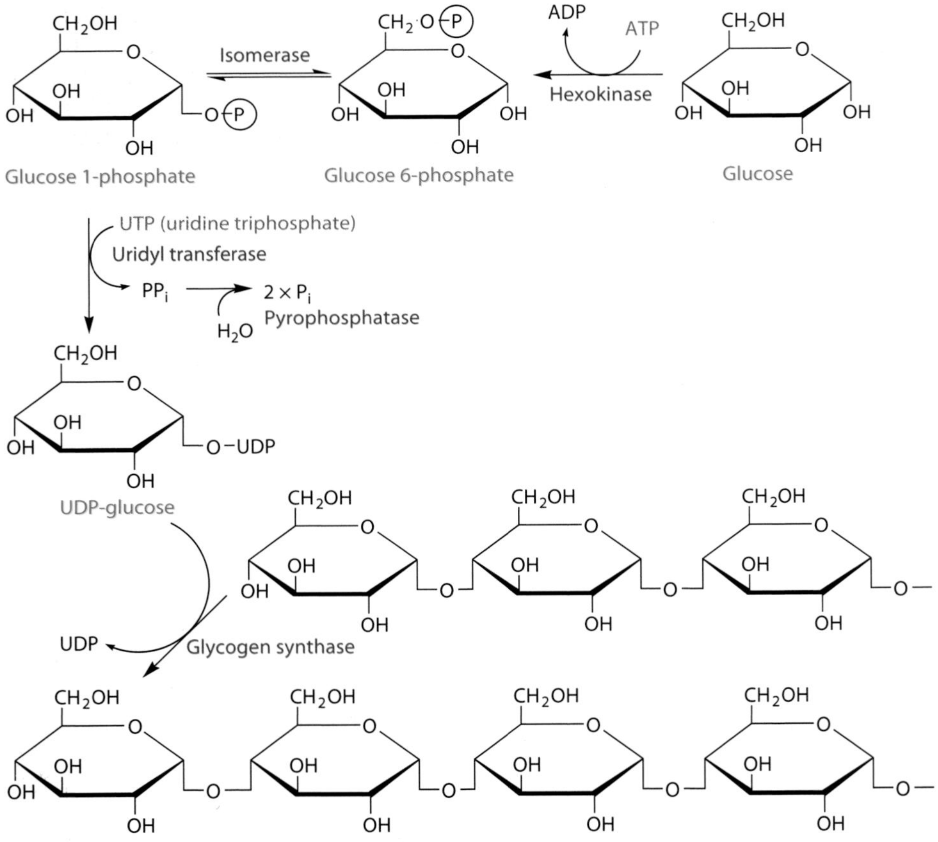

Figure 5.37 The synthesis of glycogen.

adipose tissue, and, of course, it cannot be sustained—once glycogen has been depleted the rapid loss of water (and weight) will cease.

5.6.3.1   *Glycogen utilisation*

In the fasting state, glycogen is broken down by the removal of glucose units one at a time from the many free ends of the molecule. The reaction is a phosphorolysis—cleavage of the glycoside link between two glucose molecules by the introduction of phosphate (Figure 5.9). The product is glucose 1-phosphate, which is isomerised to glucose 6-phosphate. In the liver, glucose 6-phosphatase catalyses the hydrolysis of glucose 6-phosphate to free glucose, which is exported for use especially by the brain and red blood cells.

Muscle cannot release free glucose from the breakdown of glycogen, since it lacks glucose 6-phosphatase. However, as shown in Figure 5.38, muscle glycogen can be an indirect source of blood glucose in the fasting state. Glucose 6-phosphate from muscle glycogen undergoes glycolysis to pyruvate (Figure 5.10), which is then transaminated to alanine. Alanine is exported from muscle and taken up by the liver for use as a substrate for gluconeogenesis (Section 5.7).

Glycogen phosphorylase stops cleaving α1→4 links four glucose residues from a branch point, and a debranching enzyme catalyses the transfer of a three glucosyl unit to the free end of another chain. The α1→6 link is then hydrolysed by a glucosidase, releasing glucose.

The branched structure of glycogen means that there are a great many points at which glycogen phosphorylase can act; in response to stimulation by adrenaline, there is a very rapid rise in blood glucose as a result of phosphorolysis of glycogen (Section 10.3.2.1).

Endurance athletes require a slow release of glucose 1-phosphate from glycogen over a period of hours, rather than a rapid release. There is some evidence that this is achieved better from glycogen that is less branched, and therefore has fewer points at which

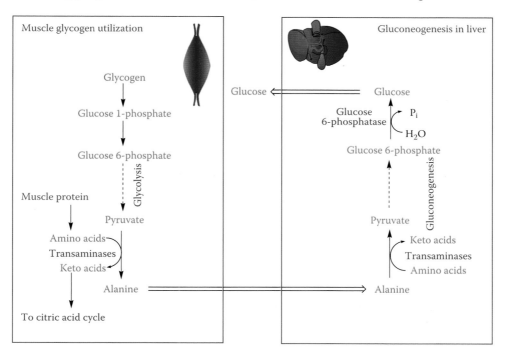

Figure 5.38 Indirect utilisation of muscle glycogen to maintain blood glucose.

glycogen phosphorylase can act. The formation of branch points in glycogen synthesis is slower than the formation of α1→4 links, and this has been exploited in the process of 'carbohydrate loading' in preparation for endurance athletic events. The athlete exercises to exhaustion, when muscle glycogen is more or less completely depleted, then consumes a high carbohydrate meal, which stimulates rapid synthesis of glycogen, with fewer branch points than normal. There is little evidence to show whether this improves endurance performance or not; such improvement as has been reported may be the result of knowing that one has made an effort to improve performance rather than any real metabolic effect.

5.7   Gluconeogenesis—the synthesis of glucose from non-carbohydrate precursors

Because the brain is largely dependent on glucose as its metabolic fuel (and red blood cells and the renal medulla are entirely so), there is a need to maintain the blood concentration of glucose above about 3 mmol/L in the fasting state. If the plasma concentration of glucose falls below about 2 mmol/L there is a loss of consciousness—hypoglycaemic coma.

The plasma concentration of glucose is maintained in short-term fasting by the use of glycogen, and by releasing free fatty acids from adipose tissues, and ketone bodies from the liver, which are preferentially used by muscle, thus sparing such glucose as is available for use by the brain and red blood cells.

However, the total body content of glycogen would be exhausted within 12–18 h of fasting if there were no other source of glucose. The process of gluconeogenesis is the synthesis of glucose from non-carbohydrate precursors: amino acids from the catabolism of protein and the glycerol of triacylglycerols. It is important to note that although acetyl CoA, and hence fatty acids, can be synthesised from pyruvate (and therefore from carbohydrates), the decarboxylation of pyruvate to acetyl CoA (Figure 5.16) cannot be reversed. Pyruvate cannot be formed from acetyl CoA. Since two molecules of carbon dioxide are formed for each 2-carbon acetate unit metabolised in the citric acid cycle (Figure 5.18), there can be no net formation of oxaloacetate from acetate. Therefore, it is not possible to synthesise glucose from acetyl CoA; fatty acids and ketone bodies cannot serve as a precursor for glucose synthesis under any circumstances.

The main organ for gluconeogenesis is the liver; during prolonged starvation and at times of metabolic acidosis, when hepatic gluconeogenesis decreases, the kidney also makes a significant contribution. The key enzymes for gluconeogenesis are also expressed in small intestinal mucosal cells, but it is unclear to what extent (if at all) the small intestine may contribute to glucose production in fasting and starvation.

The pathway of gluconeogenesis is essentially the reverse of the pathway of glycolysis, shown in Figure 5.10. However, at three steps, there are separate enzymes involved in the breakdown of glucose (glycolysis) and gluconeogenesis. The reactions of pyruvate kinase, phosphofructokinase, and hexokinase cannot readily be reversed (i.e., they have equilibria which are strongly in the direction of the formation of pyruvate, fructose bisphosphate, and glucose 6-phosphate, respectively).

There are therefore separate enzymes, under distinct metabolic control, for the reverse of each of these reactions in gluconeogenesis:

- Pyruvate is converted to phosphoenolpyruvate for glucose synthesis by a two step reaction, with the intermediate formation of oxaloacetate (Figure 5.39). Pyruvate is carboxylated to oxaloacetate in an ATP-dependent reaction in which the vitamin

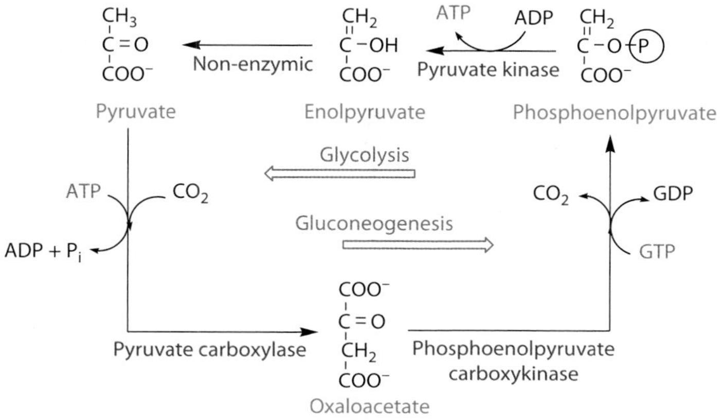

Figure 5.39 Reversal of the reaction of pyruvate kinase for gluconeogenesis: pyruvate carboxylase and phospho-enolpyruvate carboxykinase.

biotin (Section 11.12.2) is the coenzyme. This reaction can also be used to replenish oxaloacetate in the citric acid cycle when intermediates have been withdrawn for use in other pathways and is involved in the return of oxaloacetate from the cytosol to the mitochondrion in fatty acid synthesis (Figure 5.28). Oxaloacetate then undergoes a phosphorylation reaction, in which it also loses carbon dioxide, to form phospho-enolpyruvate. The phosphate donor for this reaction is GTP; this provides control of the withdrawal of oxaloacetate for gluconeogenesis if citric acid cycle activity would be impaired (Section 5.4.4).
- Fructose bisphosphate is hydrolysed to fructose 6-phosphate by a simple hydrolysis reaction catalysed by the enzyme fructose bisphosphatase.
- Glucose 6-phosphate is hydrolysed to free glucose and phosphate by the action of glucose 6-phosphatase.

The other reactions of glycolysis are readily reversible, and the overall direction of metabolism, either glycolysis or gluconeogenesis, depends mainly on the relative activities of phosphofructokinase and fructose bisphosphatase (Section 10.2.2).

Many of the products of amino acid metabolism can also be used for gluconeogenesis, since they are sources of pyruvate or one of the intermediates in the citric acid cycle, and hence give rise to oxaloacetate (Sections 5.4.4.1, 9.3.2, and Figure 5.20). The requirement for gluconeogenesis from amino acids to maintain a supply of glucose explains why there is a considerable loss of muscle in prolonged fasting or starvation, even if there are apparently adequate reserves of adipose tissue to meet energy needs.

Key points

- Energy expenditure can be measured directly by heat output from the body or indirectly by measuring oxygen consumption or the difference in the rate of loss of ^{18}O and ^{2}H from dual isotopically labelled water.
- Measurement of carbon dioxide production as well as oxygen consumption (the RQ) (and urinary excretion of urea) permits estimation of the relative amounts of fat, carbohydrate, and protein being metabolised.

- In fasting, when the major fuel is fatty acids, RQ is near 0.8; in the fed state when there is ample carbohydrate available it rises to near 1.0.
- Basal metabolic rate is the energy expenditure at rest, under controlled conditions of thermal neutrality, about 12 h after a meal; it is the energy required to maintain nerve and muscle tone, circulation and respiration, and metabolic homeostasis. It is determined by gender, age, and body weight.
- The energy cost of physical activity is expressed as the physical activity ratio (PAR) or metabolic equivalent of the task (MET)—the cost of the activity as a multiple of BMR.
- A person's overall PAL (PAR) is the sum of the PARs of individual activities × the time spent in each activity/24 h.
- Diet-induced thermogenesis is the increase in metabolic activity after a meal; it is mainly the energy cost of synthesising reserves of triacylglycerol and glycogen as well as increased protein synthesis.
- From the composition of adipose tissue it is possible to calculate that there will be a change of 33 g in body weight per MJ energy imbalance per day. In practice the weight change is less than this because of adaptation to increased or decreased food intake.
- In the fed state, there is an ample supply of metabolic fuel, and reserves of fat and glycogen are formed; these are used in the fasting state to ensure a supply of fuel for tissues.
- The brain and central nervous system are largely reliant on glucose, and red blood cells and renal medulla wholly so; in the fasting state, muscle does not utilise glucose but metabolises fatty acids released from adipose tissue reserves and ketone bodies synthesised by the liver.
- Glycolysis is the pathway by which glucose is oxidised to 2 mol of the 3-carbon compound pyruvate. There is a net yield of 7 mol of ATP per mol of glucose metabolised.
- In maximum exertion, glycolysis can proceed anaerobically, with reduction of pyruvate to lactate; the net yield is then 2 mol ATP per mol of glucose oxidised. Resynthesis of glucose from lactate in the liver is ATP expensive; oxygen debt is the increased oxygen consumption associated with increased metabolic activity to provide the ATP needed.
- The pentose phosphate pathway provides an alternative to part of the pathway of glycolysis; it is the pathway for synthesis of ribose, and also for the production of NADPH.
- Favism, due to impaired activity of glucose 6-phosphate dehydrogenase in the pentose phosphate pathway, impairs the ability of red blood cells to reduce glutathione, and hence impaired ability to reduce H_2O_2, leading to haemolytic crisis in response to metabolic stress.
- Pyruvate is oxidised to acetyl CoA in a multi-step reaction for which thiamin (vitamin B_1) provides the coenzyme. The reaction is irreversible.
- The acetate moiety of acetyl CoA, arising from pyruvate oxidation, the oxidation of fatty acids, and some amino acids, undergoes oxidation in the citric acid cycle, with a yield of 10 mol of ATP per mol of acetate.
- The citric acid cycle also provides the main pathway for the interconversion of 4- and 5-carbon compounds arising from amino acid metabolism, and the provision of substrates for gluconeogenesis.

- In the fed state, fatty acids are available to tissues from chylomicrons and VLDL, by the action of lipoprotein lipase in capillary blood vessels. In the fasting state, fatty acids are provided by hydrolysis of adipose tissue triacylglycerol, catalysed by hormone-sensitive lipase.
- The uptake of fatty acids into the mitochondrion for oxidation requires formation of acyl carnitine, and the process is regulated by the availability of free CoA inside the mitochondrion.
- The β-oxidation of fatty acids proceeds by the stepwise removal of 2-carbon units as acetyl CoA, with a yield of 4 mol of ATP per acetyl CoA formed.
- Ketone bodies are synthesised in the liver in the fasting state to provide a metabolic fuel for muscle, to spare glucose. In prolonged starvation the brain can utilise ketone bodies to some extent.
- Fatty acids are synthesised in the fed state from acetyl CoA exported from the mitochondria as citrate. Fatty acid synthetase is a large multi-enzyme complex; the final product is palmitate (C16:0) and none of the intermediate compounds is released. Longer chain fatty acids are synthesised from palmitate in the endoplasmic reticulum and mitochondria.
- Unsaturated fatty acids are synthesised by dehydrogenation of saturated fatty acids. Mammals can only insert double bonds between C-9 and the carboxyl group of a fatty acid; there is a dietary requirement for ω3 and ω6 polyunsaturated fatty acids, although precursors can undergo chain elongation and further desaturation.
- Triacylglycerol synthesis from fatty acids is relatively ATP expensive.
- Chylomicrons carry newly absorbed lipids from the small intestine to tissues; the liver clears chylomicron remnants.
- VLDL is assembled in the liver, containing triacylglycerol from chylomicron remnants and formed from newly synthesised fatty acids. In the circulation, it loses lipids and gains proteins, becoming intermediate density, then LDL.
- LDL transports cholesterol to tissues and acquires cholesterol from HDL. It is normally cleared by receptor-mediated uptake in the liver. The LDL receptor is downregulated by a high intracellular concentration of free cholesterol, and chemically modified (oxidised) LDL is not recognised by the liver receptor. It is taken up by macrophage scavenger receptors. Lipid engorged macrophages infiltrate the blood vessel endothelium, forming fatty streaks that develop into atherosclerotic plaque.
- HDL collects surplus cholesterol from peripheral tissues, returning it to the liver (either directly or by transfer to LDL) for catabolism and excretion.

Further resources on the CD

The energy balance computer simulation program in the virtual laboratory on the CD.

chapter six

Diet and health
Nutrition and chronic non communicable diseases

Patterns of disease and mortality differ around the world and one of the factors that can be correlated with many of the differences is diet, although there are obviously other environmental (and genetic) factors involved. This chapter is concerned with the ways in which we can gather evidence that diet is, or may be, a factor in the development of chronic non-communicable diseases (especially atherosclerosis and coronary heart disease, and cancer), and how we can use these findings to produce guidelines for a prudent or healthful diet.

At one time, these diseases were known as diseases of affluence because they were seen mainly in affluent Western countries and mainly amongst the wealthier sections of society. Increasingly, they are becoming major causes of morbidity and premature death in developing countries and are more common amongst the poorer, rather than wealthier, sections of society in developed countries. They are diseases associated with a nutrition transition, from a traditional diet in which total food was often only marginally adequate, to one in which a super-abundant amount of food is available, with increased intake of fat (and especially saturated fat) and sugars and decreased consumption of unrefined cereals, fruit, and vegetables.

Obviously, neither undernutrition, leading to the problems discussed in Chapter 8, nor overnutrition, leading to the problems of obesity (Chapter 7) is desirable. The relative amounts of fat, carbohydrate, and protein in the diet are important, as is the mixture of different types of fat (Section 6.3.2) and carbohydrate (Section 6.3.3). Consumption of alcohol may have both beneficial and adverse effects on health (Section 6.3.5), and intakes of some vitamins and minerals above the levels that are adequate to prevent deficiency (Chapter 11) may be beneficial. A wide variety of compounds in foods that are not considered to be nutrients may also have beneficial effects (Sections 6.5.3 and 6.7).

Objectives

After reading this chapter, you should be able to

- Explain the types of evidence that link diet with the diseases of affluence.
- Describe and explain the guidelines for a prudent diet, explain the recommendations concerning dietary fat, carbohydrate, and salt, and how the message can be conveyed to the public.
- Describe and explain the interactions between nutrition and genetics and the ways in which early nutrition may affect patterns of gene expression and disease risk in later life.
- Explain what is meant by a free radical, how oxygen radicals cause tissue damage, and the main sources of oxygen radicals.
- Describe the main antioxidant nutrients and explain how they are believed to protect against cancer and heart disease.

- Describe and explain the role of homocysteine in cardiovascular disease, the role of a common polymorphism in methylene tetrahydrofolate reductase, and the apparent protective effect of folic acid.
- Describe the various protective non-nutrient compounds that are found in plant foods and explain their protective actions.

6.1 Chronic non-communicable diseases (the 'diseases of affluence')

The major causes of death in developed countries today are heart disease (atherosclerosis and coronary heart disease), hypertension (high blood pressure), stroke, and cancer. These are not just diseases of old age, although it is true to say that the longer people live, the more likely they are to develop them. Coronary heart disease is a major cause of premature death, striking a significant number of people younger than 40 years old.

As societies develop, and socioeconomic changes and improvements in general health (especially reduction in infectious diseases) result in an increase in average life expectancy to 80 years or more, so coronary heart disease becomes more prevalent, accounting for 15%–25% of deaths. In developing countries, cardiovascular disease began to emerge as a significant cause of premature death in the 1970s and 1980s; the corresponding stage in socioeconomic development in the United States was the 1920s, and somewhat later in Western Europe, where cardiovascular disease mortality mirrored that in the United States, but with a 10- to 20-year time lag. Since the 1980s, there has been a progressive fall in cardiovascular disease mortality in most developed countries, possibly reflecting changes in diet (Section 6.3).

Diet is, of course, only one of the differences between life in the developed countries of Western Europe, North America, and Australasia and that in developing countries; there are a great many other differences in environment and living conditions. In addition, genetic variation will affect susceptibility to nutritional and environmental factors (Section 6.4), and there is abundant evidence that nutritional status *in utero* and infancy affects responses to diet in adult life (Section 6.4.1).

It can be assumed that human beings and their diet have evolved together. Certainly, we have changed our crops and farm animals by selective breeding over the last 10,000 years (and more recently by genetic modification of crop plants), and it is reasonable to assume that we have evolved by natural selection to be suited to our diet. The problem is that evolution is a slow process, and there have been major changes in food availability in most countries over only a single generation. As recently as the 1930s (very recent in evolutionary terms) it was estimated that up to one third of households in Britain could not afford an adequate diet. Malnutrition was a serious problem, and the daily provision of 200 mL of milk to schoolchildren had a significant effect on their health and growth.

Foods that historically were scarce luxuries are now commonplace and available in surplus. Sugar was an expensive luxury until the middle of the 19th century; traditionally, fat was also scarce, and every effort was made to save and use all the fat (dripping) from a roast joint of meat.

There are thus two separate, but related, questions to be considered:

1. Is diet a factor in the chronic non-communicable diseases that are major causes of premature death in developed countries?
2. Might changes in average Western diets reduce the risk of developing cancer and cardiovascular disease?

6.2   *Types of evidence linking diet and chronic diseases*

The main evidence linking diet with chronic diseases is epidemiological; animal studies are used to test hypotheses derived from epidemiology to test the effects of specific nutritional changes and to investigate biological mechanisms to explain the epidemiological findings. When there is a substantial body of evidence then there can be intervention studies, in which the diets of large numbers of people are changed (e.g. by providing supplements of nutrients for which there is epidemiological evidence of a protective effect), and they are observed for 5–10 or more years, to see whether the intervention has any effect on disease incidence or mortality.

The World Health Organization has classified the strength of evidence of associations between diet and chronic non-communicable diseases as follows:

- Convincing evidence. Evidence based on epidemiological studies showing a consistent association between exposure and disease, with little or no evidence to the contrary. The evidence is based on a large number of studies, including prospective studies (Section 6.2.5), and where relevant, randomised controlled intervention trials that are large enough and continue for long enough to show consistent effects. There must also be a plausible biological explanation or mechanism.
- Probable evidence. Evidence based on epidemiological studies showing a fairly consistent association between exposure and disease, but there are defects in some of the studies, or some evidence to the contrary. Shortcomings may include studies or trials that are too short, involve too few people, or have incomplete follow-up. There is usually laboratory evidence of a plausible biological mechanism.
- Possible evidence. Evidence based mainly on cross-sectional and case-control studies (Section 6.2.4), with insufficient randomised controlled trials or prospective studies (Section 6.2.5). There is supportive evidence from laboratory and clinical investigations, but more trials are required to support the tentative associations.
- Insufficient evidence. Evidence based on a small number of studies that are suggestive, but are insufficient to establish an association between exposure and disease. There is little or no evidence from randomised controlled trials. More well-designed research is needed to support the tentative conclusions.

6.2.1   *Secular changes in diet and disease incidence*

The first type of evidence comes from studying changes in disease incidence and diet (but also other factors) over time. Table 6.1 shows the changes in diet in rural southwest Wales

Table 6.1 Secular Changes in Diet with Changes in Disease Incidence—Changes in Diet in Rural Wales Between 1870 and 1970

	1870	1970	
Protein	11	11	% of energy
Fat	25	42	% of energy
Sugar	4	17	% of energy
Starch	60	30	% of energy
Unsaturated fat	19	9	% of total fat
Cholesterol	130	517	mg/day
Dietary fibre	65	21	g/day

between 1870 and 1970. This was a century during which there was a marked decrease in hunger-related diseases and a marked increase in premature death from coronary heart disease—to the extent that in 1970, this region had one of the highest rates of coronary heart disease in Europe.

The major changes over this period were an increase in the proportion of energy derived from fat, and an increase in the proportion of dietary fat that was saturated (Section 4.3.1.1). At the same time, there was a considerable increase in cholesterol consumption (as a result of increased consumption of animal fats) and a significant decrease in the proportion of energy derived from starch, although sugar consumption increased considerably. Intake of cereal fibre also decreased. This suggests that increased intakes of fat (and especially saturated fat), cholesterol, and sugar and reduced intakes of starch and cereal fibre may be factors in the development of coronary heart disease.

A similar nutrition transition is occurring now in developing countries. There is increased overall availability of food, with increased consumption of fat (especially saturated fat) and sugars, and decreased consumption of complex carbohydrates, whole grain cereals, fruit, and vegetables. At the same time, physical activity (and hence energy requirement) is decreasing as a result of increased mechanisation in the workplace, increased mechanised transport, and low recreational activity. These changes occurred over a century or more in Western Europe and North America; they are occurring over a decade or so in many developing countries.

6.2.2   *International correlations between diet and disease incidence*

Worldwide, there are very considerable differences in mortality from cancer and coronary heart disease. Incidence of breast cancer ranges from 34/million in the Gambia to 1002/million in Hawaii and prostate cancer from 12/million in the Gambia to 912/million amongst black Americans. There is also a considerable variation in the percentage of energy derived from fat—about 10% in Bangladesh and 40% in France.

Coronary heart disease accounts for 4.8% of deaths in Japan, but 31.7% of deaths in Northern Ireland. In the Seven Countries Study conducted in the 1950s and 1960s, which was a prospective study (Section 6.2.5) in which people were followed for 15 years, the incidence of coronary heart disease was 14.4/1000 in Japan, compared with 120.2/1000 in eastern Finland; saturated fat accounted for 3% of energy intake in Japan and 22% in eastern Finland (and mean serum cholesterol was 4.3 mmol/L in Japan and 7 mmol/L in Finland).

Assuming that there are adequate and comparable data available for food consumption and disease incidence in different countries, it is possible to plot graphs such as that in Figure 6.1, which shows a highly significant positive association between fat consumption and breast cancer. It is important to note that statistical correlation does not imply cause and effect; indeed, further analysis of the factors involved in breast cancer suggest that it is not dietary fat intake, but rather adiposity, or total body fat content, that is the important factor. Significant amounts of oestrogens are formed in adipose tissue, in an uncontrolled manner, and this is a factor in the aetiology of breast cancer. Obviously, dietary fat intake is a significant factor in the development of obesity and high body fat reserves (Chapter 7).

One problem in interpreting correlations between diet and disease is that national data for food availability disguise possibly large differences between cities and rural areas. In

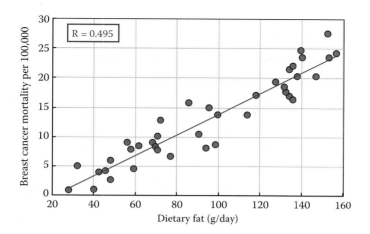

Figure 6.1 International correlation between fat intake and breast cancer in women. (From data reported by Caroll, K. K., *Cancer Research* 35: 3374–83, 1975.)

India, in the 1980s, some 17% of the rural poor had little or no visible oil or fat in their diet, whilst the urban elite received more than 30% of energy from fat; 5% of the population consumed 40% of the available fat. The food available per person in sub-Saharan Africa (excluding South Africa) fell over the period 1980–2005, but cardiovascular disease is an increasing cause of premature mortality in African cities.

Rather than looking at national data for food availability, some studies have measured plasma concentrations of nutrients or other more specific markers of intake. Figure 6.2 shows a highly significant negative correlation between mortality from coronary heart disease and the serum concentration of vitamin E, suggesting that vitamin E may be protective against the development of atherosclerosis and coronary heart disease.

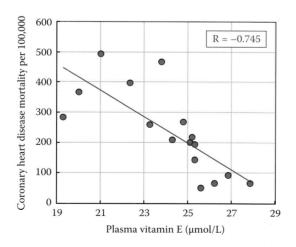

Figure 6.2 The relationship between plasma vitamin E levels and coronary heart disease. (From data reported by Gey, K. F. et al., *American Journal of Clinical Nutrition* 53: 326–34s, 1991.)

6.2.3   Studies of migrants

People who migrate from one country to another provide an excellent opportunity to study the effects of dietary and environmental factors on disease; their first-degree relatives who have not migrated provide a genetically matched control group for comparison.

Both breast and prostate cancer are rare in China and Japan, compared with the incidence of both in the United States. Studies of people who migrated from China and Japan to Hawaii or San Francisco in the 20th century showed that they had a considerably higher incidence of both cancers than their relatives at home who retained their traditional diet and lifestyle. There were similar differences in mortality from coronary heart disease.

Studies of immigrants in the mid-20th century from Poland (where gastric cancer was common, and colorectal cancer rare) to Australia (where gastric cancer is rare, and colorectal cancer more common) showed a significant increase in colorectal cancer, whilst they retained the relatively high Polish incidence of gastric cancer (although second generation Polish-Australians have the low Australian incidence of gastric cancer). This suggests that dietary or environmental factors involved in the development of colorectal cancer may act relatively late in life, whilst factors that predispose to gastric cancer act earlier in life. Infection with *Helicobacter pylori*, which was more common in Poland than in Australia, is a factor in gastric cancer. Diets high in salted and preserved meats are associated with higher incidence of gastric cancer and diets high in fat and low in non-starch polysaccharides (NSPs) are associated with higher incidence of colorectal cancer. As the incidence of gastric cancer in a population decreases, so the incidence of colorectal cancer increases.

6.2.4   Case–control studies

An alternative way of studying relationships between diet and disease is to compare people suffering from the disease with disease-free subjects who are matched for gender, ethnicity, age, lifestyle, and as many other factors as possible. Figure 6.3 shows the results of a series of such case–control studies that show that the serum concentration of β-carotene (Section 6.5.3.3) is significantly lower in people with a variety of cancers than in disease-free control subjects. Such data have been widely interpreted as suggesting that β-carotene has a protective effect against a variety of cancers; equally, it could be interpreted as suggesting that cancer affects carotene metabolism. Perhaps more importantly, the serum concentration of β-carotene reflects the consumption of fruits and

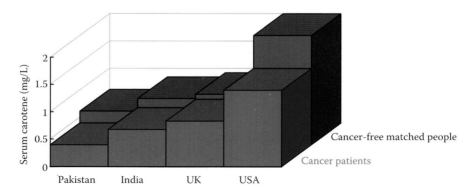

Figure 6.3 The relationship between plasma carotene and various cancers—case–control studies. (From data reported by Peto, R. et al., *Nature* 290: 201–8, 1981.)

vegetables that are rich in β-carotene (and other possibly protective compounds, Section 6.7), and β-carotene itself may be irrelevant. A diet that is rich in fruit and vegetables is likely to be relatively low in total and saturated fat (Section 6.3.2), and rich in NSPs (Sections 4.2.1.7 and 6.3.3.2).

An obvious problem here is that studies of nutritional status when people present with a disease do not give us any information about their diet at the time the disease was developing. Their diet may have changed over the years, and, of course, illness may affect what they eat now.

6.2.5 Prospective studies

The most useful epidemiological studies involve following a group of people over a long period, with assessment of their nutritional, health, and other status at the beginning of the study and at intervals thereafter. Probably the oldest such study is the UK National Survey of Health and Development, which has followed all 16,500 children born during the second week of March 1946; further cohorts were enrolled in 1970 and 2000. The Framingham Study has followed every resident of the town of Framingham, Massachusetts since 1948; the Nurses' Health Study in the United States is following some 85,000 nurses. In some such studies, blood and urine samples are stored, and diet and other records are available over a long period; thus, it is possible to measure markers of nutritional status that may not have been considered important or relevant at the start of the study.

Figure 6.4 shows the results of such a prospective study in which people were grouped according to their plasma concentration of β-carotene at the beginning of the study; those with the lowest initial concentration of serum β-carotene were more than twice as likely to die from lung cancer during the study period than those with the highest concentration. As with the case–control studies (Figure 6.3), this suggests a protective effect of β-carotene, but in this case, most of the subjects were presumably free from cancer at the beginning of the study; thus, there is not the confounding problem that the disease may have affected carotene metabolism rather than carotene affecting the chance of developing cancer. There is still the confounding problem that serum β-carotene simply reflects consumption of fruits and vegetables.

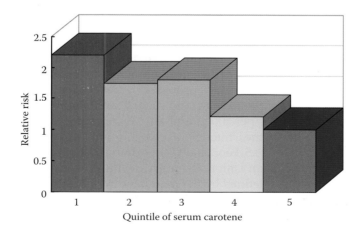

Figure 6.4 The relationship between plasma carotene and lung cancer—a prospective study. (From data reported by Peto, R. et al., *Nature* 290: 201–8, 1981.)

The European Prospective Investigation into Cancer and Nutrition (EPIC) is a multi-centre prospective study of more than half a million people in 10 European countries; to date there have been 26,000 cases of cancer and 16,000 deaths. The key findings (many of which are supported by other large prospective studies) are

- A high intake of NSPs (Section 4.2.1.7) appears to be protective against the development of colorectal polyps and their progression to cancer.
- The consumption of red meat and especially cured and processed meats increases the risk of developing colorectal cancer, whilst the consumption of fish reduces the risk.
- Alcohol consumption, obesity, and low physical activity also increase the risk of developing colorectal cancer.
- Overweight and low physical activity, together with endogenous hormones, increase the risk of developing breast cancer post-menopausally, but premenopausally, obesity is not associated with increased risk.
- There is no association between the intake of fruit and vegetables and the development of breast or prostate cancer.

6.3   Guidelines for a prudent diet

Diet is not the only factor in the development of chronic disease; many other factors, including heredity, multiple environmental factors, smoking, and exercise (or the lack of it) are also involved, as is metabolic programming in response to nutrition of the fetus *in utero* (Section 6.4.1). However, people can take decisions about diet, smoking, and exercise, whereas they can do little about the stresses of city life, environmental pollution, or the other problems of industrial society, and nothing, of course, to change their genetic makeup, which determines the extent to which they are at risk from environmental and nutritional factors (Section 6.4).

As a result of many large-scale epidemiological studies over the last half century, there is a general agreement amongst nutritionists and medical scientists about changes in the average Western diet that would be expected to reduce the prevalence of chronic disease (Table 6.2). The key changes are a reduction in the percentage of energy from fat from 40% to 30% or lower—and this reduction should be in saturated fat, not monounsaturated and polyunsaturated fats (Sections 4.3.1.1 and 6.3.2.1). The percentage of energy from carbohydrates should be increased from 42% to 55%; this should involve an increase in the consumption of starch and a reduction in the consumption of free sugars (non-milk intrinsic sugars, Section 4.2.1). These changes are summarised in Figure 6.5.

The problem is to get this 'prudent diet' message across to the public. Nutritional labelling of packaged and manufactured foods provides a great deal of information: the energy yield, fat (and saturated fat), carbohydrate (and sugars), and vitamin and mineral content, both as amount per serving, or per 100 g, and also as percentage of the reference intake (Section 11.1.1). Interestingly, in the United States, the nutrient yield must be shown per standardised serving (as defined by U.S. Food and Drug Administration) and may also be shown per 100 g, whilst in the European Union, the nutrients must be shown per 100 g and may also be shown per serving (as defined by the manufacturer). An unfortunate effect of this nutritional labelling of packaged foods is that some people seem to be unaware that fresh produce, which is not packaged and labelled, is also a source of nutrients.

Increasingly, in addition to nutritional labelling, manufacturers are being encouraged (and in some countries required) to have 'front of package' labelling that highlights the fat, saturated fat, sugar, and salt content of the food. This may take the form of a 'traffic light'

Table 6.2 Guidelines for a Prudent Diet

	% of energy
Total fat	15–30
Saturated fatty acids	<10
Polyunsaturated fatty acids	6–10
ω6 Polyunsaturated fatty acids	5–8
ω3 Polyunsaturated fatty acids	1–2
Trans-fatty acids	<1
Mono-unsaturated fatty acids	By difference
Total carbohydrate	55–75
Free sugars	<10
Protein	10–15
	Amount per day
Cholesterol	<300 mg
Sodium chloride	<5 g
Sodium	<2 g
Fruit and vegetables (excluding tubers such as potatoes, yams, and cassava)	>400 g
Dietary fibre[a]	>25 g
NSP[a]	>20 g

Source: Diet, Nutrition and the Prevention of Chronic Diseases, WHO Technical Report Series 916, WHO, Geneva 2003.

[a] This is the amount of fibre or NSP that would be provided by consuming the desirable amount of fruit and vegetables and whole grain cereals.

colour-coded label—green for low fat, saturated fat, sugar, and salt, amber for medium, and red for high. Alternatively, labels show the energy, fat, saturated fat, sugar, and salt content as the amount and as a percentage of the daily value—the amount called for by the prudent diet shown in Table 6.2, and assuming a 2000-kcal (8.4 MJ) daily energy intake. The most successful front of package labels use both schemes—traffic lights plus the amount and percentage of daily value.

Whilst such labelling helps the discriminating consumer to make healthy choices, it is relatively little help in converting the nutritional guidelines in Table 6.2 into foods. Early attempts in the 1950s and 1960s put foods into five, six, or seven groups, with the advice to eat something from each group each day. More recent public health advice shows the relative amounts of each group of foods that should be eaten. The food pyramid (Figure 6.6) has the starchy foods that should provide the main part of the diet at the base, with fruit and vegetables in the next row, then dairy produce, meat, and fish, with foods that should be

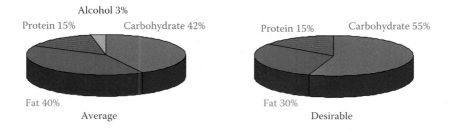

Figure 6.5 Average and desirable percentage of energy intake from different metabolic fuels.

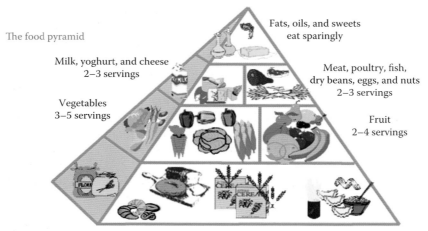

The food pyramid

Fats, oils, and sweets
eat sparingly

Milk, yoghurt, and cheese
2–3 servings

Meat, poultry, fish,
dry beans, eggs, and nuts
2–3 servings

Vegetables
3–5 servings

Fruit
2–4 servings

Bread, cereals, rice, and pasta 6–11 servings

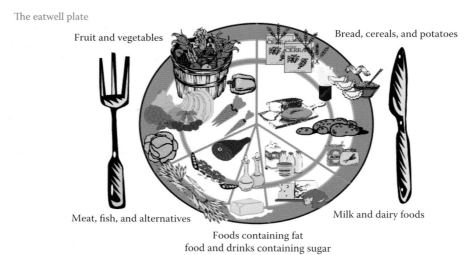

The eatwell plate

Fruit and vegetables

Bread, cereals, and potatoes

Meat, fish, and alternatives

Milk and dairy foods

Foods containing fat
food and drinks containing sugar

Choose my plate

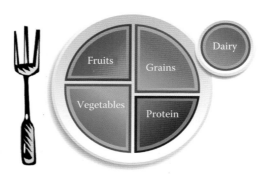

Fruits

Grains

Dairy

Vegetables

Protein

Figure 6.6 The public health message concerning a prudent diet. The food pyramid, the eatwell plate, and 'choose my plate'.

eaten sparingly (fats, oils, and sweets) at the apex. Apart from fats, oils, and sweets, there is a suggestion of how many servings of each group of foods should be consumed each day. The food pyramid has been criticised for the fact that the foods that should be eaten in least amount are shown at the top of the pyramid, implying to some people that they are the most important foods. In the UK, the Foods Standards Agency has developed the 'eatwell plate' (formerly called the balanced plate)—also shown in Figure 6.6. Here the five groups of foods (fruit and vegetables, bread, cereals, and potatoes, meat, fish, and alternatives, milk and dairy foods) and foods and drinks containing fat and sugar, are shown as sectors of the plate representing the relative amounts that should be eaten each day. Data from the UK Department of Environment, Food and Rural Affairs surveys of household purchases (which, of course, take no account of wastage) show that whilst purchases of meat, fish, and alternatives meet the guidelines, those of milk and dairy foods exceed the guidelines by 40%, and those of food and drink high in fat and sugar exceed the guidelines more than threefold. Purchases of starchy foods are only 60% of the guidelines and fruit and vegetables only 70%.

The United States has abandoned the food pyramid and now uses a simple four-sector plate for fruit, vegetables (half the plate is fruit and vegetables), grains (more than a quarter of the plate), and protein, with a separate container for dairy produce. There is no mention of fats, oils, and sugars that should be consumed in limited amounts and to have a sector labelled 'protein' (presumably to mean meat, fish, nuts, pulses, and eggs) ignores the fact that cereals, fruit, vegetables, and dairy products are all good sources of protein.

6.3.1   Energy intake

Obesity involves both an increased risk of premature death from a variety of causes and increased morbidity from conditions such as diabetes, varicose veins, and arthritis (Section 7.2.2). On the other hand, people who are significantly underweight are also at increased risk of illness as a result of undernutrition (see Chapter 8). For people whose body weight is within the desirable range, energy intake should be adequate to maintain a reasonably constant body weight, with an adequate amount of exercise. The benefits of exercise extend beyond weight control and energy balance, and include improved cardiovascular and respiratory function, muscle tone, and bone and joint health. The recommendation is to aim at 30 min of moderately vigorous exercise each day. Energy expenditure in physical activity and appropriate levels of energy intake are discussed in Section 5.1.3.

6.3.2   Fat intake

Dietary fat includes not only the obvious fat in the diet (the visible fat on meat, cooking oil, butter or margarine spread on bread), but also the hidden fat in foods. This latter may be either the fat naturally present in foods (e.g., the fat between the muscle fibres in meat, the oils in nuts, cereals, and vegetables) or fat used in cooking and manufacture of foods. There are two problems associated with a high intake of fat:

1. The energy yield of fat (37 kJ/g) is more than twice that of protein (16 kJ/g) or carbohydrate (17 kJ/g). This means that foods that are high in fat are also concentrated energy sources. It is easier to have an excessive energy intake on a high-fat diet, and hence a high-fat diet can be a factor in the development of obesity (Chapter 7).
2. There is epidemiological evidence that fat intake is correlated with premature death from a variety of conditions, including especially atherosclerosis and ischaemic heart disease, and some cancers.

Diets that provide about 30% of energy from fat are associated with the lowest risk of ischaemic heart disease. There is no evidence that a fat intake below about 30% of energy intake confers any additional benefit, although a very-low-fat diet is specifically recommended as part of treatment for severe (often genetic) hyperlipidaemia. The wide range of desirable fat intake in Table 6.2 reflects the fact that for people whose habitual fat intake is 15%–20% of energy (as in many developing countries), there is no evidence that increasing fat intake will confer any benefits, and it may well be detrimental.

6.3.2.1 The type of fat in the diet

Figure 6.7 shows the relationship between the plasma concentration of cholesterol and specifically cholesterol in plasma low-density lipoproteins (LDL, Section 5.6.2.2), and premature death from ischaemic heart disease. The main dietary factor affecting the plasma concentration of cholesterol is the intake of fat. As discussed in Section 5.6.2.1, this is because a high fat intake leads to a high concentration of chylomicrons, and then chylomicron remnants (which, like LDL, are atherogenic), in the circulation, with increased secretion of VLDL and its subsequent conversion to LDL.

Both the total intake of fat and more importantly the relative amounts of saturated and unsaturated fatty acids affect the concentration of LDL cholesterol. Figure 6.8 shows the results of a number of studies of the effects of different types of dietary fat on serum LDL cholesterol. In these studies, the effects of fats rich in saturated and polyunsaturated fatty acids were compared with a control diet containing an equivalent amount of mono-unsaturated fatty acids; thus, mono-unsaturated fatty acids appear to be neutral, but are clearly beneficial when they replace saturated fatty acids. LDL cholesterol:

- Increases by a factor related to 2× the intake of saturated fatty acids
- Decreases by a factor related to 1× the intake of polyunsaturated fatty acids
- Increases by a factor related to the square root of cholesterol intake

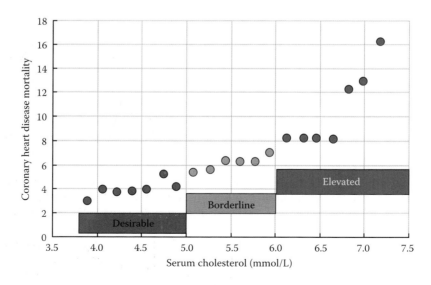

Figure 6.7 The relationship between serum cholesterol and coronary heart disease mortality. (From data reported by the Multiple Risk Factor Intervention Trial Research Group, *Journal of the American Medical Association* 248: 1465–75, 1982.)

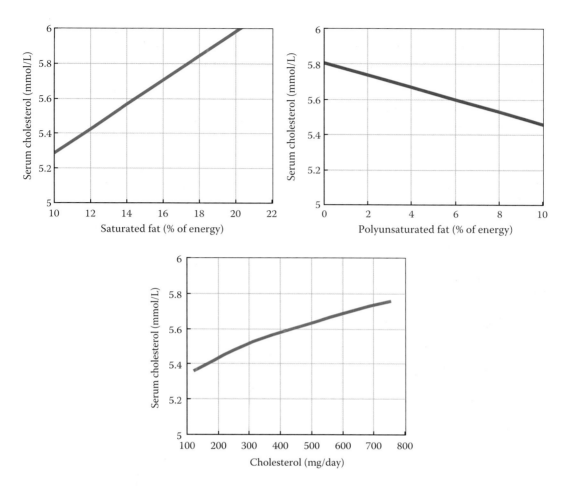

Figure 6.8 The effects of dietary saturated and polyunsaturated fatty acids (compared with mono-unsaturated fatty acids) and cholesterol on serum cholesterol. (From data reported by Keys, A. et al., *Metabolism* 14: 747–87, 1965.)

Monounsaturated and polyunsaturated fatty acids are good substrates for cholesterol esterification in cells, whilst saturated fatty acids are not. When saturated fatty acid levels are relatively high, less cholesterol is esterified in the liver; the intracellular concentration increases, repressing the synthesis of the LDL receptors. Not all saturated fatty acids have the same effect on LDL cholesterol. Myristic and palmitic acids have the greatest effect, since they down-regulate expression of the LDL receptor in the same way as does cholesterol (Section 5.6.2.2), whilst stearic (C18:0) has little effect because it is rapidly desaturated to oleic acid (Section 5.6.1.1).

Diets that are relatively rich in polyunsaturated fatty acids result in decreased synthesis of fatty acids in the liver (Section 5.6.1); this means that there is less export of lipids from the liver in very-low-density lipoproteins (Section 5.6.2.2), which are the precursors of LDL in the circulation. Polyunsaturated fatty acids (or their derivatives) act via nuclear receptors (Section 10.4) to reduce the transcription of the genes coding for acetyl CoA carboxylase and other key enzymes of fatty acid synthesis (Section 5.6.1).

In addition, the polyunsaturated fatty acids in fish oil (the ω3 series long-chain poly-unsaturated fatty acids, Section 4.3.1.1) have further protective effects. A number of studies have shown that consumption of one or two meals of oily fish per week is associated with a lower risk of cardiovascular disease. The Italian GISSI trial was a secondary prevention trial of fish oil supplements in people who had survived a myocardial infarction. After 3.5 years follow-up, there was a 20% reduction in total deaths and a 30% reduction in cardiovascular mortality. The main action of ω3 polyunsaturated fatty acids is to reduce the expression of adhesion molecules on blood platelets (so reducing the risk of blood clot formation) and on blood vessel endothelium (so reducing the adhesion of macrophages— a key step in the development of atherosclerosis). By contrast, ω6 polyunsaturated fatty acids (and especially linoleic acid) may increase the expression of adhesion molecules. The balance between ω3 and ω6 polyunsaturated fatty acids is important, and there is concern that increasing use of vegetable oils that are rich in ω6 polyunsaturated fatty acids leads to an excessively high ratio of ω6/ω3.

Epidemiological evidence suggests that a high intake of saturated fatty acids is associ-ated with impaired glucose tolerance, and the development of type II diabetes mellitus and the metabolic syndrome (Section 7.2.3). Intervention studies have shown an improve-ment in glucose tolerance and insulin sensitivity when saturated fatty acids are replaced by polyunsaturated fatty acids, although when total fat intake is more than about 37% of energy intake there is little effect.

Figure 6.9 shows the average proportions of energy from saturated, monounsaturated, and polyunsaturated fatty acids in the dietary fat in UK in the 1990s, and the desirable pro-portions. As a general rule, animal foods (meat, eggs, and milk products) are rich sources of saturated fatty acids, whilst oily fish and vegetables are rich sources of unsaturated fatty acids.

The recommendation is to reduce intake of saturated fats considerably more than just in proportion with the reduction in total fat intake. Total fat intake should be 30% of energy intake, with no more than 10% from saturated fats (compared with the average of

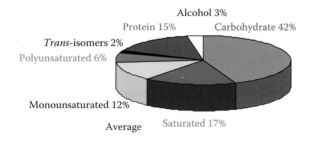

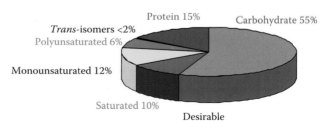

Figure 6.9 Average and desirable percentage of energy intake from different types of fat.

17% of energy from saturated fat). Average intakes of 6% of energy from polyunsaturated and 12% from monounsaturated fats match what is considered to be desirable, on the basis of epidemiological studies.

About 1%–2% of average energy intake is accounted for by the *trans*-isomers of unsaturated fatty acids (Section 4.3.1.1); ideally, they should not exceed 1%. *Trans*-fatty acids increase LDL, lower HDL, and have other effects on blood lipids that suggest an increased risk of cardiovascular disease. Meta-analysis of prospective studies involving 140,000 people suggests that a 2% increase in the proportion of energy coming from *trans*-fatty acid intake is associated with a 23% increase in coronary heart disease.

The main source of *trans*-fatty acids in the diet is from the hydrogenation of oils to produce solid fats that can be used in food manufacture, baking, and as spreads. The process involves catalytic cleavage of carbon–carbon double bonds in the fatty acids of the oil, followed by hydrogenation to form (saturated) single carbon–carbon bonds. However, some of the bonds cleaved do not undergo hydrogenation, but rather isomerise to the *trans*-form. Some food manufacturers have ceased to use hydrogenated oils, preferring instead to produce fats with suitable physicochemical properties by inter-esterification. This is a process that involves partial hydrolysis of triacylglycerols, liberating free fatty acids, followed by re-esterification under controlled conditions, to yield triacylglycerols containing the desired mixture of saturated and unsaturated fatty acids. The end product has similar physical (and hence industrial) properties to partially hydrogenated oil, but without the formation of *trans*-fatty acids. Because of the additional step of inter-esterification, the final product is, of course, more expensive.

Trans-fatty acids also occur naturally in fat from ruminants; they are synthesised by rumen bacteria and absorbed and incorporated into body fat by the animal. These seem not to be hazardous in the same way as *trans*-fatty acids formed by catalytic hydrogenation. This is probably because the main *trans*-fatty acid in ruminant fat, vaccenic acid (C18:1 *trans* ω6), is readily isomerised to conjugated linolenic acid, in which the carbon–carbon double bonds alternate with single bonds, as opposed to being separated from each other by a methylene bridge. There is some evidence of beneficial effects of conjugated linolenic acid.

6.3.3   Carbohydrate intake

If the total energy intake is to remain constant, as it should for people who are not overweight, and the proportion derived from fat is to be reduced from 40% to 30%, then the proportion derived from another metabolic fuel must be increased. It is not considered desirable to increase the proportion derived from protein above 15% of energy intake, and there is some evidence that excessively high protein intakes (greater than about 20% of energy), are associated with long-term adverse effects. This means that the proportion of energy derived from carbohydrates should increase, from 45% of energy to 55%. This should be achieved by increasing intake of starches, not sugars (Figure 6.10).

Although an intake of only 1%–2% of energy as carbohydrate is adequate to prevent ketosis (Section 5.5.3), all the available evidence is that about 55% of energy from carbohydrate is associated with optimum health. For athletes and other people with a high level of physical activity, the general consensus is that 60% of energy should come from carbohydrate, with 30% or less from fat and 10%–15% from protein.

Some early recommendations led to an increase in protein intake for people with high physical activity. However, this was not a reflection of an increased requirement for protein with increased physical activity, but rather the result of assuming that if the (then)

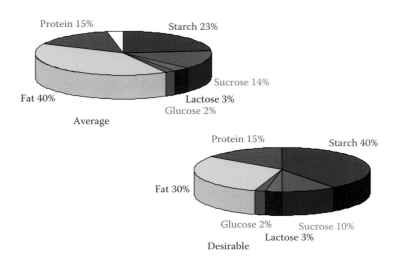

Figure 6.10 Average and desirable percentage of energy intake from different types of carbohydrate.

average protein intake was 10% of energy, people with a high energy requirement would eat more of the same foods and therefore have a higher protein intake. It was an assumed intake, not a requirement or recommendation.

6.3.3.1 Sugars in the diet

Average intakes of sugars (and especially sucrose) are generally considered to be higher than is desirable. The adverse effects of an excessive intake of sugars include

- Dental decay. Although many sugars in free solution (extrinsic sugars, Section 4.2.1) will promote the growth of oral bacteria that produce acids and cause dental decay, sucrose specifically promotes the growth of plaque-forming oral bacteria.
- Obesity. Sugars added to foods are mainly sucrose, but also increasingly high-fructose corn syrups. They increase the energy yield of the food, and increase the pleasure of eating (Section 1.4.3), so that it is relatively easy to consume an excessive amount. In addition, as discussed in Sections 5.4.1 and 10.2.2, the fructose derived from sucrose enters the pathway of glycolysis after the main regulatory point, and results in excessive synthesis of fatty acids. Under most conditions, there is little *de novo* lipogenesis from glucose because of the strict metabolic regulation of glycolysis (Section 10.2.2). When carbohydrate intake is high, it remains the preferred fuel for muscle for longer, so that there is less utilisation of triacylglycerol from adipose tissue reserves or the diet. This means that excessive carbohydrate intake can indeed lead to obesity. More importantly, the fructose derived from sucrose, and that in high-fructose corn syrups, bypasses the main regulatory step of glycolysis (Section 10.2.2), leading to production of acetyl CoA in excess of requirements for energy-yielding metabolism. The only metabolic fate for this excess acetyl CoA is synthesis of fatty acids and then triacylglycerol (Section 5.6.1). In addition, fructose does not stimulate the secretion of insulin or leptin (Section 1.4.2), nor does it suppress the secretion of ghrelin (Section 1.4.1.2); thus, it does not suppress appetite in the same way as do glucose and galactose.
- Diabetes mellitus. Sugars and other carbohydrates with a high glycaemic index (Section 4.2.1.1) lead to a higher post-prandial insulin response, which results in

increased lipogenesis and secretion of very-low-density lipoprotein from the liver (Sections 5.6.1 and 5.6.2.2). This has been associated with the development of insulin resistance and type II (non-insulin-dependent) diabetes (Sections 7.2.3 and 10.7). There is a genetic predisposition to type II diabetes, and it is difficult to determine the relative importance of heredity and sucrose consumption or the effects of sucrose *per se* and obesity.

- Atherosclerosis and coronary heart disease. There is some evidence that a high consumption of sucrose is a factor in the development of atherosclerosis and coronary heart disease, although the evidence is less convincing than that for the effects of a high (saturated) fat intake.

It is considered desirable that sucrose should provide no more than 10% of energy (compared with the current average >14%). Intakes of other sugars (mainly glucose and fructose in fruits and lactose from milk) are considered to be appropriate. However, the increasing use of high-fructose corn syrups in food and drink manufacture is a cause for concern. Corn syrup is a solution of glucose prepared by hydrolysis of maize (corn) starch that is widely used in food and beverage manufacture. Fructose is sweeter than sucrose, whilst glucose is less sweet. Isomerisation of much of the glucose to fructose increases the sweetness considerably and thus permits use of less total carbohydrate. However, as noted above, fructose enters the pathway of glycolysis after the main regulatory point (Sections 5.4.1 and 10.2.2) and results in excessive synthesis of fatty acids. The use of high-fructose corn syrups is considered to be a contributory factor in the 'epidemic' of obesity.

6.3.3.2 Undigested carbohydrates (dietary fibre and NSPs)

The residue of plant cell walls is not digested by human enzymes but provides bulk in the diet (and hence in the intestines). It is measured by weighing the fraction of foods that remains after treatment with a variety of digestive enzymes. This is what is known as dietary fibre. It is a misleading term, since not all the components of dietary fibre are fibrous; some are soluble and form viscous gels.

A more precise analytical method permits measurement of the specific polysaccharides other than starch (Section 4.2.1.7) that are the main constituents of dietary fibre; the results of such analysis are quoted as NSPs.

The two methods of analysis give different results. Measurement of NSPs in the diet gives average intakes in Britain of between 11 and 13 g/day, compared with an intake of dietary fibre of about 20 g/day, as measured by the less specific method. The difference is because dietary fibre includes lignans and other components of plant cell walls that are not carbohydrates, and are therefore not measured as NSP. NSPs (and dietary fibre) are found only in foods of vegetable origin, and vegetarians have a higher intake than omnivores.

NSPs have relatively little nutritional value in their own right, since they are compounds that are not digested or absorbed to any significant extent. Nevertheless, they are a valuable component of the diet, and some of the products of fermentation by colonic bacteria can be absorbed and utilised as metabolic fuel. Starch that is (relatively) resistant to digestion in the small intestine (Section 4.2.2.1) is a also substrate for bacterial fermentation. Non-glycaemic carbohydrates have an energy yield of 4–8 kJ/g, depending on the extent of bacterial fermentation and the extent to which the products of fermentation are absorbed.

The main products of bacterial fermentation of NSPs and resistant starch are short-chain fatty acids such as propionate and butyrate. These provide a major metabolic fuel for colon enterocytes and have an antiproliferative effect on tumour cells in culture. As noted in Section 6.2.5, there is epidemiological evidence that NSPs provide protection against the development of colorectal cancer.

Most NSPs, and especially fructose-containing oligosaccharides, have a probiotic action, promoting the growth of *Bifidobacterium* spp. that contribute to resistance of the gastrointestinal tract to colonisation by pathogenic bacteria. One of the major benefits of breast-feeding infants, compared with feeding cows' milk infant formula, is the presence of a relatively large amount of probiotic oligosaccharides in human milk, which encourages the development of a desirable intestinal microflora.

Diets low in NSPs are associated with the excretion of a small bulk of faeces, constipation, and straining whilst defecating. This has been linked with the development of haemorrhoids, varicose veins, and diverticular disease of the colon. These diseases are commoner in Western countries where people generally have a relatively low intake of NSP than in parts of the world where the intake is higher.

A number of compounds that are believed to be involved in causing or promoting cancer of the colon occur in the contents of the intestinal tract, either because they are present in foods or as a result of bacterial metabolism. They are adsorbed by cellulose and other NSPs, and so cannot interact with the cells of the gut wall but are eliminated in the faeces, thus providing protection against potential carcinogens.

Although epidemiological studies show that diets high in NSPs are associated with a low risk of colon cancer, such diets also provide relatively large amounts of fruit and vegetables and are therefore rich in vitamins C and E and carotene as well as other compounds that may have protective effects against the development of cancers. Furthermore, because they provide more fruit and vegetables and less meat, such diets are also relatively low in saturated fats, and there is evidence that a high intake of saturated fats and red and processed meat is a separate risk factor for colon cancer.

The bile salts required for the absorption of dietary fat are synthesised in the liver from cholesterol (Section 4.3.2.1). Normally about 90%–95% of the 30 g of bile salts secreted daily is reabsorbed and reutilised. NSPs adsorb bile salts; thus, they are excreted in the faeces. This means that there has to be increased synthesis *de novo* from cholesterol to replace the lost bile salts, thus reducing the total body content of cholesterol.

A total intake of about 20 g of NSPs/day is recommended (equivalent to about 25 g/day of dietary fibre). In general, this should come from fibre-rich foods—whole grain cereals and wholemeal cereal products, fruits, and vegetables—rather than supplements. This is because as well as the NSPs, these foods are valuable sources of a variety of nutrients and potentially beneficial non-nutrient compounds (Section 6.7). There is no evidence that intakes of NSPs over about 20 g/day confer any benefit, other than in the treatment of established bowel disease. Above this level of intake, it is likely that people would reach satiety (or at least feel full, or even bloated) without eating enough food to satisfy energy needs. This may be a problem for children fed on a diet that is very high in fibre—they may be physically full but still physiologically hungry.

6.3.4   Salt

There is a physiological requirement for the mineral sodium, and salt (sodium chloride) is the main dietary source of sodium. One of the basic senses of taste is for saltiness—a pleasant sensation (Section 1.4.3.1). However, average intakes of salt in Western countries are considerably higher than the physiological requirement for sodium. Most people are apparently able to cope with this excessive intake adequately by excreting the excess, but people with a genetic predisposition to develop high blood pressure are sensitive to the amount of sodium in their diet. About 10% of the population are salt sensitive, and there is a relationship between sodium intake and the increase in blood pressure that occurs with increasing age. As shown in Table 6.2, salt intake should not exceed 5 g/day (or 2 g of sodium). Obesity (Chapter 7) and alcohol (Section 6.3.5) probably have a greater effect on blood pressure than does salt intake. Nevertheless, reduction of salt intake is a major goal of public health nutrition.

6.3.5   Alcohol

A high intake of alcoholic drinks can be a factor in causing obesity, both as a result of the energy yield of the alcohol itself and also because of the relatively high carbohydrate content of many alcoholic beverages. People who satisfy much of their energy requirement from alcohol frequently show vitamin deficiencies because they are meeting their energy needs from drink and therefore not eating enough foods to provide adequate amounts of vitamins and minerals. Deficiency of vitamin B_1 (Section 11.6.3) is a problem amongst heavy drinkers, at least partly because alcohol inhibits the absorption of the vitamin.

In moderate amounts, alcohol has an appetite-stimulating effect and may also help the social aspect of meals. Furthermore, there is good epidemiological evidence that modest consumption of alcohol is protective against atherosclerosis and coronary heart disease. However, alcohol has harmful effects in excess, not only in the short term, when drunkenness may have undesirable consequences, but also in the longer term.

Figure 6.11 shows the relationship between alcohol consumption and mortality from various causes—it is a classical 'J-shaped' curve, with a protective effect of modest consumption compared with abstinence, but a sharp increase in mortality with excessive consumption.

Opinions differ as to whether the protective effect of modest alcohol consumption is due to the alcohol itself or some other constituent of alcoholic beverages. Figure 6.12 shows that there are differences between the effects of wine, beer, and spirits, regardless of the amount of alcohol consumed. Some studies have shown the same protective of red wine and de-alcoholised wine, suggesting that alcohol is not the protective factor; the various polyphenols in red wine may well have an antioxidant action (Section 6.7.2.3).

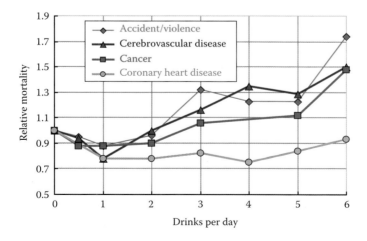

Figure 6.11 The effects of habitual alcohol consumption on mortality from various causes. (From data reported by Boffetta, P., Garfinkel, L., *Epidemiology* 1: 342–8, 1990.)

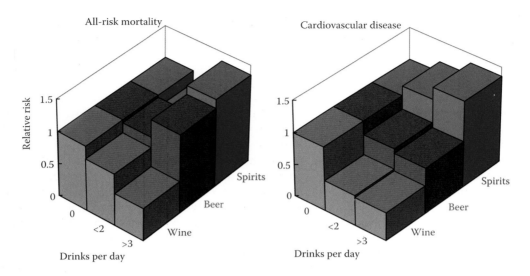

Figure 6.12 The effects of different alcoholic beverages on mortality. (From data reported by Grøbbæk, M. et al., *British Medical Journal* 310: 1165–9, 1995.)

One problem in interpreting the data on alcohol consumption is that those who consume no alcohol will include not only those who for religious or other reasons choose to abstain from alcohol but also those whose health has already been damaged by excessive consumption.

Habitual excess consumption of alcohol is associated with long-term health problems, including loss of mental capacity, liver damage, cancer of the oesophagus, and hypertension. Continued abuse can lead to physical and psychological addiction. The infants of mothers who drink more than a very small amount of alcohol during pregnancy are at risk of congenital abnormalities, and heavy alcohol consumption during pregnancy can result in the fetal alcohol syndrome—low birth weight and lasting impairment of intelligence as well as congenital deformities.

The guidelines on alcohol intake are summarised in Table 6.3, and the alcohol content of beverages in Table 6.4. The difference between the daily and weekly prudent upper limits

Table 6.3 Prudent Upper Limits of Alcohol Consumption

Royal College of Physicians	
Men	21 units (= 168 g alcohol)/week
Women	14 units (= 112 g alcohol)/week
UK Department of Health	
Men	4 units (= 32 g alcohol)/day
Women	3 units (= 24 g alcohol)/day

Table 6.4 Amounts of Beverages Providing 1 Unit of Alcohol

8 g absolute alcohol
1/2 pint of beer (300 mL)
1 glass of wine (100 mL)
Single measure of spirits (25 mL)

of alcohol consumption reflects the greater danger of binge drinking (the whole week's intake in one evening) compared with more modest consumption through the week.

6.4 Nutritional genomics: interactions between diet and genes

The discipline of nutrigenetics is the study of the effects of genotype on nutrient requirements and hence how genetics is involved in the effects of diet on health. The discipline of nutrigenomics is the study of how nutrients interact with genes and the nutritional control of gene expression.

Although diet and other environmental factors are important in the aetiology of chronic diseases, genetics is an important factor in both cancer and cardiovascular disease. In many cases, the genetic factor influences the extent to which an individual is sensitive to the long-term health effects of the diet; there is a considerable interaction between genes and diet. The long-term aim of nutritional genomic research is to identify which people are likely to be susceptible to the adverse effects of, for example, saturated fat intake and which are not, and so to be able to develop individualised nutritional advice.

When a variant of a gene is found relatively widespread in the population, it is known as a genetic polymorphism (as opposed to rare variants or mutations that are the cause of classical inborn errors of metabolism affecting only a very small number of people). A number of genetic polymorphisms affect the extent to which different metabolic and nutritional insults affect health:

- About 10% of the population are sensitive to the hypertensive effect of excessive salt intake (Section 6.3.4).
- About 10% of the population are genetically at risk of iron overload (Sections 4.5.3.1 and 11.15.2.3) as a result of polymorphisms in the HFE gene (responsible for detecting iron status), hepcidin, or the transferrin receptor.
- Polymorphisms of various apo-proteins of the plasma lipoproteins, and of LDL receptor and cholesterol ester transfer protein account for much of the variance in atherosclerosis (Section 5.6.2).
- Polymorphisms of the insulin receptor substrate (Section 10.7) explain much of the inherited susceptibility to type II diabetes mellitus.
- Polymorphisms of the vitamin D receptor explain much of the susceptibility to osteoporosis (Section 11.3.3).
- Polymorphisms of methylene tetrahydrofolate reductase are associated with elevated blood homocysteine and a higher than normal requirement for folic acid, a factor in neural tube defects and cardiovascular disease (Sections 6.6.1.1 and 11.11).
- A number of polymorphisms occur in the untranscribed regions of genes, affecting the extent of gene expression rather than the activity of the protein product.

6.4.1 Epigenetic modifications—the fetal origins of adult disease

Unlike polymorphisms, which are inherited, epigenetic modifications are changes to the genome that do not involve changes to the base sequence of DNA (Section 9.2.1), but methylation of cytosine residues that results in changes in the extent to which a gene is expressed. This is part of the normal process of cell and tissue differentiation in development, the silencing of some genes and switching on of others.

The first clue that nutrition *in utero* may affect health in later life came from studies conducted by Barker and coworkers during the late 20th century, and the theory of the fetal origins of adult disease is also known as the Barker hypothesis. They had detailed records of the birth weights and lengths of infants born in rural Hertfordshire during the early 20th century and were able to trace and follow up many of these people in late middle age. The key finding was that moderately low birth weight (at the lower end of the normal range) is associated with a greater risk of obesity, diabetes mellitus, and the metabolic syndrome (Section 7.2.3) in later life. Modest undernutrition *in utero*, leading to relatively low birth weight, leads to metabolic changes—adaptation to low energy and nutrient availability by increasing metabolic efficiency. These metabolic changes are imprinted in the genome by changes in DNA methylation; the individual has a persistently thrifty phenotype and high metabolic efficiency. The consequence of this is that the affected person gains weight readily, and develops obesity and the associated metabolic consequences in later life if adequate food is available.

6.5   Free radicals, oxidative damage, and antioxidant nutrients

Early epidemiological studies of vitamin E and cardiovascular disease (Figure 6.2) and of β-carotene and various cancers (Figures 6.3 and 6.4) led to a hypothesis that one of the factors in the aetiology of cardiovascular disease, cancer, autoimmune diseases, and some neurodegenerative diseases, is that the initiating factor is tissue damage (to lipids, proteins, or DNA) caused by free radicals. The apparent protective effects of vitamin E and β-carotene suggested that compounds that can quench free radicals may be protective. The main tissue damaging radicals are oxygen radicals (sometimes known as reactive oxygen species), and it is usual to talk of oxidative damage as a result of radical action and to consider protective compounds to be antioxidants.

Free radicals are highly reactive, unstable, molecular species that have an unpaired electron in the outermost shell. They exist for only an extremely short time, of the order of nanoseconds (10^{-9} s) or less, before they react with another molecule, either gaining or losing a single electron, to achieve a stable configuration. However, this in turn generates another radical; thus, radical reactions are self-perpetuating. To show that a compound is a free radical, its chemical formula is shown with a dot (•) to represent the unpaired electron. For example, the hydroxyl radical is $•OH$, superoxide is $•O_2^-$, and nitric oxide is $NO•$.

If two radicals react together, each contributes its unpaired electron to the formation of a new, stable configuration. This means that the chain reaction, in which reaction of radicals with other molecules generates new radicals, is quenched. Because radicals are short-lived and present in low concentrations in cells, it is rare for two radicals to react together in this way.

Some radicals are relatively stable. This applies especially to those that have aromatic rings or conjugated double-bond systems. An unpaired electron can be delocalised through such a system of double bonds, and the resultant radical is less reactive and longer lived than most radicals. Compounds that are capable of forming stable radicals are important in quenching radical chain reactions. Vitamins C (Sections 6.5.3.4 and 11.14) and E (Sections 6.5.3.5 and 11.4) and β-carotene (Section 6.5.3.3) form stable radicals and are generally regarded as having a protective antioxidant action.

6.5.1   Tissue damage by oxygen radicals

Radicals may interact with any compounds present in the cell, and the result may be initiation of cancer, heritable mutations, atherosclerosis, and coronary heart disease or

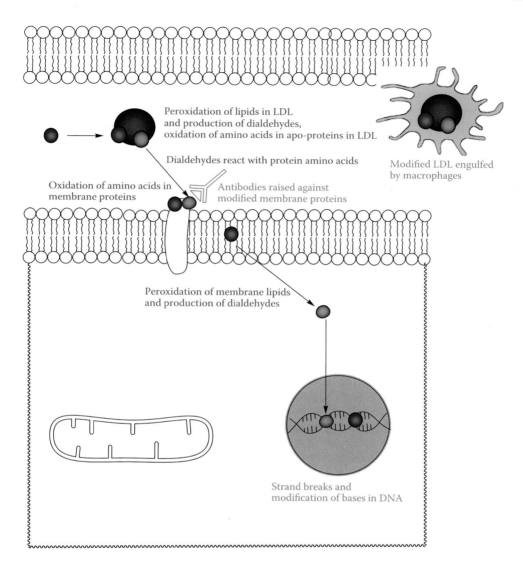

Figure 6.13 Tissue damage caused by oxygen radicals.

autoimmune disease. As shown in Figure 6.13, the most important, and potentially damaging, actions of free radicals are

1. With DNA in the nucleus (Section 9.2.1), causing chemical changes to the nucleic acid bases or breaks in the DNA strand. This damage may result in heritable mutations if the damage is to ovaries or testes or the induction of cancer in other tissues. Whilst much damage to DNA is detected and repaired by the DNA repair system in cells, some will escape detection.
2. With individual amino acids in proteins. This results in a chemical modification of the protein, which may therefore be recognised as foreign by the immune system, leading to the production of antibodies against the modified protein that will also

react with the normal, unmodified body protein. This can be a cause of autoimmune disease. Some modified amino acids (e.g. dihydroxyphenylalanine) are capable of undergoing non-enzymic redox cycling, resulting in the production of more oxygen radicals.

3. With unsaturated fatty acids in cell membranes. This leads to the formation of dialdehydes, which react with DNA, causing chemical modification, and hence may result in either heritable mutations or initiation of cancer. Dialdehydes can also react with amino acids in proteins, leading to modified proteins that stimulate the production of auto-antibodies.

4. With unsaturated fatty acids or amino acids in plasma lipoproteins (Section 5.6.2). Oxidised low-density lipoprotein is not recognised by the LDL receptors in the liver, but is taken up by scavenger receptors in macrophages. Macrophage uptake of LDL is unregulated, and the cells become engorged with lipid. These lipid-rich macrophages (called foam cells because of their microscopic appearance) then infiltrate the epithelium of blood vessel walls, leading to the development of fatty streaks, and eventually atherosclerosis.

6.5.2 Sources of oxygen radicals

As shown in Figure 6.14, ionising radiation such as X-rays, the radiation from radioactive isotopes and ultraviolet from sunlight cause lysis of water to yield hydroxyl radicals. In addition, oxygen radicals arise in the body in four main ways:

6.5.2.1 Reoxidation of reduced flavins

The reoxidation of reduced flavin coenzymes (Sections 2.4.1.2 and 3.3.1.2) involves formation of a number of radicals as transient intermediates, although the final products are not radicals. Because radicals are unpredictable, some always escape from the normal reaction sequence. Overall, some 3%–5% of the 30 mol of oxygen consumed by an adult each day is converted to oxygen radicals rather than undergoing complete reduction to water in the mitochondrial electron transport chain (Section 3.3.1.2). There is thus a total daily formation of some 1.5 mol of reactive oxygen species that are potentially able to cause damage to tissues.

6.5.2.2 The macrophage respiratory burst

Macrophages provide an important protection against invading micro-organisms, which they engulf, kill, and digest. The cytotoxic action of macrophages is due to production of halogen and oxygen radicals. This means that even a mild infection can lead to a considerable increase in the total radical burden in the body, which can be detected by an increase in the products of lipid peroxidation in the bloodstream. Radical damage to cell membranes may be an important factor in the aetiology of the protein-energy deficiency disease kwashiorkor (Section 8.5.1); infection is a common precipitating factor in under-nourished children.

Stimulation of macrophages leads to a considerable increase in the consumption of glucose (the respiratory burst), which is metabolised by the pentose phosphate pathway (Section 5.4.2), leading to increased production of NADPH. The respiratory burst oxidase (NADPH oxidase) is a flavoprotein that transfers electrons from NADPH onto cytochrome b_{558}, which then reduces oxygen to superoxide. The reaction is
$$NADPH + 2\,O_2 \rightarrow NADP^+ + 2\,{}^{\bullet}O_2^- + 2H^+.$$

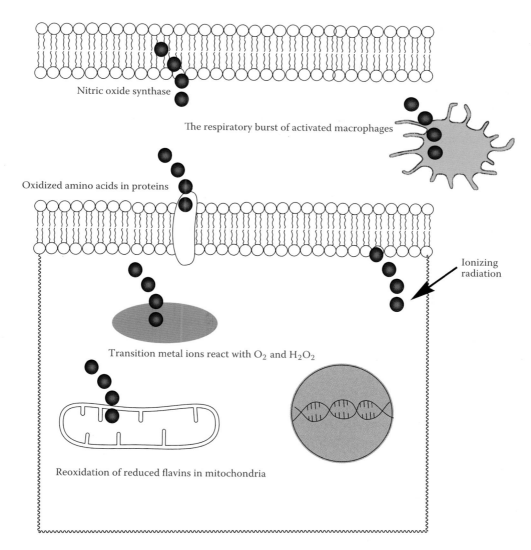

Figure 6.14 Sources of oxygen radicals.

The respiratory burst oxidase is a trans-membrane multi-enzyme complex that is activated in response to

- Complement fragment C_{5a}, which arises from the antibody–antigen reaction
- Peptides containing N-formyl-Met-Leu-Phe, which may be bacterial or arise from the mitochondria of damaged tissue
- Cytokines and other signalling molecules released in response to infection, including platelet activating factor, leukotrienes, and interleukins

6.5.2.3   Formation of nitric oxide

Production of nitric oxide ($NO^\bullet$), by hydroxylation of arginine, is a part of normal cell signalling. In addition to being a radical, and hence potentially damaging in its own right, nitric oxide can react with superoxide to form peroxynitrite, which in turn decays to yield the more damaging hydroxyl radical. Nitric oxide was first discovered as the endothelium-derived relaxation factor, and this loss of nitric oxide by reaction with superoxide may be an important factor in the development of hypertension.

6.5.2.4 *Non-enzymic formation of radicals*

A variety of transition metal ions react with oxygen or hydrogen peroxide in solution generating hydroxyl radicals: $M^{n+} + H_2O_2 \rightarrow M^{(n+1)+} + {}^\bullet OH + OH^-$. Physiologically important ions include iron, copper, cobalt, and nickel.

Metal ions are not normally present in free solution to any significant extent but are bound to transport proteins (in plasma) or storage proteins and enzymes (in cells). Thus, iron is bound to transferrin (in plasma) and haemosiderin and ferritin in tissues, copper is bound to ceruloplasmin in plasma, and metallothionein in plasma binds a wide variety of metal ions. The adverse effects of iron overload (Sections 4.5.3.1 and 11.15.2.3) are the result of free iron ions, not bound to storage proteins, undergoing non-enzymic reactions to produce oxygen radicals.

6.5.3 *Antioxidant nutrients and non-nutrients— protection against radical damage*

Apart from avoidance of exposure to ionising radiation, there is little that can be done to prevent the formation of radicals, since they are the result of normal metabolic processes and responses to infection. There are, however, a number of mechanisms to minimise the damage done by radical action. Since the important radicals are oxygen radicals, and the damage done is oxidative damage, the protective compounds are known collectively as antioxidants.

Compounds such as vitamins C and E, β-carotene, and ubiquinone (Section 3.3.1.2) are radical trapping antioxidants. Vitamin E can form the stable tocopheroxyl radical by reaction with the lipid peroxides formed by interaction with oxygen radicals with unsaturated fatty acids in cell membranes and plasma lipoproteins. As shown in Figure 6.15, the tocopheroxyl radical is relatively stable because of resonance isomerism—the lone electron can be at any one of three positions in the molecule. The tocopheroxyl radical persists long enough in the lipid phase of the cell membrane or plasma lipoprotein to interact with ascorbate (vitamin C) in the plasma or cytosol. It is reduced back to tocopherol, at the expense of vitamin C being oxidised to monodehydroascorbate. Monodehydroascorbate is also stable and persists long enough to undergo enzymic reduction back to ascorbate or a non-enzymic reaction between 2 mol of monodehydroascorbate to yield ascorbate and dehydroascorbate. Dehydroascorbate may either be reduced to ascorbate or undergo non-enzymic reaction to diketogulonate, which enters pathways of carbohydrate metabolism (Figure 6.16).

6.5.3.1 *Superoxide dismutase, peroxidases, and catalase*

Superoxide is a substrate for the enzyme superoxide dismutase, which catalyses the reaction

$$ {}^\bullet O_2^- + H_2O \rightarrow O_2 + H_2O_2. $$

In turn, hydrogen peroxide is removed by catalase and a variety of peroxidases:

$$ 2\,H_2O_2 \rightarrow 2\,H_2O + O_2. $$

As a further protection, many of the reactions in the cell that generate superoxide or hydrogen peroxide occur in the peroxisomes—intracellular organelles that also contain superoxide dismutase, catalase and peroxidases.

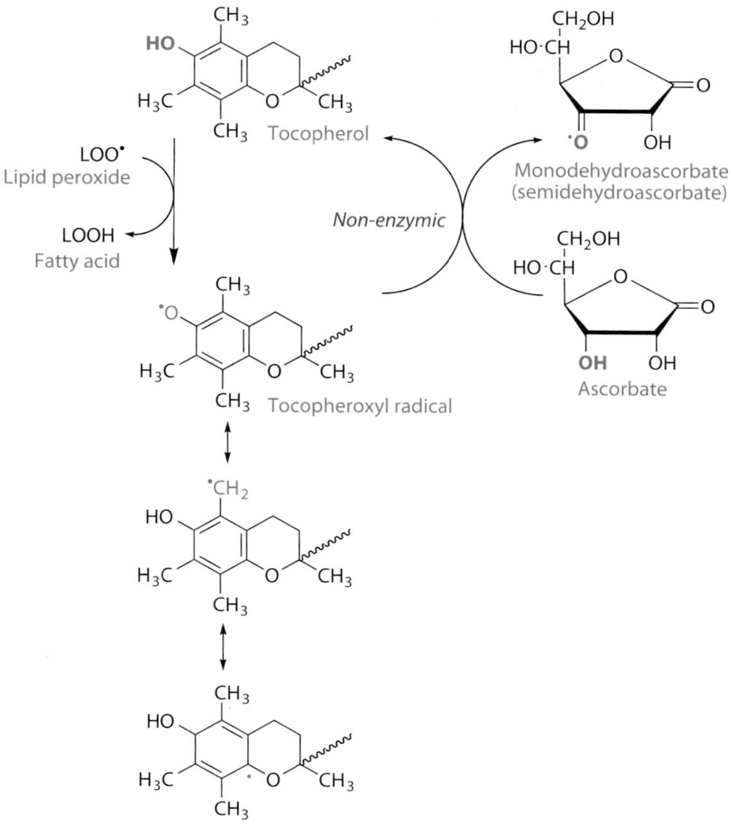

Figure 6.15 The antioxidant role of vitamin E and resonance stabilisation of the tocopheroxyl radical.

6.5.3.2 *Glutathione peroxidase*

Lipid peroxides formed by radical action on unsaturated fatty acids in membranes and low-density lipoprotein can be reduced to unreactive alcohols, and hydrogen peroxide can be reduced to water, by the enzyme glutathione peroxidase. The reaction involves the oxidation of the tripeptide glutathione (γ-glutamyl-cysteinyl-glycine, GSH) to the disulphide-linked GSSG. In turn, oxidised glutathione is reduced back to the active peptide by glutathione reductase (Figure 5.15).

Glutathione reductase has selenium at the catalytic site, as a selenocysteine residue (Section 11.15.2.5). This explains the role of selenium as an antioxidant nutrient; in selenium deficiency there is impaired activity of glutathione peroxidase, although once requirements have been met there is no increase in glutathione reductase activity or antioxidant protection with increased intakes of selenium. Glutathione reductase is a flavoprotein and is especially sensitive to riboflavin (vitamin B_2) depletion; measurement of glutathione reductase activation by its coenzyme added *in vitro* is a method of assessing riboflavin status (Sections 2.7.3 and 11.7).

6.5.3.3 *β-Carotene and other carotenes*

The epidemiological evidence (e.g., Figures 6.3 and 6.4) shows that high blood levels of β-carotene are associated with low incidence of a variety of cancers, and suggests that

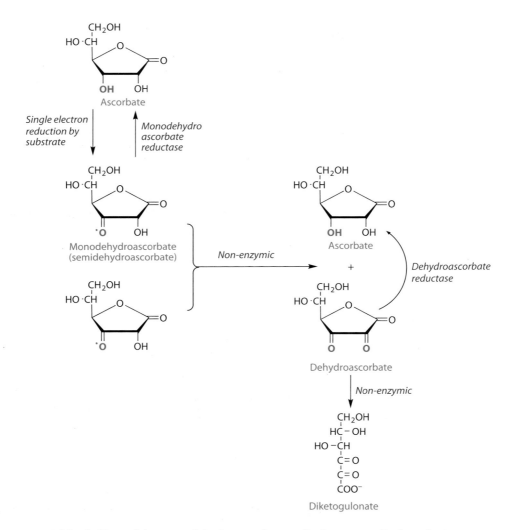

Figure 6.16 Metabolism of the monodehydroascorbate radical to non-radical products.

β-carotene may be protective, although the plasma concentration of β-carotene simply reflects the intake of fruit and vegetables. As shown in Figure 6.17, β-carotene (and other carotenes) can form a stable radical because the lone electron can be delocalised throughout the conjugated carbon–carbon double bond system.

There have been two large intervention trials with β-carotene to protect against lung cancer. The α-tocopherol β-carotene (ATBC) was conducted in Finland with a large group of smokers, who were given supplements of β-carotene, α-tocopherol (vitamin E), both, or neither. The results were reported in 1994. The vitamin E arm of the study showed no effect. The β-carotene intervention gave the opposite result to what was expected. More of those people taking the β-carotene supplements died from lung cancer than those taking placebo (Figure 6.18). There were also more deaths from bladder and gastric cancer, but fewer from other cancers, amongst those taking the supplements.

The second trial, the Carotene and Retinol Efficacy Trial (CARET), used both β-carotene and preformed vitamin A in two groups of people at risk of developing lung

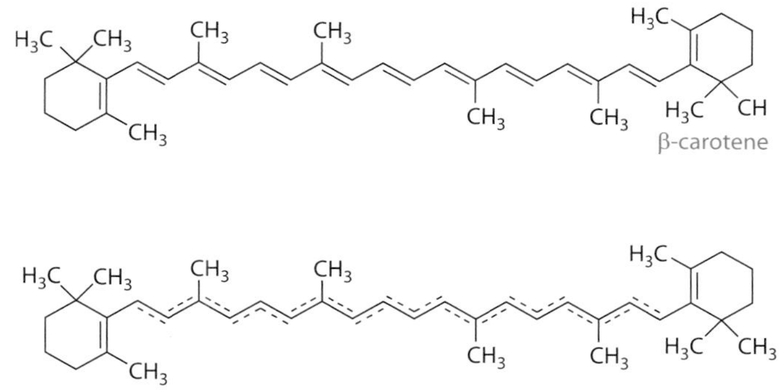

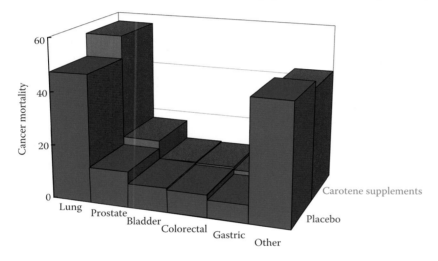

Figure 6.17 The delocalisation of a lone electron in the conjugated double-bond system of β-carotene.

Figure 6.18 The effects of β-carotene supplementation on death from lung and other cancers. (From data reported by the Alpha-Tocopherol Beta-Carotene Cancer Prevention Study Group, *New England Journal of Medicine* 330: 1029–35, 1994.)

cancer—smokers and people exposed to industrial asbestos dust. This trial was started in 1993 and was terminated prematurely in 1996 because of a 46% excess mortality from lung cancer amongst those taking the supplements.

Although β-carotene has a radical-trapping antioxidant action at low partial pressures of oxygen (as are found in most tissues), at higher partial pressures of oxygen (for example, in the lungs), it loses its antioxidant action and, especially at high concentrations, becomes an autocatalytic pro-oxidant. Following these two intervention trials of β-carotene in smokers, the UK Food Standards Agency has specifically recommended that smokers should not take carotene supplements.

6.5.3.4   *Vitamin C—an antioxidant and a pro-oxidant*

As shown in Figure 6.15, vitamin C can act at the surface of cells or lipoproteins to reduce the tocopheroxyl radical back to tocopherol, forming the stable monodehydroascorbate radical. It can also react with superoxide and hydroxyl radicals:

$$\text{Ascorbate} + {}^{\bullet}\text{O}_2^- + \text{H}^+ \rightarrow \text{H}_2\text{O}_2 + \text{monodehydroascorbate}$$

$$\text{Ascorbate} + {}^{\bullet}\text{OH} + \text{H}^+ \rightarrow \text{H}_2\text{O} + \text{monodehydroascorbate.}$$

The resultant monodehydroascorbate can then undergo enzymic reduction back to ascorbate, or a non-enzymic reaction between 2 mol of monodehydroascorbate to yield ascorbate and dehydroascorbate (Figure 6.16). Although ascorbate has a protective role in the reactions shown above, it can also be a source of oxygen radicals, and hence potentially damaging:

$$\text{Ascorbate} + \text{O}_2 \rightarrow {}^{\bullet}\text{O}_2^- + \text{monodehydroascorbate}$$

$$\text{Ascorbate} + \text{Cu}^{2+} \rightarrow \text{Cu}^+ + \text{monodehydroascorbate; Cu}^+ + \text{H}_2\text{O}_2 \rightarrow \text{Cu}^{2+} + {}^{\bullet}\text{OH} + \text{OH}^-.$$

It is unlikely that high intakes of vitamin C will result in significant radical formation, since once intake increases above about 100–120 mg/day, the vitamin is excreted quantitatively in the urine. However, there is some evidence that vitamin C supplements increase coronary heart disease mortality in diabetics; like excessively high concentrations of glucose, vitamin C can glycate proteins, including LDL (Section 10.7.1).

6.5.3.5 *Intervention trials with vitamin E*

The epidemiological evidence (e.g., that shown in Figure 6.2) suggests that vitamin E may be protective against coronary heart disease, and Figure 6.15 shows a plausible biological mechanism for a radical trapping antioxidant action of vitamin E. One of the early randomised placebo-controlled intervention trials of vitamin E as a protective agent against cardiovascular disease was the Cambridge Heart Antioxidant (CHAOS) study. As shown in Figure 6.19, the results were unexpected. There was the expected decrease in non-fatal myocardial infarctions amongst those taking the vitamin E supplements, which is good news, since each non-fatal infarction causes damage to heart muscle that cannot be repaired. However, there was an increase in the number of fatal infarctions, and an

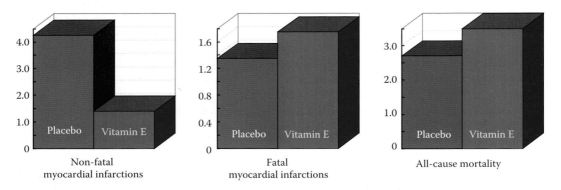

Figure 6.19 The effect of vitamin E supplementation in the Cambridge Heart Antioxidant Study. (From data reported by Stephens, N. G. et al., *Lancet* 347: 781–6, 1996.)

- Slowing the translation of cytochrome P_{450} mRNA, with no effect on transcription (Sections 9.2.2.1 and 9.2.3)
- Increasing the clearance of potential carcinogens and metabolites by induction of glutathione *S*-transferases

6.7.2.2   *Glucosinolates*

Glucosinolates (Figure 6.27) occur in brassicas (cabbage, cauliflower, broccoli, Brussels sprouts) and some other plants. The enzyme myrosinase in vacuoles in the plant cell is released when cells are damaged; it catalyses cleavage of glucosinolates to yield a variety of isothiocyanates, thiocyanates, and nitriles plus the aglycone. Intestinal bacteria have a similar enzyme, thus glucosinolates from cooked vegetables yield similar products.

Like the allyl sulphur compounds in *Allium* spp., the aglycones of glucosinolates lower the activity of microsomal cytochrome P_{450} by

- Direct enzyme inhibition
- Down-regulation of enzyme synthesis—it is not known whether this is at the level of transcription or translation

They also increase the clearance of potential carcinogens and metabolites by induction of glutathione *S*-transferases and quinone reductase.

There is a potential hazard associated with excessive consumption of brassicas—a number of the glucosinolates have a goitrogenic action, reducing synthesis of the thyroid hormones (Section 11.15.3.3). Two mechanisms are involved:

1. Thiocyanate (SCN⁻) competes with iodide for tissue uptake and is goitrogenic when iodine intakes are marginal.
2. Oxazolidine-2-thiones (e.g. goitrin, Figure 6.23) inhibit thyroxine synthesis by inhibition of iodination of mono-iodotyrosine to di-iodotyrosine. They are goitrogenic regardless of iodine nutritional status.

Goitre is a well-known problem in cattle fed on brassicas, but there is no evidence of reduced thyroid hormone status in people consuming, e.g. 150 g sprouts/d for several

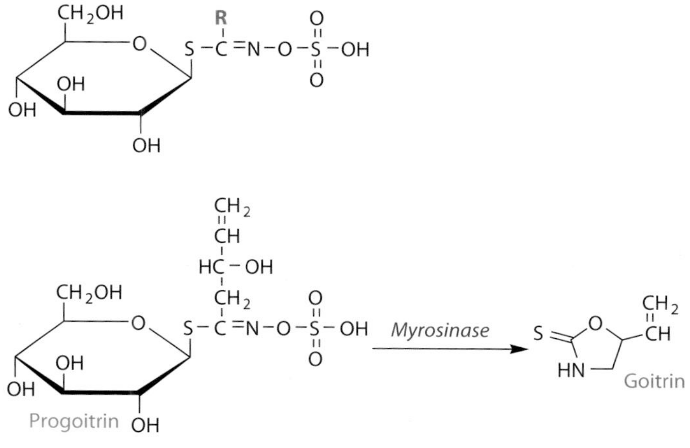

Figure 6.27 The general structure of glucosinolinates and the formation of goitrin from progoitrin.

weeks. However, iodine deficiency goitre was a problem in the Netherlands (a country that cannot be considered to be upland, over limestone soil, or inland, the usual criteria for iodine deficiency, Section 11.15.3.3) until the introduction of iodide enrichment of salt at the beginning of the 20th century. The traditional Dutch diet included a considerable amount of sauerkraut (fermented cabbage)—to such an extent that during the 16th and 17th centuries, when seafarers from most countries suffered from scurvy (vitamin C deficiency, Section 11.14.3) during long voyages of exploration, the Dutch mariners did not.

6.7.2.3 *Flavonoids*

There are six main groups of flavonoids (Figure 6.28) in plants; most occur as glycosides (with a variety of sugars) and are hydrolysed to aglycones by digestive enzymes. They serve both to protect plants against attack and as the pigments of many plants (especially the anthocyanin pigments of berry fruits). They were at one time considered to be vitamins (vitamin P), although there is no evidence that they are dietary essentials. During the 1970s, they were considered to be potential mutagens and carcinogens because they are polyphenols and can undergo redox cycling with the production of oxygen radicals. Since the 1990s, they have been considered as potentially protective antioxidants because they can form relatively stable radicals that persist long enough to undergo reaction to non-radical products. Indeed, on a molar basis, their antioxidant action is 1.5–5-times greater than that of vitamin C, although they are less well absorbed from foods. However, they are still potentially capable of forming oxygen radicals by non-enzymic reaction, and some inhibit the absorption of inorganic iron (Section 4.5.3.1).

The flavonoids are also inhibitors of phase I detoxication reactions and activators of phase II reactions. In addition, they can form inactive complexes with a number of carcinogens.

Epidemiological evidence suggests a beneficial effect of a high intake of flavonoids with respect to cardiovascular disease (accounting for perhaps 8% of the international variation in coronary heart disease), although there is no epidemiological evidence of a negative association with cancer. Intakes of flavonoids are estimated to be around 23 mg/day, of which almost half comes from tea; onions, apples, and red wine are also good

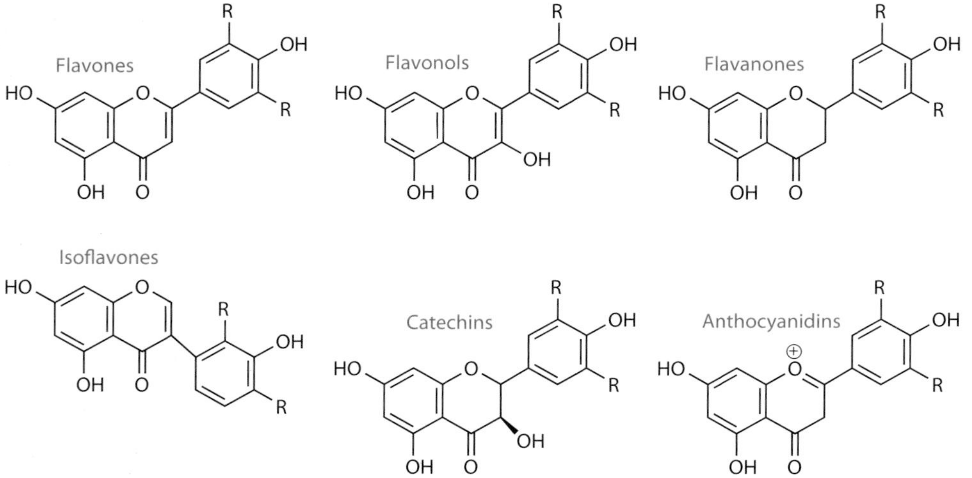

Figure 6.28 The major classes of flavonoids.

sources. Catechins are found mainly in tea and red wine and grapes; flavanones in citrus fruits and anthocyanins in red wine and grapes.

6.7.3   *Phytoestrogens*

A number of compounds that are widely distributed in plants as glycosides and other conjugates have weak oestrogenic action, although they are not chemically steroids. They all have two hydroxyl groups that are in the same position relative to each other as the hydroxyl groups in oestradiol (Figure 6.29); thus, they bind to oestradiol receptors. The amounts present in plants increase in response to microbial and insect attack, suggesting that they function as antimicrobial or antifungal agents in plants. Legumes, especially soya beans, are rich sources. Phytoestrogens undergo entero-hepatic recycling and are metabolised by intestinal bacteria; thus, there may be considerable inter-individual variation in the pattern of active metabolites that is absorbed.

The phytoestrogens produce typical and reproducible oestrogen responses, with an activity 1/500–1/1000 of that of oestradiol. They may be agonistic or antagonistic to oestradiol when both are present at the target tissue (isoflavones are mainly antagonistic, lignans are mainly agonistic). They compete with oestradiol for receptor binding, but the phytoestrogen–receptor complex does not undergo normal activation; thus, it has only a weak effect on the hormone response element of DNA (Section 10.4).

Phytoestrogens also reduce circulating free oestradiol because they increase the synthesis of sex hormone binding globulin in liver, by stabilising the mRNA, rather than true induction of gene expression. This means that more hormone is bound to globulin, and therefore, less is available for uptake into target tissues. Vegetarians have higher levels of circulating sex hormone binding globulin than do omnivores, presumably because of their higher intake of phytoestrogens. The correlation between adiposity and breast cancer is almost certainly due to synthesis of oestradiol in adipose tissue; enterolactone, and some

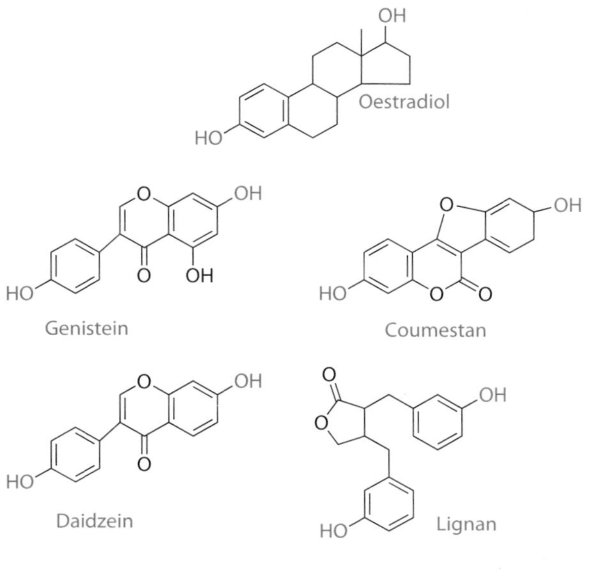

Figure 6.29 Phytoestrogens—non-steroidal compounds that have two hydroxyl groups in the correct orientation to bind to the oestradiol receptor.

of the other flavonoid phytoestrogens, inhibit aromatase, the key enzyme of oestradiol synthesis, and will therefore reduce production of oestradiol in adipose tissue.

In Japan, where the traditional diet contains relatively large amounts of phytoestrogens from soya products, there is a low incidence of cancer of the breast and prostate as well as an unexpectedly low incidence of osteoporosis (Section 11.15.1.2), despite lower peak bone density of Japanese compared with European or American women. Whilst some prospective and case–control studies show a protective effect of soya consumption with respect to breast cancer, others do not.

6.7.4   Miscellaneous actions of phytochemicals

Salicylates are irreversible inhibitors of cyclo-oxygenase and hence inhibit the synthesis of thromboxane A_2 and have an anticoagulant action. They occur in many fruits (and red wine) in amounts similar to the dose of aspirin recommended to prevent excessive blood clotting in patients at risk of thrombosis.

Allyl sulphur compounds (Section 6.7.2.1) in garlic inhibit platelet coagulation and again have a potentially beneficial effect with respect to thrombosis.

Terpenes (Figure 6.30) such as limonene (in peel oil of citrus fruits, and aromatic oils of caraway, dill, etc.), myrecene (in nutmeg), and zingiberine (in ginger) are poly-isoprene derivatives that inhibit isoprenylation of the P21-*ras* oncogene product; isoprenylation is essential for action of the ras protein, which is known to be associated with pancreatic cancer.

Genistein (but not other phytoestrogens) inhibits cell proliferation by inhibiting the tyrosine kinase activity of the epithelial growth factor receptor.

Nitrate is actively secreted in saliva and inhibits the growth of *Helicobacter pylori*, the bacterium that is the causative agent of gastric ulcers and is probably also important in the aetiology of gastric cancer. In smokers, thiocyanate competes with nitrate for secretion in saliva; this may explain how smoking exacerbates gastric ulcers. The average dietary intake of nitrates is about 70 mg/day (beetroot is an especially rich source), compared with endogenous production of 1 mg/kg body weight/day. However, endogenous production may increase 20-fold in response to inflammation and immune stimulus because of increased formation and oxidation of nitric oxide.

There is, however, epidemiological evidence that high consumption of cured and salted meat products, in which nitrate is used, is associated with an increased risk of gastric cancer. This is largely due to the reduction of nitrate to nitrite during the curing process. In the acid conditions of the stomach, nitrite can react non-enzymatically with amines in foods, forming carcinogenic nitrosamines. A high intake of nitrate from drinking water (the result of leaching fertilisers into rivers) followed by reduction of nitrate to nitrite by intestinal bacteria has been associated with the development of methaemoglobinaemia in infants.

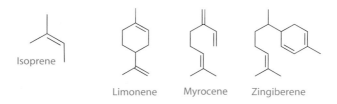

Figure 6.30 Some terpenes found in foods.

It is unclear at what level of intake the beneficial effects of nitrate intake are exceeded by its adverse effects.

Key points

- Evidence that diet is a factor in the aetiology of chronic diseases comes from various types of epidemiological study, supported by plausible biological mechanisms, but controlled intervention trials are needed to test any hypotheses developed from epidemiological data and mechanistic studies.
- For people whose weight is within the desirable range, energy intake should be adequate to maintain reasonably constant body weight, with a desirable level of physical activity.
- Fat should provide no more than 30% of energy.
- Saturated fatty acids raise serum cholesterol, and polyunsaturated lower it, compared with mono-unsaturated fatty acids.
- The balance between ω3 and ω6 polyunsaturated fatty acids is important.
- Saturated fatty acids should provide no more than 10% of energy intake. *Trans*-isomers of unsaturated fatty acids should provide no more than 1% of energy.
- The reduction in fat intake should be balanced by increased carbohydrate intake, up to 55% of energy—mainly as starches. Free sugars should provide no more than about 10% of energy intake.
- Undigested carbohydrates (resistant starch and NSPs or dietary fibre) have a number of potential health benefits, and higher intakes are associated with lower risk of colorectal cancer.
- About 10% of the population are sensitive to the hypertensive effects of salt, and salt intakes should not exceed 5 g/day.
- Moderate alcohol consumption may provide health benefits, but habitual intake should not exceed 4 units/day for men or 3 units per day for women.
- Genetic polymorphisms may explain the differences in sensitivity to various dietary and metabolic factors implicated in the aetiology of chronic diseases.
- Free radicals are highly reactive molecular species with an unpaired electron. Oxygen radicals can cause damage to nucleic acids, lipids, and proteins, leading to mutation, initiation of cancer, development of autoimmune disease, and atherosclerosis and coronary heart disease.
- Oxygen radicals are formed in the normal re-oxidation of reduced flavins, the macrophage respiratory burst, as a result of nitric oxide synthesis, in a variety of non-enzymic reactions of metal ions, and as a result of lysis of water by ionising radiation.
- Protection against radical damage is provided by enzymes that reduce superoxide, hydrogen peroxide, and lipid peroxides as well as vitamins C and E, and β-carotene, which form relatively stable radicals that persist long enough to undergo reaction to non-radical products.
- Epidemiological studies suggest that β-carotene is protective against various cancers, but intervention trials have shown increased death from lung cancer amongst people taking β-carotene supplements. This is mainly because β-carotene is an antioxidant at low partial pressure of oxygen, but an oxidant at high partial pressures of oxygen, as occur in the lungs.
- Epidemiological studies suggest that vitamin E is protective against atherosclerosis and coronary heart disease, but many intervention studies have shown increased death amongst people taking vitamin E supplements. This is mainly because the

stable vitamin E radical can penetrate deeper into tissues and plasma lipoproteins, and cause more damage.

- A number of intervention trials have shown increased mortality amongst people taking antioxidant supplements. This may be because excessive antioxidant action impairs the signalling function of radicals, especially in initiating apoptosis.
- Elevated plasma homocysteine is a risk factor for atherosclerosis and cardiovascular disease; homocysteine has atherogenic actions, may lead to production of free radicals, and has a procoagulant action.
- A common polymorphism of methylene tetrahydrofolate reductase is associated with both increased risk of cardiovascular disease and also elevated plasma homocysteine. Supplements of folic acid lower plasma homocysteine and some intervention trials show an improvement of intermediate markers of cardiovascular risk, although there is no significant reduction in total mortality.
- A variety of other compounds found in plant foods, not normally considered to be nutrients, may provide protection in various ways against the development of chronic disease.

chapter seven

Overweight and obesity

If the intake of metabolic fuels (i.e. the total intake of food) is greater than is required to meet energy expenditure, the result is storage of the excess, largely as triacylglycerol in adipose tissue. This chapter is concerned with the problems associated with excessive accumulation of body fat: overweight and obesity, which are serious public health problems worldwide. There has been a considerable increase in the prevalence of obesity in all countries over the last three decades, to the extent that WHO talks of a global epidemic of obesity. In 2005, it was estimated that, for the first time in human history, there were more overweight and obese people in the world than those who were hungry and underfed. By 2013, some 13% of the world's population were undernourished, whilst 22% were overweight and 7.5% were obese. Many developing countries have the problems of undernutrition (Chapter 8) and overnutrition at the same time. Perhaps more seriously, metabolic programming (Section 6.4.1) as a result of marginal undernutrition *in utero* and in early life is a major factor in the development of obesity and the metabolic syndrome (Section 7.2.3) in later life.

Objectives

After reading this chapter you should be able to

- Explain what is meant by desirable body weight, calculate body mass index (BMI), and determine whether or not it is within the desirable range.
- Describe the methods that are available to determine body fat content and its distribution.
- Describe the health hazards associated with overweight and obesity and explain the association between obesity and insulin resistance in the metabolic syndrome and the development of type II diabetes mellitus.
- Explain the causes of obesity and describe the methods available for its treatment.

7.1 Desirable body weight

Figure 7.1 shows the results of one of the early prospective studies to determine desirable ranges of weight. 750,000 people were classified by weight, then followed for 15 years. Those who were most overweight were twice as likely to die as those whose weight was around the average.

People who were significantly below average weight at the beginning of the study were also more at risk of premature death. However, this may be because those people who were significantly underweight were already seriously ill (Section 8.4), rather than implying that a moderate degree of underweight is undesirable or poses any health hazards.

7.1.1 Body mass index

Many of the early studies of overweight and premature mortality used relatively complex tables of weight for height, sometimes also corrected for skeletal frame size. A simpler

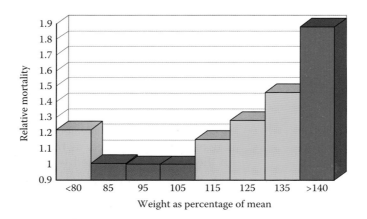

Figure 7.1 Excess mortality with obesity. (From data reported by Garfinkel, L., *Cancer* 58: 1826–9, 1986.)

solution is to calculate the body mass index (BMI), sometimes also called Quetelet's index, after the 19th century Belgian mathematician who first demonstrated its usefulness. BMI is calculated from the weight (in kg) divided by the square of the height (in meters)—i.e. BMI = weight (kg)/height^2 (m). The desirable range, associated with optimum life expectancy, is between 20 and 25. Values of BMI below 18.5 are associated with undernutrition (Chapter 8); there is no evidence that a moderate degree of underweight (BMI 18.5–20) is associated with any adverse outcomes. Table 7.1 and Figure 7.2 show the classification of overweight and obesity by BMI.

The adult ranges of BMI are not applicable to children. Figure 7.3 shows the 25th, 50th, and 75th centile of BMI with age between 2 and 20 years.

Many people gain weight as they grow older. There is some evidence, albeit disputed, that a modest increase in BMI (by 1 unit per decade) may be associated with better health in old age. Figure 7.4 shows the upper and lower limits of the acceptable (if not strictly desirable) range of BMI at different ages.

Although BMI provides a useful way of assessing weight relative to height, and for most people, a high BMI reflects excessive adipose tissue, it does not provide useful information for people like bodybuilders, whose high BMI is due to increased muscle mass, not adipose tissue.

Table 7.1 Classification of Overweight and Obesity by BMI

	BMI	Excess weight (kg)	Percentage of desirable weight
Desirable	20–25	–	100
Acceptable but not desirable	25–27	<5	100–110
Overweight	25–30	5–15	110–120
Obese	30–40	15–25	120–160
Severely obese	>40	>25	>160

Note: BMI = weight (kg)/height^2 (m).

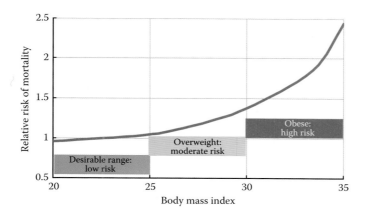

Figure 7.2 Excess mortality with obesity as defined by BMI.

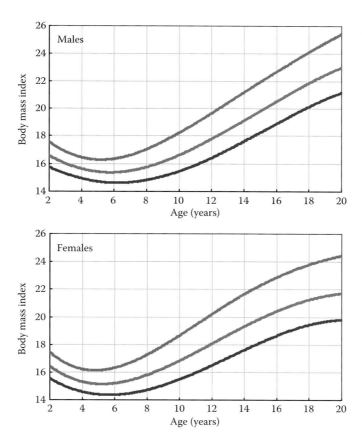

Figure 7.3 Ranges of BMI for ages 2–20 years. The curves show the 75th centile (red), 50th centile (green), and 25th centile (blue). (From U.S. Centers for Disease Control and Prevention data.)

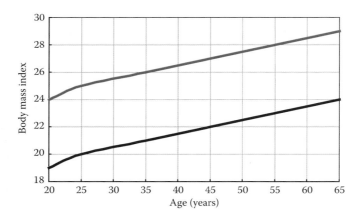

Figure 7.4 Upper and lower limits of acceptable (if not desirable) ranges of BMI with age.

7.1.2   Estimation of body fat

The important factor for health is the proportion of body weight that is fat. This is termed adiposity. A number of techniques are available for assessing adiposity, although most of them are research techniques and are not appropriate for routine screening of the general public.

7.1.2.1   Determination of body density

The density of body fat is 0.9 g/mL, whilst that of the fat-free body mass is 1.10 g/mL. This means that if the density of the body can be measured, then the proportion of fat and lean tissue can be calculated.

Density is determined either by weighing in air and again totally submerged in water or by measuring the volume of the body by its displacement of water when submerged. Neither procedure is particularly pleasant for the experimental subject, and considerable precision is necessary in the measurements. A body density of 1.08 g/cm^3 represents a very low body fat content of 8.3%, whilst a density of 1 g/cm^3 represents a very high body fat content of 43%. Whilst direct determination of body density is the standard, against which all the other techniques discussed below must be calibrated, it is clearly a research technique and not appropriate for general use.

7.1.2.2   Determination of total body water or potassium

The fat content of the body can be determined by estimating the fat-free mass of the body. This can be done by measuring total body water (fat-free tissue is 73% water) by giving a dose of water labelled with ^{2}H or ^{18}O and then measuring the dilution of the label in plasma, urine, or saliva. As discussed in Section 5.1.2, the different rates of loss of label from ^{2}H and ^{18}O can be used to estimate total carbon dioxide production, and hence total energy expenditure, over a period of 1–3 weeks. However, there is no significant difference in the rate of loss of either label in the short time that is required for equilibration of the test dose with total body water.

Alternatively, the total body content of potassium can be measured. Potassium occurs only in the fat-free mass of the body, and the radioactive isotope ^{40}K occurs naturally. It is a weak γ-emitter, and total body potassium can be determined by measuring the γ-radiation of the appropriate wavelength emitted by the body. This requires total enclosure in a shielded whole body counter for about 15 min to achieve adequate precision, and because of this, and the cost of the equipment required, again this is purely a research technique.

7.1.2.3   *Imaging techniques*

Fat, bone, and lean tissues absorb X-rays and ultrasound to different extents and respond to magnetic resonance (MR) imaging differently. This means that an X-ray, ultrasound, or MR image will permit determination of the amounts of different tissues in the body, by measuring the areas (or volumes if scanning techniques are used) occupied by each type of tissue. Such imaging techniques permit determination not only of the total amount of fat in the body, but also its distribution. It is adipose tissue within the abdominal cavity, rather than subcutaneous adipose tissue, that is the main health hazard (Section 7.2.2.1).

7.1.2.4   *Measurement of whole body electrical conductivity and impedance*

Fat is an electrical insulator, whilst lean tissue, being a solution of electrolytes, will conduct an electric current. If electrodes are attached to the hand and foot, and an extremely small alternating electric current (typically 80 μA at 50 MHz) is passed between them, measurement of the fall in voltage permits calculation of the conductivity or impedance of the body. The percentage of fat and lean tissue can be calculated from equations based on a series of studies in which this technique has been calibrated against direct determination of density (Section 7.1.2.1).

Measurement of either total body electrical conductivity (TOBEC) or bio-electrical impedance (BIE) have been used mainly in research, but many gyms and fitness centres now have the equipment to measure body fat in this way.

7.1.2.5   *Measurement of skinfold thickness*

Where equipment is not available to determine body fat by electrical conductivity or impedance, the thickness of subcutaneous adipose tissue is measured as an index of total body fat content, using standardised calipers that exert a moderate pressure (10 g/mm^2 over an area of 20–40 mm^2). For greatest precision, the mean of the skinfold thickness at four sites is calculated:

1. Over the triceps, at the midpoint of the upper arm
2. Over the biceps, at the front of the upper arm, directly above the cubital fossa, at the same level as the triceps site
3. Subscapular, just below and laterally to the angle of the shoulder blade, with the shoulder and arm relaxed
4. Supra-iliac, on the mid-axillary line immediately superior to the iliac crest

The desirable ranges of mean skinfold thickness are for men, 3–10 mm and for women, 10–22 mm. However, the important factor for health is intra-abdominal fat (Section 7.2.2.1), which cannot be estimated from skinfold thickness. A combination of skinfold measurements with measurement of the ratio of waist/hip circumference gives an indication of the relative amounts of subcutaneous and intra-abdominal fat.

7.2   *The problems of overweight and obesity*

Overweight and obesity are a major problem in most developed countries (Figure 7.5), and in developing countries, there are problems of both obesity and undernutrition.

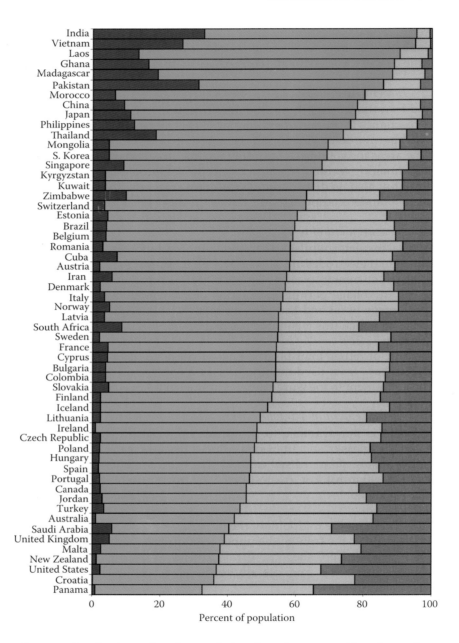

Figure 7.5 Overweight, obesity, and underweight in selected countries. Blue shows the percentage of the population of each country significantly underweight (see Chapter 8), green, the percentage within the desirable range of BMI 20–25, orange, the percentage overweight (BMI 25–30), and red, the percentage obese (BMI > 30). (From World Health Organization data.)

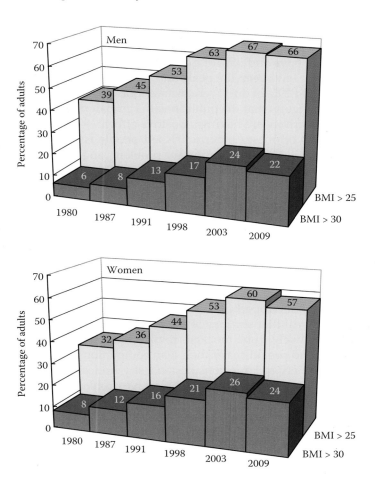

Figure 7.6 The increasing prevalence of overweight and obesity in UK, 1980–2009. (From UK Department of Health data.)

There is a worrying increase in the prevalence of overweight and obesity, to the extent that the World Health Organization talks of an epidemic of obesity. As shown in Figure 7.6, the prevalence of obesity amongst men in Britain increased fourfold and that amongst women more than threefold, between 1980 and 2003. It is ironic that in 1980 the UK Department of Health was sufficiently worried by the problem of obesity that a major target of the *Health of the Nation* policy document was to halve the prevalence of obesity within a decade. In fact, it doubled in this time. The rapid increase in overweight and obesity has slowed, and there was a small drop in the prevalence of obesity between 2003 and 2009 (the most recent year for which data are available). Nevertheless, two thirds of men and over half of all women in Britain are overweight and 22% of men and 24% of women are obese. This rapid increase in the prevalence of overweight and obesity has occurred in most countries, although there is evidence that, as in Britain, the rate of increase is slowing in many countries, suggesting either that public health campaigns are having an effect or that the increased mortality associated with obesity has killed a significant number of people.

Childhood obesity is a major cause for concern. In the UK in 1995 24% of boys and 25% of girls were overweight, and 11% of boys and 12% of girls were obese. By 2004, this had increased to 33% of boys and 35% of girls overweight and 19% of boys and 18.5% of girls obese. This seems to have been the peak, and by 2006 (the last year for which data are available), 31% of boys and 29% of girls were overweight, with 17% of boys and 15% of girls obese. This reduction suggests that the public health campaigns promoting healthy eating and increased physical activity are having a positive effect.

Worldwide, the ratio of obese/undernourished people is 1.4/1. In developing countries, undernutrition is still the more important problem, and the ratio is 0.7/1, whilst in developed countries, obese people outnumber underweight people by 11.8/1.

7.2.1   Social problems of obesity

Historically, a moderate degree of overweight was considered desirable; when food was scarce, fatness was a visible sign of wealth. There was also a survival advantage in having reserves of fat to survive periods of food shortage or famine. As food supplies, at least in developed countries, have become more assured, perceptions have changed. Fatness is no longer regarded as a sign of wealth. Indeed, obesity is more common amongst lower socioeconomic groups in developed countries, although in developing countries, it is still mainly confined to the wealthier sections of the population. No longer are the overweight envied; rather, they are likely to be mocked, reviled, and made deeply unhappy by the unthinking comments and prejudices of their lean companions.

Because Western society at large considers obesity undesirable, and fashion emphasises slimness, many overweight and obese people have problems of a poor self-image and low self-esteem. Obese people are certainly not helped by the all-too-common prejudice against them, the difficulty of buying clothes that will fit, and the fact that they are often regarded as a legitimate butt of crude and cruel humour. This may lead to a sense of isolation and withdrawal from society, and may frequently result in increased food consumption for comfort—thus resulting in yet more weight gain, a further loss of self-esteem, further withdrawal, and more eating for compensation.

The psychological and social problems of the obese spill over to people of normal weight as well. There is continual advertising pressure for 'slimness', and newspapers and magazines are full of propaganda for slimness and 'diets' for weight reduction. This may be one of the factors in the development of major eating disorders such as anorexia nervosa and bulimia (Section 1.4.5).

7.2.2   The health risks of obesity

The major causes of premature death associated with obesity are

- Cancer, especially breast, prostate and colorectal cancers
- Atherosclerosis, coronary heart disease, high blood pressure, and stroke
- Complications of type II diabetes mellitus
- Respiratory diseases

In addition to the diseases caused by, or associated with, obesity, obese people are considerably more at risk of death during surgery and of postoperative complications. There are three main reasons for this:

1. Surgery is longer and more difficult when the surgeon has to cut through large amounts of subcutaneous and intra-abdominal adipose tissue.
2. Induction of anaesthesia is more difficult when veins are not readily visible through subcutaneous adipose tissue, and maintenance of anaesthesia is complicated by the solubility of anaesthetic agents in fat; thus, there is a large buffer pool in the body, and adjustment of the dose is difficult.
3. Most importantly, anaesthesia depresses lung function (as does being in a supine position), in all people. Obese people suffer from impaired lung function under normal conditions, largely as a result of adipose tissue in the upper body segment; total lung capacity may be only 60% of that in lean people, and the mechanical workload on the respiratory muscles may be twice that of lean people. Therefore, they are especially at risk during surgery.

Because of their impaired lung function, obese people are more at risk of respiratory distress, pneumonia, and bronchitis than are lean people. In addition, excess body weight is associated with increased morbidity from such conditions as

- Arthritis of the hips and knees, associated with the increased stress on weight-bearing joints. In addition, there is increased synthesis of nitric oxide in response to leptin action, and this has been implicated in the destruction of cartilage. Rheumatoid arthritis may also be exacerbated in obese people, as a result of the immunodulatory inflammatory actions of leptin.
- Varicose veins and haemorrhoids, associated with increased intra-abdominal pressure and possibly due more to a low intake of dietary fibre (Sections 4.2.1.7 and 6.3.3.2) and hence straining on defecation, rather than directly a result of obesity.
- Obesity in childhood and adolescence is associated with lower bone mineral density and increased risk of developing osteoporosis (Section 11.15.1.2) in later life.

7.2.2.1   The distribution of excess adipose tissue

The adverse effects of obesity are due not only to the excessive amount of body fat but also to its distribution in the body. Measurement of the waist/hip ratio provides a convenient way of defining two patterns of adipose tissue distribution:

1. Predominantly in the upper body segment (thorax and abdomen)—the classical male pattern of obesity, sometimes called apple-shaped obesity
2. Predominantly in the lower body segment (hips)—the classical female pattern of obesity, sometimes called pear-shaped obesity

It is the male pattern of abdominal obesity that is associated with the major health risks. In most studies of coronary heart disease, there is a threefold excess of men compared with women, a difference that persists even when the data are corrected for such risk factors as blood pressure, cholesterol in low-density lipoproteins, BMI, smoking, and physical activity. However, if the data are corrected for the waist/hip ratio, there is only a 1.4-fold excess of men over women.

Figure 7.7 shows the effects of body weight and waist/hip ratio on the prevalence of diabetes in women, and Figure 7.8 shows that increased intra-abdominal (visceral) fat is associated with insulin resistance (and hence ultimately the development of diabetes) even in people whose BMI is within the desirable range.

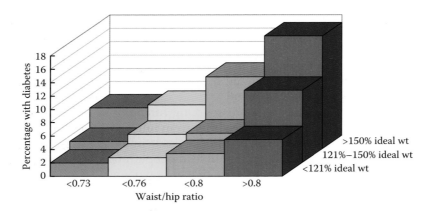

Figure 7.7 The effects of obesity and abdominal adiposity on the prevalence of diabetes. (From data reported by Hartz, A. J. et al., *American Journal of Epidemiology* 119: 71–80, 1984.)

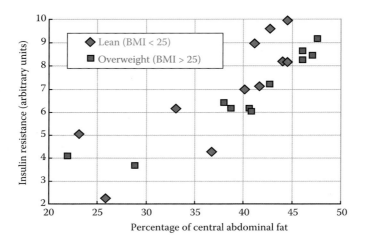

Figure 7.8 The effect of abdominal adiposity in lean and obese subjects on insulin resistance. (From data reported by Wilkin, T. J., Chapter 4 in *Adult obesity: a paediatric challenge*, Voss, L. D. & Willkin, T. J., Eds., Taylor & Francis, London, 2003.)

Visceral adipose tissue is metabolically more active than subcutaneous adipose tissue. It is drained by the hepatic portal vein, going directly to the liver where non-esterified fatty acids stimulate production and release of glucose. The non-esterified fatty acids released from subcutaneous adipose tissue mainly act as a source of metabolic fuel to muscle and other tissues, with the liver only clearing the remainder. Visceral adipose tissue produces less leptin than does subcutaneous adipose tissue; thus, abdominal fat will have less effect than subcutaneous fat on long-term regulation of food intake and energy expenditure (Section 1.4.2).

Subcutaneous and visceral adipose tissue have different embryological origins; subcutaneous adipose tissue develops from white adipocyte precursors, whilst visceral adipose tissue develops from brown adipose tissue precursors. This suggests that the original function of visceral adipose tissue was thermogenesis to maintain body temperature

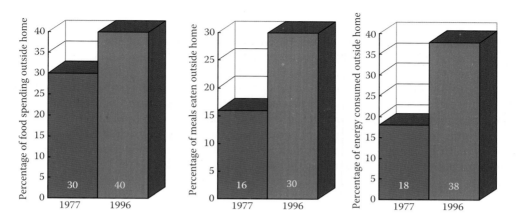

Figure 7.9 U.S. food consumption away from home. (From data reported by Critser, G., *Fatland: How Americans became the fattest people in the world*, Penguin Books, London, 2003.)

7.3.3 Control of appetite

Most people manage to balance their food intake with energy expenditure remarkably precisely. Indeed, even people who are overweight or obese are in energy balance when their weight is more or less constant. As discussed in Section 1.4.2, leptin is central to the control of both food intake and energy expenditure, and there are a number of mechanisms involved in short-term control of food intake, with regulation of both hunger and satiety.

Very rarely, people are overweight or obese as a result of a physical defect of the appetite control centres in the brain (Section 1.4)—for example, some tumours can cause damage to the satiety centre; thus, the patient feels hunger, but not the sensation of satiety, and has no physiological cue to stop eating. A very small number of children who are pathologically obese have defects in their leptin receptors or downstream signalling from the leptin receptor; thus, that they have little or no control over their appetite and energy expenditure.

More commonly, obesity can be attributed to a psychological failure of appetite control. At its simplest, this can be blamed on the variety of attractive foods available. People can easily be tempted to eat more than they need, and it may take quite an effort of willpower to refuse a choice morsel. Even when hunger has been satisfied, the appearance of a different dish can stimulate appetite. Experimental animals, which normally do not become obese, can be persuaded to overeat and become obese by providing them with a 'cafeteria' array of attractive foods.

A number of studies comparing severely obese people with lean people have shown that they do not respond to the normal cues for hunger and satiety. Rather, in many cases, it is the sight of food that prompts them to eat, regardless of whether they are 'hungry' or not. If no food is visible, they will not feel hungry; conversely, if food is still visible they will not feel satiety. There have been no similar studies involving more moderately overweight people; thus, it is not known whether this failure of appetite regulation is a general problem or whether it only affects severely obese people with BMI > 40.

7.3.4   How obese people can be helped to lose weight

In considering the treatment of obesity, two different aspects of the problem must be considered:

1. The initial problem, which is to help the overweight or obese person to reduce his or her weight to within the desirable range, where life expectancy is maximum.
2. The long-term problem of helping the now lean person to maintain desirable body weight. This is largely a matter of education, increasing physical activity, and changing eating habits. The same guidelines for a prudent diet (Section 6.3) apply to the slimmed-down, formerly obese, person as to anyone else.

The aim of any weight reduction regime is to reduce the intake of food to below the level needed for energy expenditure, so that body reserves of fat will have to be used. The theoretical maximum possible rate of weight loss is 230 g/MJ energy imbalance per week; for a person with an energy expenditure of 10 MJ/day, total starvation would result in a loss of 2.3 kg/week. In practice, the rate of weight loss is lower than this theoretical figure because of the changes in metabolic rate and energy expenditure that occur with changes in both body weight and food intake (Section 5.2).

Very often, the first 1 or 2 weeks of a weight-reducing regime are associated with a very much greater loss of weight than this. Obviously, this cannot be due to loss of fat. It is due to loss of the water associated with glycogen (Sections 4.2.1.6 and 5.2). Although it is not sustained, the initial rapid rate of weight loss can be extremely encouraging for the obese person. The problem is to ensure that he or she realises that it will not, and indeed cannot, be sustained. It also provides excellent advertising copy for less than totally scrupulous vendors of slimming regimes, who make truthful claims about the weight loss in the first week or two and omit any information about the later weeks and months needed to achieve goal weight.

7.3.4.1   Starvation

More or less, total starvation has been used in a hospital setting to treat seriously obese patients, especially those who are to undergo elective surgery. Vitamins and minerals have to be supplied (Chapter 11) as well as fluid, but an obese person can lose weight at about the predicted rate of 2–2.5 kg/week if starved completely. There are two major problems with total starvation as a means of rapid weight loss:

1. The problem of enforcement. It is very difficult to deprive someone of food and to prevent them finding more or less devious means of acquiring it—by begging or stealing from other patients, visitors, and hospital volunteers, or even by walking down to the hospital shop or out-patients' cafeteria.
2. As much as half the weight lost in total starvation may be protein from muscle and other tissues, to provide a source of amino acids for gluconeogenesis to maintain blood glucose (Section 5.7). This is not desirable; the metabolic stress of surgery causes a considerable loss of protein (Section 9.1.2.3), and it would be highly undesirable to start this loss before surgery.

7.3.4.2   Very low-energy diets

Many of the problems associated with total starvation can be avoided by feeding a very low energy intake, commonly 1–1.5 MJ/day, in specially formulated meal replacements that provide adequate intakes of vitamins and minerals. Such regimes have shown excellent results in the treatment of severe obesity. There is very much less loss of tissue protein than in total starvation, and people feel less hungry than if they are starved completely.

If very low-energy diets are used together with a programme of exercise, the rate of weight loss can be close to the theoretical maximum of 2–2.5 kg/week. Such diets should probably be regarded as a treatment of last resort, for people with a serious problem of obesity that does not respond to more conventional diet therapy. These diets do not provide appropriate education in changes to diet for long-term maintenance of reduced weight.

7.3.4.3 Conventional diets

For most people, the problem is not one of severe morbid obesity, but a more modest excess body weight. Even for people who have a serious problem of obesity, it is likely that less drastic measures than those discussed above will be beneficial. The aim is to reduce energy intake to below expenditure and so ensure the utilisation of adipose tissue reserves. To anyone who has not tried to lose weight, the answer would appear to be simply to eat less. Obviously it is not so simple; a vast array of diets, slimming regimes, and special foods is available.

The ideal approach to the problem of obesity and weight reduction would be to provide people with the information they need to choose an appropriate diet for themselves. This is not easy. It is not simply a matter of reducing energy intake, but of ensuring at the same time that intakes of protein, vitamins, and minerals are adequate. The preparation of balanced diets, especially when the total energy intake is to be reduced, is a skilled task, and a major function of the professional dietitian. Furthermore, there is the problem of long-term compliance with dietary restrictions—the diet must not only be low in energy and high in nutrients, it must also be attractive and pleasant to eat in appropriate amounts.

A simple way of helping people to select an appropriate diet for weight reduction is to offer three lists of foods:

1. Energy-dense foods that should be avoided. These are generally foods rich in fat and sugar but providing little in the way of vitamins and minerals. Such foods include oils and fats, fried foods, fatty cuts of meat, cakes, biscuits, etc., and alcoholic beverages. They should be eaten sparingly, if at all.
2. Foods that are relatively high in energy yield, but also good sources of protein, vitamins, and minerals. They should be eaten in moderate amounts.
3. Foods that are generally rich sources of vitamins and minerals, high in starch and non-starch polysaccharides (dietary fibre), and low in fat and sugars (i.e., nutrient dense). These can be eaten (within reason) as much as is wanted.

An alternative method is to provide people with a series of meal plans and menus, designed to be nutrient-dense and energy-low and providing sufficient variety from day to day to ensure compliance. To make this less rigid and prescriptive, it is easy to provide a list of foods with 'exchange points', permitting one food to be substituted for another. At its simplest, such a list would give portions of foods with approximately the same energy yield. A more elaborate exchange list calculates 'points' for foods based on their energy yield, nutrient density, and total or saturated fat content. The consumer is given a target number of 'points' to be consumed each day, depending on gender, physical activity, and the amount of weight to be lost and can make up a diet to meet this target. An advantage of this is that foods that might be considered forbidden in a simple energy-counting diet can be permitted—but a single portion may constitute a whole day's points.

An interesting variant of the exchange points system also allocates (negative) points to physical activity, thus promoting physical activity as well as sound eating habits.

An alternative to providing meal plans and menus or exchange lists of foods and 'points' and leaving the client to prepare his or her own meals is to provide ready-prepared meals from a suitable menu, calculated to be low in energy density but of high nutrient density. These may be available from supermarkets or may be delivered (frozen) to the home.

7.3.4.4 Very low carbohydrate (ketogenic) diets

From time to time, there is a fashion for very low carbohydrate diets for weight reduction, typically allowing less than 20 g of carbohydrate per day in the initial stages, but with unlimited fat and protein. Such diets are effective, but the subjects become ketotic and feel unwell. Three factors explain the efficacy of such diets:

1. In response to a high-protein diet, there is a considerable increase in the rate of whole body protein turnover, which is ATP-expensive (Section 9.2.3.3), resulting in increased energy expenditure.
2. A high-protein intake decreases the expression of neuropeptide Y in the hypothalamic appetite control centres (Section 1.4.1.1), thus, decreasing hunger.
3. To maintain an adequate supply of glucose for the central nervous system and red blood cells, there has to be considerable gluconeogenesis from amino acids; again this is ATP-expensive (Section 5.7), resulting in increased energy expenditure.

Although very-low-carbohydrate diets are effective for weight loss, they are unlikely to be useful for long-term maintenance of desirable body weight, and they run counter to all advice on what constitutes a prudent diet (Section 6.3). Not only are they undesirably high in fat, but there is also some evidence that excessively high intakes of protein may pose long-term health hazards.

7.3.4.5 Low glycaemic index diets

Carbohydrates with a low glycaemic index (Section 4.2.1.1) lead to a slower increase in blood glucose after a meal and hence to less insulin secretion. As a result, there is less synthesis of fatty acids and triacylglycerol (Section 5.6.1).

Although sucrose has a low glycaemic index, because it yields 1 mol of glucose and 1 mol of fructose and so has less effect on blood glucose than an equivalent amount of glucose, it is misleading to consider it to be beneficial in the same way as low glycaemic starches are beneficial because of the effect of fructose in increasing fatty acid synthesis (Section 6.3.3.1).

7.3.4.6 High-fibre diets

One of the problems raised by many people who are restricting their food intake is that they continually feel hungry. Quite apart from true physiological hunger, the lack of bulk in the gastrointestinal tract may be a factor here. This problem can be alleviated by increasing the intake of dietary fibre or non-starch polysaccharide (Sections 4.2.1.7 and 6.3.3.2)—increased consumption of whole grain cereal products, fruits, and vegetables. Such regimes are certainly successful and again represent essentially a more extreme version of the general advice for a prudent diet (Section 6.3). Soluble non-starch polysaccharides (plant mucilages and gums) increase the viscosity of the intestinal contents and slow the absorption of the products of digestion, thus effectively decreasing the glycaemic index of a meal.

It is generally desirable that the dietary sources of non-starch polysaccharides should be ordinary foods rather than 'supplements'. However, as an aid to weight reduction, a number of preparations of dietary fibre are available. Some of these are more or less ordinary foods, but containing added fibre, which gives texture to the food and increases the feeling of fullness and satiety. Some of the special slimmers' soups, biscuits, etc., are of this type. They are formulated to provide about one third of a day's requirement of protein, vitamins, and minerals, but with a low energy yield. They are supposed to be taken in place of one meal each day, and to aid satiety, they contain carboxymethylcellulose or another non-digested polysaccharide.

7.3.4.7   *Alternating food restriction and free consumption*

It was noted in Section 5.2 that energy requirements fall as body weight falls. While much of this is obligatory, there is also an element of metabolic adaptation to a low energy intake—increased metabolic efficiency and decreased protein turnover (Section 9.2.3.3). There is some evidence that this metabolic adaptation can be avoided by alternating a few days of food restriction with a day or two during which a larger amount of food is consumed, then returning to food restriction. Whilst this may work for some people, its success will depend on the amount of food eaten during the 'free' days. It is unlikely to entrain the sound dietary habits that are required for long-term maintenance of weight loss.

7.3.4.8   *'Diets' that probably would not work*

Weight reduction depends on reducing the intake of metabolic fuels, but ensuring that the intake of nutrients is adequate to meet requirements. Equally important is the problem of ensuring that the weight that has been lost is not regained—in other words, eating patterns must be changed after weight has been lost to allow for maintenance of a body weight with a well-balanced diet.

There is a bewildering array of different diet regimes on offer to help the overweight and obese to lose weight. Some of these are based on sound nutritional principles and provide about half the person's energy requirement, with adequate amounts of protein, vitamins, and minerals. They permit a sustained weight loss of about 1–1.5 kg/week.

Other 'diets' are neither scientifically formulated nor based on sound nutritional principles, and indeed frequently depend on pseudo-science to attempt to give them some validity. They frequently make exaggerated claims for the amount of weight that can be lost and rarely provide a balanced diet. Publication of testimonials from 'satisfied clients' cannot be considered to be evidence of efficacy, and publication in a book that is a bestseller or in a magazine with wide circulation cannot correct the underlying flaws of many of these diets.

Diets that are not based on sound science or on misinterpretation of science, include

- The Beverley Hills diet, based on the unfounded belief that enzymes from certain fruits (pineapple, mango, etc.) are required to digest foods and that undigested food in the gastrointestinal tract leads to obesity.
- The blood group diet, based on the unfounded belief that blood groups evolved at different times, and the diet prevalent at the time a person's blood group evolved is optimum for health and weight control.

- The cabbage soup diet, which advocates consumption of large amounts of home-made cabbage soup with a very limited range of other foods; this is likely to be nutritionally inadequate in many respects.
- The combining diet. This is a system of eating based on the unfounded concept that carbohydrates and proteins should not be eaten at the same meal. It ignores the fact that almost all carbohydrate-rich foods also contain significant amounts of protein (see Figure 9.3). In any case, in the absence of adequate carbohydrate, protein is oxidised as a metabolic fuel (i.e., to provide energy) and therefore not available for tissue building. Also called food combining or Hay diet.
- Various detox diets, based on the unfounded belief that weight gain is the result of accumulation of toxins in the body, and a period of fasting and strict avoidance of such supposed toxins as caffeine and food additives is beneficial. Various herbal supplements are often included in 'detox diets', with little or no evidence of efficacy. Proponents claim that the sensation of lightheadedness that occurs after a few days of more or less complete fasting is the result of toxins being released.
- The duvet diet, based on the observation that sleep deprivation leads to increased secretion of the hormones cortisol and ghrelin (which stimulate appetite) and reduced secretion of leptin (which reduces appetite). By extrapolation, it is assumed that increasing the time spent sleeping will reduce appetite and food intake and so permit weight loss. There is no evidence of efficacy.
- The macrobiotic diet. This is a system of eating associated with Zen Buddhism. It consists of several stages, finally reaching Diet 7, which is restricted to cereals. Cases of severe malnutrition have been reported on this diet. It involves the Chinese concept of *yin* (female) and *yang* (male), whereby foods and even different vitamins (indeed, everything in life) are predominantly one or the other and must be balanced.
- The pH diet, based on balancing the intake of acid- and base-forming foods, again with little or no scientific basis.
- The zone diet, based on the unfounded belief that each meal should comprise a fixed proportion of macronutrients: 40% carbohydrate, 30% fat, and 30% protein.

Some diets permit almost unlimited consumption of only a very limited number of foods (the cabbage soup diet mentioned above is an extreme example). The idea is that if someone is permitted to eat as much they wish of only a very limited range of foods, even desirable and much liked foods, they will end up eating very little because even a favourite food soon palls if this is all that is permitted. In practice, these diets do neither good nor harm. People get so bored that they give up before there can be any significant effect on body weight, or any adverse effects of a very unbalanced diet. This is all to the good—if people did stick to such diets for any length of time, they might well encounter problems of protein, vitamin, and mineral deficiency.

7.3.4.9 Slimming patches

The basal metabolic rate is controlled to a considerable extent by the thyroid hormone tri-iodothyronine, and iodine deficiency (Section 11.15.3.3) results in impaired synthesis of thyroid hormone, a low metabolic rate, and ready weight gain. Pathological overactivity of the thyroid gland results in increased synthesis and secretion of thyroid hormone and an increased basal metabolic rate, with weight loss.

The synthesis of thyroid hormone is regulated, and in the absence of thyroid disease, provision of additional iodine does not increase hormone secretion except in people who were iodine deficient. Nevertheless, there are people who market various iodine-rich preparations to aid weight loss. Foremost amongst these are the so-called slimming patches, which contain seaweed extract as a source of iodine that is supposed to be absorbed from a small patch applied to the skin. There is no evidence that such patches have any beneficial effect at all, and indeed, in a number of cases that have been taken to court the patches have been shown to contain very little, if any, iodine anyway—at least partly because iodine is volatile and is lost in the manufacture of the patches.

7.3.4.10   Sugar substitutes

The average consumption of sugar is higher than is considered desirable (Section 6.3.3.1), and omitting sugar from tea and coffee would make a significant contribution to reduction of energy intake—a teaspoon of sugar is 5 g of carbohydrate and thus provides 80 kJ—in each of 6 cups of tea or coffee a day, two spoons of sugar would thus account for some 960 kJ—almost 10% of the average person's energy expenditure. Quite apart from this obvious sugar, there is a great deal of sugar in beverages—for example, a 330 mL can of lemonade provides 20 g of sugar (=320 kJ).

Because many people like their tea and coffee sweetened, and to replace the sugar in lemonades, etc., a number of intense sweeteners are used as sugar substitutes. These are synthetic chemicals that are very much sweeter than sugar, but are not metabolic fuels. Even those that can be metabolised (for example, aspartame, which is an amino acid derivative) are taken in such small amounts that they make no significant contribution to intake. All of these compounds have been extensively tested for safety, but as a result of concerns about possible hazards, some are not permitted in some countries, although they are widely used elsewhere.

One of the most successful of intense sweeteners is sucralose (trichlorosucrose). It is about 600 times sweeter than sucrose, twice as sweet as saccharine, and three times as sweet as aspartame. It is not absorbed or metabolised. It is commonly supplied mixed with maltodextrins and other bulking agents; thus, it can be used on a volume-equivalent basis to replace sucrose, and because it is stable to heat, it can be used to replace sugar in baking.

Sugar alcohols such as sorbitol (Section 4.2.1.3) are poorly absorbed from the small intestine, and therefore have only about half the energy yield of other carbohydrates. Unlike intense sweeteners, they can be used in the manufacture of jam, sweets, and other foods, where they provide the same bulk and have the same osmotic preservative effect as sugars, but at half the energy yield.

7.3.4.11   Fat substitutes

In addition to low-fat versions of conventional foods (e.g. leaner cuts of meat used in manufactured foods and minced meat; skimmed and semi-skimmed milk, and cheese and yoghurt made from skimmed or semi-skimmed milk), there are a number of fat substitutes available for food manufacture. Some of these are based on modified starch or protein and are used in the manufacture of very low fat spreads (to replace butter or margarine) and salad dressings and dips. Fatty acid esters of sucrose (Olestra™ or Olean™) can be used for frying foods in the same way as oils and fats that are fatty acid esters of glycerol, but they are not hydrolysed by digestive enzymes, and thus have no nutritional value.

7.3.4.12   Pharmacological treatment of obesity

A number of compounds act either to suppress the activity of the hunger centre in the hypothalamus or to stimulate the satiety centre. Sometimes this is an undesirable side-effect of drugs used to treat disease and can contribute to the undernutrition seen in chronically ill people (Section 8.4). As an aid to weight reduction, especially in people who find it difficult to control their food intake, drugs that suppress appetite may be useful.

A number of compounds that have been used as appetite suppressants, including amphetamine (highly addictive and now a controlled drug): fenfluramine (and the D-isomer, dexfenfluramine), phentermine, diethylpropion, and mazindol have been withdrawn from the market because of problems of psychiatric disturbance and possible addiction. The combination of phentermine and fenfluramine was withdrawn in the 1990s, after a number of reports associating it with cardiac damage, although the problems were later associated with fenfluramine, and phentermine is still used, albeit with the danger of addiction and abuse. Rimonabant was withdrawn in 2009 because of an association with severe depression and an increase in suicide. Sibutramine was withdrawn in 2010 because of an association with cardiovascular events and strokes.

Topiramate, an anti-convulsant medication used to treat epilepsy and migraine, leads to appetite suppression as a side-effect. It has been licenced for use as an appetite suppressant drug, in combination with phentermine. Zonisamide is another anti-convulsant drug that leads to weight loss and appetite suppression as a side-effect. Three clinical trials of its use in treating obesity seem to have been conducted; two appear not to have reported any results (suggesting lack of efficacy or safety) and the third reported better weight loss than with placebo, but with no statistics reported; thus, it is not possible to evaluate its efficacy. Bupropion is an antidepressant and is used to aid smoking cessation. There is some evidence of efficacy for weight loss, and it is undergoing clinical trials in combination with zonisamide.

The South African succulent plant *Hoodia gordonii* has been traditionally used by the San people of the Kalahari to stave off hunger, and a steroid glycoside has been isolated from the plant that has an anorectic action in experimental animals. However, there is no evidence from clinical trials that it is effective for weight reduction in human beings, and it is doubtful how much of the active ingredient survives first-pass metabolism in the liver. Controversially, when the active steroid glycoside was first isolated from hoodia, the plant was patented by the South African Council for Scientific and Industrial Research. Subsequently, when licences were granted to a major pharmaceutical company to exploit hoodia, the terms included payment of royalties to the San people for the plant, which is endangered and on the list of plants prohibited from international trade without a specific licence from the Convention on International Trade in Endangered Species (CITES). Two major international companies have released their rights to exploit hoodia because of lack of evidence of efficacy and the difficulty of either synthesising the active compound or ensuring the safety and activity of extracts from the plant. Despite the lack of evidence, supplements of (or purporting to contain) hoodia are widely marketed with claims to reduce appetite and lower blood pressure.

A number of compounds have been marketed as 'carbohydrate blockers', which are supposed to act by inhibiting amylase (Section 4.2.2.1), thus reducing the digestion of starch. There is no evidence that they are effective, and none has been licenced for pharmaceutical use. Similarly, there is no evidence of efficacy of compounds that are marketed as 'fat burners', which are supposed to increase the rate at which fat is metabolised; if they were effective, they would increase metabolic rate to such an extent that the consumer would have a persistent fever.

Inhibitors of pancreatic lipase (Section 4.3.2) reduce lipid digestion and absorption, and some (e.g. Xenical®) have been licenced for use in morbidly obese patients who have made a serious effort to lose weight by more conventional means. Xenical is also available over the counter is some countries under the trade name of Allitame®. The problem with the use of lipase inhibitors is that undigested fat in the gastrointestinal tract can cause discomfort, and if enough is present, foul-smelling fatty diarrhoea (steatorrhoea).

7.3.4.13 Surgical treatment of obesity

Severe obesity may be treated by surgical removal of much of the excess adipose tissue—a procedure known as liposuction. A number of further surgical treatments have also been used, but there is a considerable risk in undertaking any surgery in obese people (Section 7.2.2):

- Intestinal by-pass surgery, in which the jejunum is connected to the distal end of the ileum, thus bypassing most of the small intestine where the digestion and absorption of food occurs (Section 4.1). The resultant malabsorption means that the subject can, and indeed must, eat a relatively large amount of food, but will only absorb a small proportion. There are severe side effects of intestinal by-pass surgery, including persistent foul-smelling diarrhoea and flatulence and failure to absorb medication, as well as problems of mineral and vitamin deficiency. This procedure has been more or less abandoned in most centres.
- Gastroplasty and partial gastric by-pass, in which the physical capacity of the stomach is reduced to half or less. This limits the amount of food that can be consumed at any one meal. Whilst the results of such surgery appear promising, long-term follow-up suggests that some patients experience serious side-effects, including micronutrient deficiencies. However, gastroplasty and gastric bypass may have a beneficial effect beyond that from reducing the physical capacity of the stomach. If the gastric fundus is removed then the secretion of the appetite stimulating hormone ghrelin (Section 1.4.1.2) is significantly reduced.

7.3.4.14 Help and support

Especially for the severely obese person, weight loss is a lengthy and difficult experience. Friends and family can be supportive, but frequently specialist help and advice are needed. To a great extent, this is the role of the dietitian and other health-care professionals. In addition, there are a number of organisations, normally of formerly obese people, who can offer a mixture of professional nutritional and dietetic advice together with practical help and counselling. The main advantage of such groups is that they provide a social setting, rather than the formal setting of the dietitian's office in an out-patient clinic, and fellow members have experienced similar problems. Many people find the sharing of the problems and experiences of weight reduction extremely helpful.

Key points

- Obesity is a major problem of public health in developed countries, and increasingly so in developing countries; worldwide, there are now more overweight and obese people than undernourished.
- BMI provides a convenient way of classifying ranges of body weight. There is a considerable increase in premature mortality amongst people who are obese (BMI > 30).
- Various ways can be used to assess the total body fat content, but only imaging techniques permit differentiation between subcutaneous fat and visceral (inter-organ) fat. Excess visceral fat poses a more serious threat to health than does subcutaneous fat.

- Obese people are more likely to suffer from a range of physical illnesses and to experience social problems; they are more at risk of death during surgery.
- Abdominal obesity leads to the development of insulin resistance and the metabolic syndrome, which develops into type II diabetes mellitus.
- Obesity is associated with chronic low-grade inflammation and increased oxidative stress.
- The underlying cause of obesity is a low level of physical activity coupled with plentiful availability of food, especially food that is high in fat and sugars. High-fructose consumption may be a contributor to excessive synthesis of fatty acids.
- Effective treatment of obesity requires not only energy restriction to lose weight, but changes to diet habits and physical activity to maintain reduced weight. The most successful slimming regimes are those that are somewhat more restricted versions of the general advice for a prudent diet.

chapter eight

Protein-energy malnutrition
Problems of undernutrition

If the intake of metabolic fuels is lower than is required to meet energy expenditure, the body's reserves of fat, carbohydrate (glycogen), and protein are used. Undernutrition may develop because of inadequate food intake (due to lack of food or pathological disorders of appetite), increased metabolic rate as a result of cancer and other chronic diseases, or malabsorption. Especially in lean people, who have small reserves of body fat, there can be a large loss of tissue protein (to provide substrates for gluconeogenesis) when food intake is inadequate. As the deficiency continues, there is increasing loss of tissue, until eventually essential tissue proteins are catabolised as metabolic fuels—a process that obviously cannot continue for long.

Objectives

After reading this chapter, you should be able to

- Explain what is meant by protein-energy malnutrition, and differentiate between marasmus and kwashiorkor
- Explain why marasmus can be considered to be the predictable outcome of prolonged negative energy balance
- Describe the groups of people in developed countries who are at risk of protein-energy malnutrition
- Describe the features of cachexia, and explain how it differs from marasmus
- Describe the features of kwashiorkor, and explain how it differs from marasmus

8.1   Problems of deficiency

Human beings have evolved in a hostile environment in which food has always been scarce. Only in the past half-century has there been a surplus of food, and in much of sub-Saharan Africa, food is still in short supply. There is a twofold difference in the food available per head of population between the wealthiest and poorest countries. In some developing countries, there is only some 8.2 MJ available per person, and this does not take account of wastage of food through spoilage and damage by pests.

Although food available per head of population has increased in most countries, in many sub-Saharan African countries, it has decreased over the past decade. The increased yields of food crops resulting from the green revolution of the late 20th century have been overcome by increased population, severe adverse weather (both droughts and floods, sometimes in the same year in different regions of the world), and increasing use in developed countries of food crops (especially maize, sugar cane, and soya) for production of biofuels as an alternative to the use of oil. Almost one in seven of the world's population (a total of just over 1 billion people) suffer from food insecurity—even if their foods needs are met now, this cannot be guaranteed throughout the year. One hundred and eighty million children worldwide are undernourished, and up to 210 million people are at risk of undernutrition. Nevertheless, despite the increase in population, the percentage of people undernourished worldwide has decreased from 19% in 1990 to 12% in 2012.

Figure 8.1 shows the numbers of people who are so undernourished that they have a body mass index (BMI) <17; whilst most of these people are in developing countries, a significant number of people in developed countries are also undernourished.

Figure 8.2 shows the increase in the world's population from 1 billion in 1800 to the present 6.5 billion, and the predicted increase through the present century until it stabilises around 11–12 billion by 2100. Most of this increase will be in developing countries that

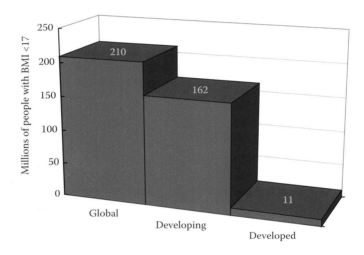

Figure 8.1 Numbers of people with BMI less than 17. (From United Nations Food and Agriculture Organization data.)

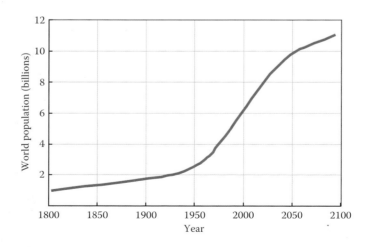

Figure 8.2 World population growth 1800–2100. (From World Health Organization data.)

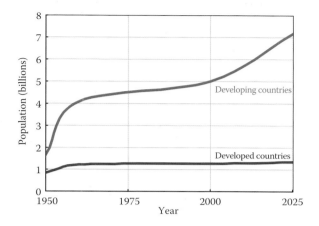

Figure 8.3 Population growth in developed and developing countries 1950–2025. (From World Health Organization data.)

already suffer from malnutrition and food shortages (Figure 8.3). It is difficult to see how food production can be increased to match this increase in population.

Deficiency of individual nutrients is also a major problem—the total amount of food may be adequate to satisfy hunger, but the quality of the diet is inadequate. Deficiencies of vitamin A (Section 11.2.4), iron (Sections 11.15.2.3 and 11.16), and iodine (Section 11.15.3.3) are major public health problems worldwide and are priority targets for the World Health Organization. Deficiency of vitamins B_1 (Section 11.6.3) and B_2 (Section 11.7.3) continues to be a problem in parts of Asia and Africa, and selenium deficiency (Section 11.15.2.5) is a significant problem in large areas of China, and elsewhere.

8.2 Protein-energy malnutrition

The terms *protein-energy malnutrition* and *protein-energy deficiency* are used to mean a general lack of food, as opposed to specific deficiencies of vitamins or minerals (discussed in Chapter 11). The problem is not one of protein deficiency, but rather a deficiency of metabolic fuels. Indeed, there may be a relative excess of protein, in that protein that might be used for tissue protein replacement, or for growth in children, is being used as a fuel because of the deficiency of energy intake.

This was demonstrated in a series of studies in India in the early 1980s. Children whose intake of protein was marginally adequate were given additional carbohydrate (as sugary drinks). They showed an increase in growth, and the deposition of new body protein. This was because their previous energy intake was inadequate; increasing their energy intake both spared dietary protein for the synthesis of tissue proteins and also provided an adequate energy source to meet the high energy cost of protein synthesis (Section 9.2.3.3). After the need for water, the body's first requirement, at all times, is for an adequate source of metabolic fuels. Only when energy requirements have been met can dietary protein be used for tissue protein synthesis.

The severity of protein-energy malnutrition in adults can be assessed from the BMI (the ratio of weight, in kg, to height², in m, Section 7.1.1), as shown in Table 8.1.

Table 8.1 Classification of Protein-Energy Malnutrition by BMI

BMI	
20–25	Desirable range
18.5–20	Underweight but acceptable
17–18.4	Moderate protein-energy malnutrition
16–17	Moderately severe protein-energy malnutrition
<16	Severe protein-energy malnutrition

Note: BMI = weight (kg)/height^2 (m).

Table 8.2 Classification of Protein-Energy Malnutrition in Children

	No oedema	Oedema
60%–80% of expected weight for age	Underweight	Kwashiorkor
<60% of expected weight for age	Marasmus	Marasmic-kwashiorkor

There are two extreme forms of protein-energy malnutrition:

1. Marasmus can occur in both adults and children and occurs in vulnerable groups of the population in developed countries as well as in developing countries.
2. Kwashiorkor only affects children, and has only been reported in developing countries. The distinguishing feature of kwashiorkor is that there is fluid retention, leading to oedema, together with fatty infiltration of the liver.

Protein-energy malnutrition in children can be classified by both the deficit in weight compared with what would be expected for age and also the presence or absence of oedema, as shown in Table 8.2. The most severely affected group, and therefore the priority group for intervention, are those suffering from marasmic kwashiorkor—they are both severely undernourished and also oedematous.

8.2.1 Detection of malnutrition in adults

The British Association for Parenteral and Enteral Nutrition (BAPEN) has developed a screening tool to detect malnutrition in adults—the Malnutrition Universal Screening Tool (MUST). Scores are given for the following:

- The patient's current BMI
  - BMI ≥ 20, score = 0
  - BMI 18.5–20, score = 1
  - BMI < 18.5, score = 2
- Any unintentional weight loss over the last 3–6 months
  - <5%, score = 0
  - 5%–10%, score = 1
  - >10%, score = 2
- An additional score of 2 is added for an acute disease effect and if there has been, or is likely to be, no food intake for more than 5 days.

These scores are then summed to calculate the overall risk of malnutrition, which determines the appropriate course of action:

- Score = 0. There is a low risk of malnutrition, and no action need be taken, although repeated screening will be required weekly in hospital, monthly in care homes, and annually for people living in the community who are at special risk (especially those aged over 75).
- Score = 1. There is a medium risk of malnutrition, and the patient needs to be observed. In hospitals and care homes, this means taking a record of food and fluid intake for 3 days. For people living in the community, there should be a repeated screen in 1–6 months, and appropriate dietary advice may be required.
- Score = 2. There is a high risk of malnutrition, and treatment is necessary. This will generally be referral to a dietitian to encourage better eating, although supplemental feeding and food fortification may be required. In extreme cases, intravenous feeding may also be required.

8.3   Marasmus

Marasmus is a state of extreme emaciation; the name is derived from the Greek for wasting. It is the predictable outcome of prolonged negative energy balance, with severe depletion of all body energy reserves.

Not only have fat reserves been exhausted, but there is wastage of muscle as well, and as the condition progresses there is loss of protein from the heart, liver, and kidneys, although as far as possible, essential tissue proteins are protected. Protein synthesis is energy expensive (Section 9.2.3.3), and in marasmus, there is a considerable reduction in the rate of protein synthesis, although catabolism continues at the normal rate (Section 9.1.1). The amino acids released by the catabolism of tissues proteins are substrates for gluconeogenesis to maintain a supply of glucose for the brain and red blood cells (Section 5.7). Those that cannot be used for gluconeogenesis are metabolised as metabolic fuels or used for ketone body synthesis to provide fuel for muscle (Section 5.5.3).

As a result of the reduced protein synthesis, there is a considerable impairment of immune responses; thus, undernourished people are more at risk from infections than those who are adequately fed. Diseases that are minor childhood illnesses in developed countries can often prove fatal to undernourished children in developing countries. Measles is commonly cited as the cause of death, although it would be more correct to give the true cause of death as malnutrition.

One of the proteins secreted by the liver, which is most severely affected by protein-energy malnutrition, is the plasma retinol binding protein, which transports vitamin A from liver stores to its sites of action (Section 11.2.2.2). As a result, there are clinical signs of vitamin A deficiency; although there may be adequate reserves in the liver, they cannot be mobilised because of a lack of the binding protein.

A more serious effect of protein-energy malnutrition is impairment of cell proliferation in the intestinal mucosa. The villi are shorter than usual, and in severe cases the intestinal mucosa is almost flat. This results in a considerable reduction in the surface area of the intestinal mucosa, and hence a reduction in the absorption of such nutrients as are available from the diet. As a result, diarrhoea is a common feature of protein-energy malnutrition. Thus, not only does the undernourished person have an inadequate intake of food, but the absorption of what is available is impaired, compounding the problem.

Undernutrition also results in reduced muscle strength and increased fatigability, leading to inactivity and inability to work and may also predispose to falls. Reduced strength of the respiratory muscles predisposes to chest infections, and impairs recovery from chest infections as well as leading to a poor prognosis under general anaesthesia. At the same time, inactivity predisposes to sores and thromboembolism, impaired thermogenesis leads to hypothermia, and reduced protein synthesis impairs wound healing. Even when not accompanied by physical illness, undernutrition causes apathy, depression, self-neglect, hypochondriasis, loss of libido, and deterioration in social interactions.

8.3.1   Causes of marasmus and vulnerable groups of the population

In developing countries, the cause of marasmus is either a chronic shortage of food or the more acute problem of famine, where there will be very little food available at all. All too frequently, famine comes after a long-term shortage of food; thus, its effects are all the more rapid and serious. Even when food is available in the markets, its cost is beyond the reach of many.

A lack of food is unlikely to be a problem in developed countries, although the most socially and economically disadvantaged in the community are at risk. In Britain, 2% of adults have a BMI < 18.5, and one survey showed that 40% of consecutive hospital admissions were at least mildly undernourished. A study by the Royal College of Physicians in 2002 found that 3% of men and 6% of women who were living in their own homes were significantly undernourished. For people living in care homes the situation was considerably worse, with 16% of men and 15% of women significantly undernourished. Overall, it is estimated that there are 2 million undernourished people in the UK (3% of the population), and the cost to the National Health Service of treating malnutrition and its clinical sequelae is in excess of £7 billion per year.

Three further factors may cause undernutrition: disorders of appetite, impairment of the absorption of nutrients, and allergic responses to and intolerance of foods.

8.3.1.1   Malabsorption

Any clinical condition that impairs the absorption of nutrients from the intestinal tract will lead to undernutrition, despite an apparently adequate intake. Obviously, major intestinal surgery will result in a reduction in the amount of intestine available for the digestion and absorption of nutrients. Here the problem is known in advance, and precautionary measures can be taken: a period of intravenous feeding to supplement normal food intake and careful counselling by a dietitian to ensure adequate nutrient intake despite the problems.

A variety of infectious diseases can cause malabsorption and diarrhoea. In many cases, this lasts only a few days and so has no long-term consequences. However, some intestinal parasites can cause long-lasting diarrhoea and damage to the intestinal mucosa, leading to malnutrition if the infection persists for too long.

8.3.1.2   Food intolerance and allergy

The problem of disaccharide intolerance was discussed in Section 4.2.2.2. Food allergies, involving an immune response and the production of antibodies, as opposed to intolerance, which does not, result from the absorption of relatively large intact peptides derived from dietary proteins (Section 4.4.3.2). Allergic reactions to foods may include dermatitis, eczema, and urticaria, asthma, allergic rhinitis, muscle pain, rheumatoid arthritis, and migraine as well as effects on the gastrointestinal tract. In severe cases, exposure to a food can cause potentially fatal anaphylactic shock. These reactions are likely to impair the sufferer's appetite and may contribute to undernutrition. There can be serious damage to the intestinal mucosa, leading to severe malabsorption, and hence malnutrition despite an apparently adequate intake of food. Allergy to nut proteins (and especially peanuts) has become a common problem, and other common allergens include cow's milk, eggs, shellfish, strawberries, and kiwifruit; laws in many countries now require that potential allergens from a standard list that may be present in the food must be declared on the label.

In general, once the offending food has been identified, the patient's condition has stabilised, and body weight has been restored, continuing treatment is relatively easy, although avoidance of some common foods may provide significant problems. It is the identification of the offending food that provides the greatest problem and frequently calls for lengthy investigations, maintaining the patient on a very limited range of foods, then gradually introducing additional foods, until the offending item is identified.

Patients with food intolerances or allergies are generally extremely ill after they have eaten the offending food, and this may persist for several days. Even after the offending foods have been identified, and the patient's condition has been stabilised, there may be continuing problems of appetite and eating behaviour.

Coeliac disease is an allergy to one specific protein in wheat and some other cereals—the gliadin fraction of gluten. There is a gradient in the prevalence of coeliac disease across Europe, with the lowest rates in the Middle East, where wheat was first introduced as a dietary staple, and the highest in Ireland, where wheat only became a major food in the late 19th century.

There is a considerable loss of intestinal mucosa in coeliac disease and flattening of the intestinal villi, so that the appearance of the intestine is similar to that seen in marasmus. This reduction in the absorptive surface of the intestine leads to persistent fatty diarrhoea (steatorrhoea) and a failure to absorb nutrients. The result is undernutrition, and severe emaciation can occur in patients with untreated coeliac disease. Once the diagnosis is established, and the immediate problems of undernutrition have been dealt with, treatment is by avoidance of all wheat, barley, and rye-based products; oats are also sometimes a problem. In practice, this is less easy than it sounds—apart from the obvious foods, such as bread and pasta, wheat flour is used in a great many food products. There is therefore a need for counselling from a dietitian, and careful reading of labels for lists of ingredients. A number of products have the symbol of the Coeliac Society on the label to show that they are known to be free from gluten, and therefore safe for patients to eat, and many supermarkets now have a shelf or aisle of gluten-free breads, cakes, biscuits, and pasta. Gluten-free bread is also increasingly widely available in restaurants and hotels.

8.4   Cachexia

Patients with advanced cancer, HIV infection and AIDS, and a number of other chronic diseases are frequently undernourished. Physically, they show all the signs of marasmus, but there is considerably more loss of body protein than occurs in starvation. The condition is called cachexia, from the Greek for 'in a poor condition'. A number of factors contribute to the problem:

- The patients are extremely sick, and because of this, appetite may be impaired.
- Many of the drugs used in chemotherapy can cause nausea, loss of appetite, and alteration of the senses of taste and smell (Section 1.4.3.1), so that foods that were appetising are now unappetising or even aversive.
- Chemotherapy and radiotherapy inhibit cell division, leading to reduced cell proliferation in the intestinal mucosa, villous atrophy, and malabsorption.

- There is a considerable increase in basal metabolic rate, to the extent that patients are described as being hypermetabolic.
- A number of cytokines increase the rate of breakdown of tissue protein. This is a major difference from marasmus, in which protein synthesis is reduced, but catabolism in unaffected.

8.4.1   Hypermetabolism in cachexia

Many tumours metabolise glucose anaerobically to release lactate. This is then used for gluconeogenesis in the liver; there is a cost of 4 mol of ATP and 2 mol of GTP for each mol of glucose reformed from lactate (Figure 5.13), and hence, there has to be an increased rate of metabolism in the liver to provide this ATP and GTP. Figure 8.4 shows the increase in glucose cycling in hypermetabolic patients with advanced cancer.

The cytokines secreted in response to many tumours and in inflammatory disease stimulate mitochondrial uncoupling proteins (Section 3.3.1.5), leading to thermogenesis and hence increased oxidation of metabolic fuels. An increase in body temperature of 1°C is equivalent to a 13% increase in metabolic rate.

Hormone-sensitive lipase in adipose tissue (Sections 5.3.2 and 10.5.1) is activated by a small proteoglycan produced by tumours that cause cachexia. This results in increased liberation of fatty acids from adipose tissue, with re-esterification to triacylglycerols (which are exported in VLDL, Section 5.6.2.2) in the liver—futile cycling of lipids. The esterification of fatty acids requires 6 mol of ATP per mol of triacylglycerol formed (Section 5.6.1.2).

8.4.2   Increased protein catabolism in cachexia

As in marasmus, protein synthesis is impaired as a result of low availability of ATP. In addition, there is a considerable depletion of individual amino acids, resulting in an incomplete mixture of amino acids available for protein synthesis, for three main reasons:

1. Many tumours have a high requirement for glutamine and leucine.
2. There is increased utilisation of alanine and other amino acids as a result of the stimulation of gluconeogenesis by tumour necrosis factor.
3. Interferon-γ induces indoleamine dioxygenase and depletes tissue pools of tryptophan.

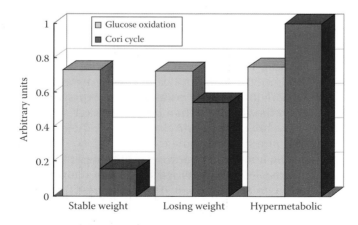

Figure 8.4 Glucose cycling in patients with cancer cachexia.

Unlike marasmus, cachexia is characterised by an increase in the rate of protein catabolism as well as reduced synthesis. Tumor necrosis factor causes increased protein catabolism, by increasing both the expression of ubiquitin and the activity of the ubiquitin-dependent protease (Section 9.1.1.1). The proteoglycan produced by tumours that cause cachexia also stimulates protein catabolism—in this case, the mechanism is unknown.

8.5 Kwashiorkor

Kwashiorkor was first described in Ghana, in west Africa, in 1932—the word is the Ga name for the condition. In addition to the wasting of muscle tissue, loss of intestinal mucosa (leading to diarrhoea) and impaired immune responses seen in marasmus, children with kwashiorkor show a number of characteristic features that distinguish this disease:

- Fluid retention, and hence severe oedema, associated with a decreased concentration of plasma proteins. The puffiness of the limbs, due to the oedema, masks the severe wasting of muscles.
- Enlargement of the liver due to the accumulation of abnormally large amounts of fat in the liver, to the extent that instead of its normal reddish-brown colour, the liver is pale yellow when examined at *post-mortem* or during surgery. The metabolic basis for this fatty infiltration of the liver is not known. It is the enlargement of the liver that causes the paradoxical 'pot-bellied' appearance of children with kwashiorkor; together with the oedema, they appear, from a distance, to be plump, yet they are starving.
- Characteristic changes in the texture and colour of the hair. This is most noticeable in African children—instead of tightly curled black hair, children with kwashiorkor have sparse, wispy hair, which is less curled than normal and poorly pigmented—it is often reddish or even grey.
- A sooty, sunburn-like skin rash.
- A characteristic expression of deep misery.

8.5.1 Factors in the aetiology of kwashiorkor

The underlying cause of kwashiorkor is an inadequate intake of food, as is the case for marasmus. Kwashiorkor traditionally affects children aged between 3 and 5 years. In many societies, a child continues to suckle until about this age, when the next child is born. As a result, the toddler is abruptly weaned, frequently onto very unsuitable food. In some societies, children are weaned onto a dilute gruel made from whatever is the local cereal; in others, the child may be fed on the water in which rice has been boiled—it may look like milk, but has little nutritional value. Sometimes, the child is given little or no special treatment but has to compete with the rest of the family for its share from the stew pot. A small child has little chance of getting an adequate meal under such conditions, especially if there is not much food for the whole family anyway.

There is no satisfactory explanation for the development of kwashiorkor rather than marasmus. At one time, it was believed that it was due to a lack of protein, with a more or less adequate intake of energy. However, analysis of the diets of children suffering from kwashiorkor shows that this is not so. Furthermore, children who are protein deficient have a slower rate of growth and are therefore stunted (Section 9.1.2.2); as shown in Figure 8.5, children with kwashiorkor are less stunted than those with marasmus. Finally, many of the signs of kwashiorkor, and especially the oedema, begin to improve early in treatment, when the child is still receiving a low protein diet (Section 8.5.2).

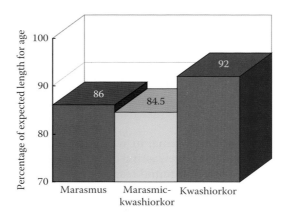

Figure 8.5 Stunting of growth in kwashiorkor, marasmus, and marasmic-kwashiorkor.

Very commonly, an infection precipitates kwashiorkor in children whose nutritional status is inadequate, even if they are not yet showing signs of malnutrition. Indeed, paediatricians in developing countries expect an outbreak of kwashiorkor a few months after an outbreak of measles.

The most likely precipitating factor is that, superimposed on general food deficiency, there is a deficiency of the antioxidant nutrients such as zinc, copper, carotene, and vitamins C and E (Section 6.5.3). The macrophage respiratory burst in response to infection leads to the production of oxygen and halogen radicals as part of their cytotoxic action (Section 6.5.2.2). The added oxidant stress of an infection may well trigger the sequence of events that leads to the development of kwashiorkor.

8.5.2 Rehabilitation of malnourished children

The intestinal tract of the malnourished child is in a very poor state. This means that the child is not able to deal at all adequately with a rich diet, or a large amount of food. Rather, treatment begins with small frequent feeding of liquids—a dilute sugar solution for the first few days, followed by diluted milk, and then full strength milk. This may be achieved by use of a nasogastric tube so that the dilute solution can be provided at a slow and constant rate throughout the day and night. Where such luxuries are not available, the malnourished infant is fed from a teaspoon, a few drops at a time, more or less continually.

Once the patient has begun to develop a more normal intestinal mucosa (when the diarrhoea ceases), ordinary foods can gradually be introduced. Recovery is normally rapid in children, and they soon begin to grow at a normal rate.

Key points

- Although food available per head of population has increased in most countries (apart from sub-Saharan Africa), undernutrition remains a problem, and predicted population growth is unlikely to be matched by further increases in food production.
- Protein-energy malnutrition is a lack of total food, and not specifically of protein.
- Marasmus is the predictable outcome of prolonged energy depletion: loss of adipose tissue reserves and wasting of muscle as a result of decreased protein synthesis.

- Cachexia in chronic diseases resembles marasmus, but in addition, there is hypermetabolism and increased protein catabolism.
- Kwashiorkor involves oedema as well as wasting; the trigger to develop kwashiorkor in an undernourished child is probably radical damage, superimposed on general undernutrition.

chapter nine

Protein nutrition and metabolism

The need for protein in the diet was demonstrated early in the 19th century, when it was shown that animals fed only on fats, carbohydrates, and mineral salts were unable to maintain their body weight and showed severe wasting of muscle and other tissues. It was known that proteins contain nitrogen (mainly in the amino groups of their constituent amino acids, Section 4.4.1), and methods for measuring the total amount of nitrogenous compounds in foods and excreta were soon developed. It is obvious that a growing child or animal requires a dietary intake of protein to increase the total protein content of the body with growth. However, it was not until the middle of the 20th century that it became clear why an adult also requires a daily intake of protein. There is continual catabolism and replacement of tissue proteins. In the fasting state between meals, proteins are catabolised to provide amino acids for gluconeogenesis (Section 5.7), and in the fed state, amino acids in excess of immediate requirements for protein synthesis are not stored, but are catabolised and used as metabolic fuel.

Objectives

After reading this chapter, you should be able to

- Explain what is meant by the terms nitrogen balance and dynamic equilibrium.
- Describe the processes involved in tissue protein catabolism.
- Explain the basis for current recommendations for protein intake, and for essential and non-essential amino acids.
- Explain what is meant by protein nutritional value or quality, and why it is of little importance in most diets.
- Describe the processes involved in protein synthesis, desribe in outline the flow of information from DNA → RNA → protein, and explain the energy cost of protein synthesis.
- Describe and explain the pathways by which the amino nitrogen of amino acids is metabolised and explain the importance of transamination.
- Describe and explain the metabolism of ammonia and the synthesis of urea.
- Describe the metabolic fates of the carbon skeletons of amino acids.

9.1   Nitrogen balance and protein requirements

Figure 9.1 shows an overview of protein metabolism; in addition to the dietary intake of about 90 g of protein, a considerably larger amount, up to 200 g, of endogenous protein is secreted into the intestinal lumen. This endogenous protein consists of digestive enzymes, albumin, and other proteins, the proteins in shed intestinal mucosal cells, and mucin in the protective mucus that is secreted throughout the gastrointestinal tract for protection of cells against the actions of digestive enzymes. There is a small faecal loss equivalent to about 10 g of protein/day; the remainder is hydrolysed to free amino acids and small

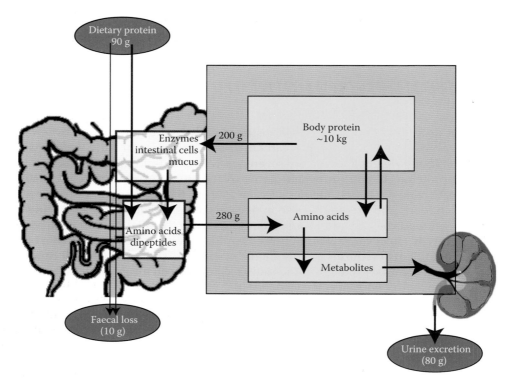

Figure 9.1 An overview of protein metabolism.

peptides that are absorbed (Section 4.4.3.2); thus, the total amount of amino acids and small peptides absorbed is more than twice the dietary intake of protein. The faecal loss of nitrogen is partly composed of undigested dietary protein, but the main contributors are intestinal bacteria and shed mucosal cells, which are only partially broken down, and mucin in mucus secreted by intestinal mucosal goblet cells (Figure 4.2). Mucin is especially resistant to enzymic hydrolysis and contributes a considerable proportion of inevitable losses of nitrogen, even on a protein-free diet.

There is a small pool of free amino acids in the body, in equilibrium with proteins that are being catabolised and synthesised. A small proportion of this amino acid pool is used for synthesis of a variety of specialised metabolites (including hormones and neurotransmitters, purines, and pyrimidines). An amount of amino acids equivalent to that absorbed from the dietary intake is oxidised, with the carbon skeletons being used for gluconeogenesis (Sections 5.7 and 9.3.2) or as metabolic fuels and the nitrogen being excreted, mainly as urea (Section 9.3.1.4).

The state of protein nutrition, and the overall state of body protein metabolism, can be determined by measuring the dietary intake of nitrogenous compounds and the output of nitrogenous compounds from the body. Although nucleic acids contain nitrogen (Sections 9.2.1 and 9.2.2), protein is the major dietary source of nitrogenous compounds, and measurement of total nitrogen intake gives a good estimate of protein intake. Nitrogen constitutes 16% of most proteins, and therefore the protein content of foods is calculated based on milligrams of nitrogen × 6.25, although for some foods with an unusual amino acid composition, other factors are used.

sources of protein. With diets based largely on cassava, there is a more serious problem in meeting protein requirements.

9.1.2.1   Protein requirements for physical activity and body building

Some early calculations of protein requirements and desirable levels of intake showed an increasing protein intake for people with a high energy expenditure in occupational work or sport (Section 6.3.3.1). There is no evidence that higher physical activity increases protein requirements. Rather, it was assumed that as physical activity, and so energy requirement, increased, more of the same types of food, typically providing 10% of energy from protein, would be eaten. Therefore, the protein intake would increase with energy expenditure, but this was not a higher requirement for protein, simply the result of practical nutrition.

Similarly, there is little evidence that sportspeople and body builders have a higher requirement for protein than would be met by eating normal foods. The American Dietetic Association position paper on nutrition and athletic performance makes a protein recommendation for endurance and strength-trained athletes of 1.2–1.7 g/kg body weight, with the statement that 'These recommended protein intakes can generally be met through diet without the use of protein or amino acid supplements. Energy intake sufficient to maintain body weight is necessary for optimal protein use' (American College of Sports Medicine and American Dietetic Association of Dietitians of Canada, 2009).

Even in children recovering from protein-energy malnutrition (Chapter 8), who have a high rate of net protein synthesis, total synthesis is two to three times greater than the net gain in body protein. Protein synthesis is energy expensive (Section 9.2.3.3), and for increased muscle protein synthesis in response to training, the need is for energy rather than protein. There is little evidence that the various protein supplements widely marketed to athletes permit any greater increase in muscle protein synthesis than ordinary foods would. There is also the concern that some of these sports supplements may contain undeclared ingredients, including steroid hormones, which may increase tissue protein synthesis, but are banned substances in competitive sport.

9.1.2.2   Protein requirements of children

Because children are growing, and increasing the total amount of protein in the body, they have a proportionally greater requirement for protein than do adults (Table 9.3). A

Table 9.3 Safe Levels of Protein Intake for Children and Adolescents

Age (years)	Safe level of intake, g/kg body weight/day
0.5	1.31
1	1.14
1.5	1.03
2	0.97
3	0.90
4–6	0.87
7–10	0.92
11–14	0.90 (male)
	0.89 (female)
15–18	0.87 (male)
	0.84 (female)

Source: Protein and Amino Acid Requirements in Human Nutrition, WHO Technical
Reports Series 935, World Health Organization, Geneva, 2007.

growing child should be in positive nitrogen balance. However, the need for protein for growth is relatively small compared with the requirement for protein turnover. Children in Western countries consume more protein than is needed to meet their requirements, but in developing countries, protein intake may well be inadequate to meet the requirement for growth.

A protein-deficient child will grow more slowly than one receiving an adequate intake of protein—this is stunting of growth. The protein-energy deficiency diseases, marasmus, and kwashiorkor (Sections 8.3 and 8.4) result from a general lack of food (and hence metabolic fuels), not a specific deficiency of protein. Nevertheless, many children in developing countries are stunted because their diet provides a more or less adequate energy intake but inadequate protein.

9.1.2.3   *Protein losses in trauma and infection—requirements for convalescence*

One of the metabolic reactions to a major trauma, such as a burn, a broken limb, or surgery, is an increase in the net catabolism of tissue proteins. As shown in Table 9.4, apart from the loss of blood associated with injury, as much as 750 g of protein (about 6%–7% of the total body content) may be lost over 10 days. Even prolonged bed rest results in a considerable loss of protein because there is atrophy of muscles that are not used. Muscle protein is catabolised as normal, but without the stimulus of exercise, less is replaced.

This protein loss is mediated by the hormone cortisol, which is secreted in response to stress, and the cytokines that are secreted in response to trauma; four mechanisms are involved:

1. Induction of tryptophan dioxygenase and tyrosine transaminase by cortisol and some cytokines. This results in depletion of the tissue pools of these two amino acids, leaving an unbalanced mixture that cannot be used for protein synthesis (Section 9.2.3.2).
2. In response to cytokine action, there is an increase in metabolic rate, leading to an increased rate of oxidation of amino acids as metabolic fuel, thus reducing the amount available for protein synthesis.
3. Some cytokines cause an increase in the rate of protein catabolism, as occurs in cachexia (Section 8.4).
4. A variety of plasma proteins synthesised in increased amount in response to cytokine action (the acute phase proteins) are richer in two amino acids, cysteine and threonine, than most tissue proteins. This leads to depletion of tissue pools of these two amino acids, again leaving an unbalanced mixture that cannot be used for protein synthesis.

Table 9.4 Protein Losses over 10 Days after Trauma or Infection

	Tissue loss	Blood loss	Catabolism	Total
Fracture of femur	–	200	700	900
Muscle wound	500–750	150–400	750	1350–1900
35% burns	500	150–400	750	1400–1650
Gastrectomy	20–180	20–10	625–750	645–850
Typhoid fever	–	–	675	685

Source: Data reported by Cuthbertson, D. P., Chapter 19, pp. 373–414, in *Human Protein Metabolism*, Vol II, Munro, H. N. and Allison, J. B. (Eds.), New York, Academic Press, 1964.

The lost protein has to be replaced during recovery, and patients who are convalescing will be in positive nitrogen balance. However, this does not mean that a convalescent patient requires a diet that is richer in protein than usual. As discussed in Section 9.1.2, average protein intakes are higher than requirements; a normal diet that provides sufficient energy will provide adequate protein to permit replacement of the losses due to illness and hospitalisation.

9.1.3   Essential amino acids

Early studies of nitrogen balance showed that not all proteins are nutritionally equivalent. More of some than others is needed to maintain nitrogen balance. This is because different proteins contain different amounts of the various amino acids (Section 4.4.1). The body's requirement is not simply for protein, but for the amino acids that make up proteins, in the correct proportions to replace the body proteins.

There are nine essential or indispensable amino acids, which cannot be synthesised in the body (Table 9.5). If one of these is provided in inadequate amounts, then regardless of the total intake of protein, it will not be possible to maintain nitrogen balance because there will not be enough of this limiting amino acid for protein synthesis to replace all losses from turnover.

For infants, a tenth amino acid, arginine, is essential. Although adults can synthesise adequate amounts of arginine to meet their requirements, the capacity for arginine synthesis is low in infants, and may not be adequate to meet the requirements for growth. Because the pathway of arginine synthesis is also the pathway for synthesis of urea for excretion of excess nitrogen (Section 9.3.1.4), infants are susceptible to hyperammonaemia if they are fed an excessively high protein intake.

Two amino acids, cysteine and tyrosine, can only be synthesised in the body from essential precursors—cysteine from methionine and tyrosine from phenylalanine. The dietary intakes of cysteine and tyrosine thus affect the requirements for methionine and phenylalanine—if more of either is provided in the diet, then less will have to be synthesised from the essential precursor.

The remaining amino acids are considered to be non-essential or dispensable; they can be synthesised from metabolic intermediates as long as there is enough total protein in the diet. If one of these amino acids is omitted from the diet, nitrogen balance can still be maintained.

Only three amino acids, alanine, aspartate, and glutamate, can be considered to be truly dispensable; they are synthesised from common metabolic intermediates (pyruvate, oxaloacetate, and α-ketoglutarate, respectively, Section 9.3.1.2).

Table 9.5 Essential and Non-Essential Amino Acids

Essential	Essential precursor	Non-essential	Semi-essential
Histidine		Alanine	Arginine
Isoleucine		Aspartate	Asparagine
Leucine		Glutamate	Glutamine
Lysine			Glycine
Methionine	Cysteine		Proline
Phenylalanine	Tyrosine		Serine
Threonine			
Tryptophan			
Valine			

The remaining amino acids are generally considered to be non-essential, but under some circumstances, the requirement may outstrip the capacity for their synthesis:

- A high intake of compounds that are excreted as glycine conjugates will increase the requirement for glycine considerably
- In response to severe trauma, there is an increased requirement for proline for collagen synthesis for healing
- In surgical trauma and sepsis, the requirement for glutamine increases—a number of studies have shown improved healing after major surgery if additional glutamine is provided

Studies of essential amino acid requirements in the 1950s were based on the amounts required to maintain nitrogen balance in young adults. Interestingly, for reasons that are not clear, these relatively short-term studies did not show a requirement for histidine. Histidine was only shown to be a dietary essential in 1975. Patients who were maintained for prolonged periods on total intravenous nutrition without histidine added to the amino acid mixture developed signs of deficiency.

More recent studies have measured the rate of whole body protein turnover, using isotopically labelled amino acids. These show that the maximum rate of protein turnover is achieved with intakes of the essential amino acids some threefold higher than are required to maintain nitrogen balance. What is not clear is whether the maximum rate of protein turnover is essential or even desirable.

Other studies have estimated essential amino acid requirements by measuring the oxidation (and hence irreversible loss) of isotopically labelled amino acids. These again suggest higher requirements than those derived from studies of nitrogen balance. However, because stable isotopes are used, the experiments involve administration of a relatively large amount of a single amino acid, which may well distort normal metabolic pools; thus, there is an excess of the test amino acid to be catabolised.

9.1.3.1 *Protein quality and complementation*

A protein that contains at least as much of each of the essential amino acids as is required will be completely useable for tissue protein synthesis, whilst one that is relatively deficient in one or more of the essential amino acids will not. More of such a protein will be required to maintain nitrogen balance or growth.

The limiting amino acid of a protein is the essential amino acid that is present in the lowest amount relative to the requirement. In animal, and most vegetable, proteins the limiting amino acid is methionine (correctly the sum of methionine plus cysteine because cysteine is synthesised from methionine, and providing adequate cysteine reduces the requirement for methionine). In cereal proteins, the limiting amino acid is lysine.

The nutritional value or quality of individual proteins depends on whether or not they contain the essential amino acids in the amounts that are required. A number of different ways of determining protein quality have been developed:

- Biological Value (BV) is the proportion of absorbed protein that is retained in the body. A protein that is completely useable (e.g., egg, human milk) has a BV of 0.9–1; meat and fish have a BV of 0.75–0.8; wheat protein 0.5; gelatin (which completely lacks tryptophan) has a BV of 0.
- Net Protein Utilisation (NPU) is the proportion of dietary protein that is retained in the body (i.e. it takes account of the digestibility of the protein). By convention, it is

measured at 10% dietary protein, at which level the experimental animal can utilise all of the protein as long as the balance of essential amino acids is correct.

- Protein Efficiency Ratio (PER) is the gain in weight of growing animals per gram of protein eaten.
- Relative Protein Value (RPV) is the ability of a test protein, fed at various levels of intake, to support nitrogen balance, compared with a standard protein.
- Chemical Score is based on chemical analysis of the amino acids present in the protein; it is the amount of the limiting amino acid compared with the amount of the same amino acid in egg protein (which is completely useable for tissue protein synthesis).
- Protein Score (or amino acid score) is again based on chemical analysis, but uses a reference pattern of amino acid requirements as the standard. This provides the basis of the legally required way of expressing protein quality in North America— the protein-digestibility corrected amino acid score (PDCAAS).

Whilst protein quality is important when considering individual foods, it is not relevant when considering total diets because different proteins are limited by different amino acids, and hence have a relative excess of others. The result of mixing different proteins in a diet is an unexpected increase in the nutritional value of the mixture. Wheat protein is limited by lysine and has a protein score of 0.6; pea protein is limited by (methionine + cysteine) and has protein score of 0.4. A mixture of equal amounts of these two individually poor quality proteins has a protein score of 0.82—as high as that of meat.

The result of this complementation between proteins that are individually of low quality is that most diets have very nearly the same protein quality, regardless of the protein quality of individual foods. The average Western diet has a protein score of 0.73, whilst the poorest diets in developing countries, with a restricted range of foods, and very little milk, meat, or fish, have a protein score of 0.6.

9.1.3.2   Unavailable amino acids and protein digestibility

Chemical analysis of the amino acid content of proteins overestimates their nutritional value because not all of the amino acids are released by digestive enzymes (Section 4.4.3) and hence available for absorption.

The most important problems arise with lysine, which can form peptide bonds from its ε-amino group to side chain carboxyl groups of aspartate and glutamate (Figure 4.22). These bonds are hydrolysed by strong acid used in chemical analysis, but are not substrates for human digestive enzymes; thus, the lysine is not available for absorption. At the same time, the presence of these cross-links inhibits the intestinal proteases; thus, several amino acids on either side of the cross-link are also not liberated.

The ε-amino group of lysine can also react non-enzymically with glucose and other carbohydrates, again rendering the amino acid unavailable for absorption. In foods, this is the basis of the non-enzymic browning reaction (Maillard reaction) that gives many cooked foods their characteristic flavour. A similar reaction occurs *in vivo* in poorly controlled diabetes mellitus, and glycation of proteins underlies many of the problems associated with poor glycaemic control (Section 10.7.1).

9.2   Protein synthesis

The information for the amino acid sequence of each of the 30–40,000 different proteins in the body is contained in the DNA in the nucleus of each cell. As required, a working copy

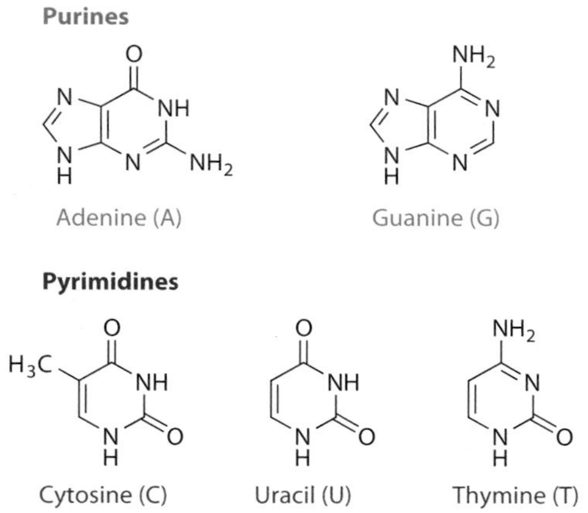

Purines

Adenine (A)   Guanine (G)

Pyrimidines

Cytosine (C)   Uracil (U)   Thymine (T)

Figure 9.4 The nucleic acid bases.

Table 9.6 Nomenclature of Nucleic Acid Bases, Nucleosides, and Nucleotides

	Base	RNA Nucleoside	RNA Nucleotide	DNA Deoxynucleoside	DNA Deoxynucleotide
A	Adenine	Adenosine	Adenylate	Deoxyadenosine	Deoxyadenylate
G	Guanine	Guanosine	Guanylate	Deoxyguanosine	Deoxyguanylate
U	Uracil	Uridine	Uridylate	–	–
T	Thymine	–	–	Deoxythymidine	Deoxythymidylate
C	Cytosine	Cytidine	Cytidylate	Deoxycytidine	Deoxycytidylate

of the information for an individual protein (the gene for that protein) is transcribed, as messenger RNA (mRNA), and this is then translated into a sequence of amino acids during protein synthesis on the ribosomes.

The information in DNA and RNA is provided by the sequence of purines and pyrimidines (the bases, Figure 9.4) along the chain. A base esterified to a sugar is a nucleoside, and the phosphorylated nucleoside is a nucleotide (Table 9.6). Both DNA and RNA are linear polymers of nucleotides. In RNA, the sugar is ribose, whilst in DNA, it is deoxyribose.

9.2.1   The structure and information content of DNA

As shown in Figure 9.5, DNA is a linear polymer of nucleotides. It consists of a backbone of deoxyribose linked by phospho-diester bonds between carbon 3 of one sugar and carbon 5 of the next. The bases of the nucleotides project from this sugar phosphate backbone. There are two strands of deoxyribonucleotides, held together by hydrogen bonds between a purine (adenine or guanine) and a pyrimidine (thymine or cytosine): adenine forms two hydrogen bonds to thymine, and guanine forms three hydrogen bonds to cytosine. Because of this hydrogen bonding, there is always an equal amount of adenine and thymine and of guanine and cytosine—the ratio of A/G equals that of C/T.

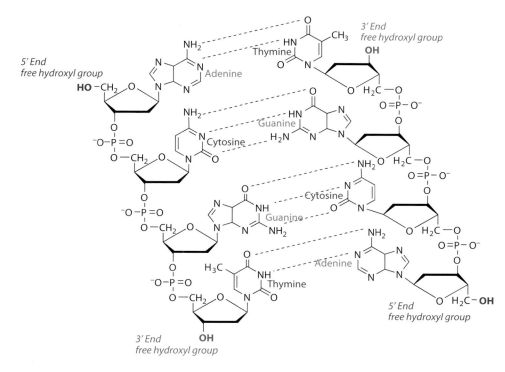

Figure 9.5 The structure of DNA.

The double-strand coils into a helix, the double helix (Figure 9.6). The two strands of a DNA molecule run in opposite directions—where one strand has a 3'-hydroxyl group at the end, on the complementary strand there is a free 5'-hydroxyl group. The information of DNA is always read from the 3' end toward the 5' end.

If stretched out, the DNA in a single cell would be about 2 m long; to fit within the nucleus, the DNA helix is supercoiled, then wound around histones (basic proteins), to

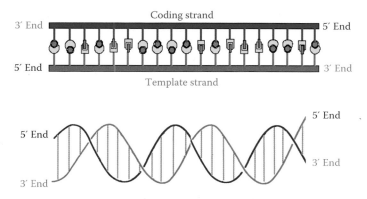

Figure 9.6 The structure of DNA–hydrogen bonding between bases and coiling of the chains to form the double helix.

form nucleosomes. There are short-linking regions between nucleosomes, which are mutation hotspots, suggesting that as well as permitting packaging of DNA, histones also protect it from damage. The chains of nucleosomes are then wound around other proteins and
folded to form chromosomes.

Only about 3%–5% of the DNA in a human cell carries information for genes; the
remainder consists mainly of

- Control regions, which promote or enhance the expression of individual genes,
  and include regions that respond to hormones and other factors that control gene
  expression (Section 10.4) as well as sites for the initiation and termination of DNA
  replication.
- Spacer regions, both between and within genes, which carry no translatable message, but serve to link those regions that do carry a translatable message. When such
  regions occur within a gene sequence, they are called introns.
- Pseudo-genes, which seem to be genes that have undergone mutation in our evolutionary past, and are now untranslatable. Presumably, these are a reminder of evolutionary history.

9.2.1.1 DNA replication

Prior to cell division, all of the DNA in the 46 chromosomes has to be replicated; each
daughter cell will have a full complement of chromosomes and genetic information. DNA
replication occurs by separating the two strands of the double helix in a relatively short
region at a time, then pairing deoxynucleotides along the separated strands to synthesise
two new strands, complementary to each original strand of DNA. This is so-called semi-
conservative replication—each new DNA molecule has one old strand and one newly synthesised strand (Figure 9.7). This process occurs at a large number of replication sites in
each chromosome at the same time.

Because each base to be incorporated into the newly synthesised DNA chain is fitted
in by hydrogen bonding to the complementary base in an existing strand of DNA, the
process has a high degree of fidelity. Nevertheless, mispairing of bases occurs about 1 in
10^7 base pairs, and if uncorrected would lead to mutations and loss of genetic information.
A separate DNA polymerase has a proofreading function; it detects a mispaired base by
distortion of the smooth shape of the newly formed regions of double helix. The offending
base is then excised and replaced by the correct one.

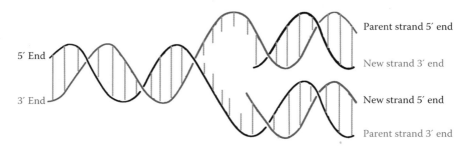

Figure 9.7 Semi-conservative replication of DNA.

9.2.1.2 The genetic code

The information in DNA, contained in a code made up of only four letters (A, G, C, and T), carries the information for the 21 different amino acids that make up the 30–40,000 different proteins that are to be synthesised. The bases are read in groups of three, rather than singly. Each group of three nucleotides is a codon—a single unit of the genetic code. Since a codon can contain any one of the four bases in each position, there are 64 possible codons, but there is a need for only 22—one for each amino acid and one to signal the end of the message.

As can be seen from Tables 9.7 and 9.8, most amino acids are coded for by more than one codon—i.e. the code is degenerate, and there are apparently redundant codons. This provides a measure of protection against mutations—in many cases, a single base change in a codon will not affect the amino acid that is incorporated into the protein, and therefore will have no functional significance.

Three codons (UAA, UAG, and UGA) do not code for amino acids but act as stop signals to show the end of the message to be translated and so terminate protein synthesis.

UGA also codes for the selenium analogue of cysteine, selenocysteine (Section 11.15.2.5). It is normally read as a stop codon, but in the presence of a specific sequence in the untranslated region of mRNA, it is read as coding for selenocysteine. Similarly, in bacteria, but not as far as is known in mammals, UAG codes for the lysine derivative pyrrolysine, again in a context-sensitive way.

Table 9.7 The Genetic Code, Showing the Codons in mRNA

Amino acid		Codon(s)
Alanine	Ala	GCU GCC GCA GCG
Arginine	Arg	CGU CGC CGA CGG AGA AGG
Asparagine	Asn	AAU AAC
Aspartic acid	Asp	GAU GAC
Cysteine	Cys	UGU UGC
Glutamic acid	Glu	GAA GAG
Glutamine	Gln	CAA CAG
Glycine	Gly	GGU GGC GGA GGG
Histidine	His	CAU CAG
Isoleucine	Ile	AUU AUC AUA
Leucine	Leu	UUA UUG CUU CUC CUA CUG
Lysine	Lys	AAA AAG
Methionine	Met	AUG
Phenylalanine	Phe	UUU UUC
Proline	Pro	CCU CCC CCA CCG
Serine	Ser	UCU UCC UCA UCG AGU AGC
Threonine	Thr	ACU ACC ACA ACG
Tryptophan	Trp	UGG
Tyrosine	Tyr	UAU UAC
Valine	Val	GUU GUC GUA GUG
STOP		UAA UAG UGA[a]

[a] UGA also codes for selenocysteine in a specific context.

Table 9.8 The Genetic Code, Showing the Codons in mRNA

First base	Second base				Third base
	U	C	A	G	
U	Phe	Ser	Tyr	Cys	U
U	Phe	Ser	Tyr	Cys	C
U	Leu	Ser	STOP	STOP[a]	A
U	Leu	Ser	STOP	Trp	G
C	Leu	Pro	His	Arg	U
C	Leu	Pro	His	Arg	C
C	Leu	Pro	Gln	Arg	A
C	Leu	Pro	Gln	Arg	G
A	Ile	Thr	Asn	Ser	U
A	Ile	Thr	Asn	Ser	C
A	Ile	Thr	Lys	Arg	A
A	Met	Thr	Lys	Arg	G
G	Val	Ala	Asp	Gly	U
G	Val	Ala	Asp	Gly	C
G	Val	Ala	Glu	Gly	A
G	Val	Ala	Glu	Gly	G

[a] UGA also codes for selenocysteine in a specific context.

9.2.2 Ribonucleic acid (RNA)

In RNA, the sugar is ribose, rather than deoxyribose as in DNA, and RNA contains the pyrimidine uracil where DNA contains thymine (Figure 9.8). There are four main types of RNA in the cell:

1. Messenger RNA (mRNA) is synthesised in the nucleus, as a copy of one strand of DNA (the process of transcription, Section 9.2.2.1). After some editing of the message, it is transferred into the cytosol, where it binds to ribosomes. The information carried by the mRNA is then translated into the amino acid sequence of the protein.
2. Ribosomal RNA (rRNA) is part of the structure of the ribosomes on which protein is synthesised (Section 9.2.3.2).
3. Transfer RNA (tRNA) provides the link between mRNA and the amino acids required for protein synthesis on the ribosome (Section 9.2.3.1).
4. Micro RNA (miRNA), which regulates the expression of many genes.

9.2.2.1 Transcription to form messenger RNA (mRNA)

In the transcription of DNA to form mRNA (Figure 9.9), a part of the desired region of DNA is separated from its protective proteins, uncoiled, and the two strands of the double helix are separated. A copy of one DNA strand (the template strand) is then synthesised by binding the complementary nucleotide triphosphate to each base of DNA in turn, followed by condensation to form the phospho-diester link between ribose moieties. The sequence of bases in the resultant RNA is thus identical to that in the coding strand of DNA, except that where DNA contains thymidine, RNA contains uridine.

Upstream of the region of DNA that contains a gene there is a promoter region, which includes the sequence TATA. Transcription factors bind to this TATA box, resulting in

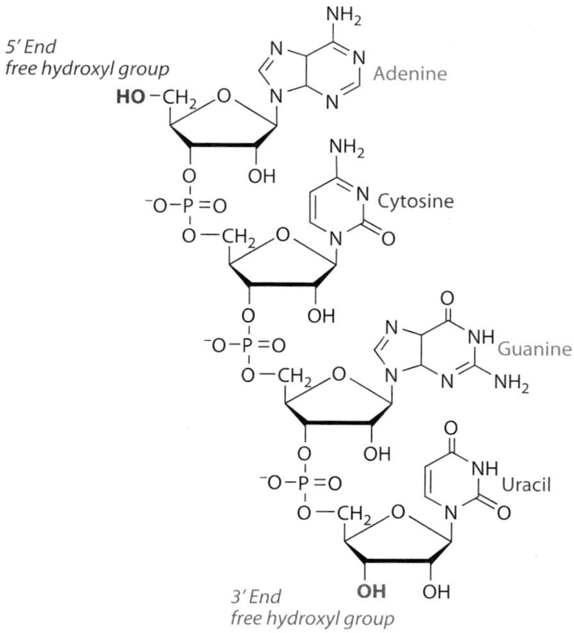

Figure 9.8 The structure of RNA.

activation of RNA polymerase, and the initiation of transcription of some 25–30 base pairs downstream from the TATA box. Much of the non-coding DNA that was described above as pseudo-genes consists of regions that were once genes, but, having lost their TATA boxes or their promoter regions, are now untranscribable.

Further control regions (enhancer regions and hormone response elements) may be found upstream, downstream, or in the middle of a gene. These act to increase the rate at which the gene is transcribed.

The primary transcript is a complete copy of the template strand of DNA, and undergoes post-transcriptional processing:

- The 5' end of the RNA is blocked by addition of the unusual base 7-methyl-guanosine triphosphate. This is called the 'cap' and has a role in the initiation of protein synthesis (Section 9.2.3.2). The 5' end of the RNA is the first to be synthesised, and the cap is added before transcription has been completed.
- A tail of up to 250 adenosine residues is added to the 3' end of the RNA, after the termination codon. This poly-A tail stabilises the mRNA and provides protection against hydrolysis by RNase in the cytosol. It is also useful to molecular biologists, since mRNA can readily be isolated by binding the poly-A tail to a suitable probe.
- Introns are regions of the DNA within a gene that do not carry coding information for the protein to be synthesised. The final step in RNA processing is to excise the introns and splice together the coding regions (exons) to provide a continuous sequence that will be translated. In a number of cases, there may be alternative ways of splicing the same primary transcript in different tissues—the same gene can give rise to different proteins as a result of removing different introns and sometimes also removing exons.

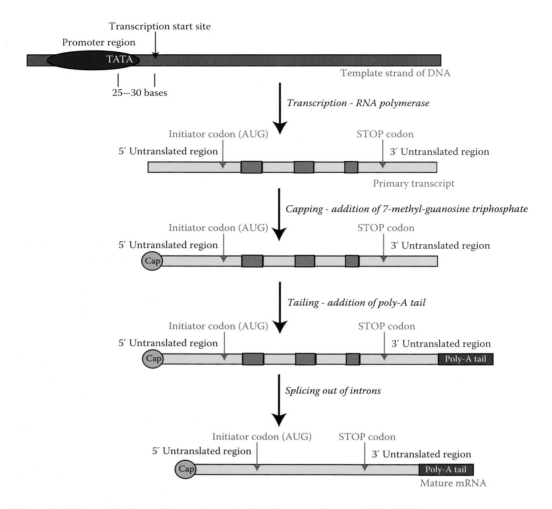

Figure 9.9 Transcription and post-transcriptional processing to yield mRNA.

9.2.3   Translation of mRNA—the process of protein synthesis

The process of protein synthesis consists of translating the message carried by the sequence of bases on mRNA into amino acids, and then forming peptide bonds between the amino acids to form a protein. This occurs on the ribosome, and requires a variety of enzymes as well as specific transfer RNA (tRNA) molecules for each amino acid.

Micro-RNA (miRNA) are small (22 nucleotide) non-coding RNA molecules that are encoded either by the gene for the protein involved or by introns in that gene. They base-pair with complementary regions in the mRNA and act either to repress translation or to target the mRNA for catabolism. The human genome contains more than 1000 miRNA species, and the expression up to 60% of all genes may be controlled by miRNA.

9.2.3.1   Transfer RNA (tRNA)

The key to translating the message carried by the codons on mRNA into amino acids is transfer RNA (tRNA). There are 56 different types (species) of tRNA in the cell. They all

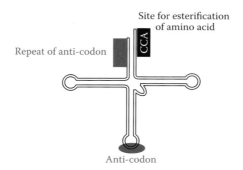

Figure 9.10 Transfer RNA.

have the same general structure, RNA twisted into a cloverleaf shape and consisting of some 70–90 nucleotides (Figure 9.10). About half the bases in tRNA are paired by hydrogen bonding, which maintains the shape of the molecule. The 3′ and 5′ ends of the molecule are adjacent to each other as a result of this folding.

The different species of tRNA have many regions in common with each other, and all have a –CCA tail at the 3′ end, which reacts with the amino acid. Two regions are important in providing the specificity of the tRNA species:

1. The anti-codon, a sequence of three bases at the base of the cloverleaf. The bases in the anti-codon are complementary to the bases of the codon of mRNA, and each species of tRNA binds specifically to one codon, or, in some cases, two closely related codons for the same amino acid.
2. The region at the 5′ end of the molecule, which repeats the information contained in the anti-codon.

Amino acids bind to activating enzymes (amino acyl-tRNA synthetases), which recognise both the amino acid and the appropriate tRNA molecule. The first step is reaction between the amino acid and ATP, to form amino acyl AMP, releasing pyrophosphate. The amino acyl AMP then reacts with the –CCA tail of tRNA to form amino acyl-tRNA, releasing AMP.

The specificity of these enzymes is critically important to the process of translation. Each enzyme recognises only one amino acid but will react with all the various tRNA species that carry an anti-codon for that amino acid. Mistakes are extremely rare. The easiest possible mistake would be the attachment of valine to the tRNA for isoleucine, or vice versa because of the close similarity between the structures of these two amino acids (Figure 4.19). However, it is only about once in every 3000 times that this mistake occurs. Amino acyl-tRNA synthetases have a second active site that checks that the correct amino acid has been attached to the tRNA, and if not, hydrolyses the newly formed bond, releasing tRNA and the amino acid.

9.2.3.2 *Protein synthesis on the ribosome*

The ribosome consists of two subunits, composed of RNA and a variety of proteins. It permits the binding of the anti-codon region of amino acyl tRNA to the codon on mRNA and aligns the amino acids for formation of peptide bonds. As shown in Figure 9.11, the ribosome binds to mRNA and has two tRNA binding sites. One, the P site, contains the growing peptide chain, attached to tRNA, whilst the other, the A site, binds the next amino acyl tRNA to be incorporated into the peptide chain.

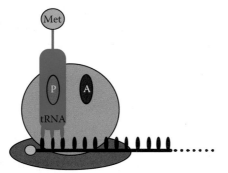

1. Initiation: methionyl tRNA binds to P site

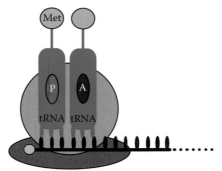

2. Second aminoacyl tRNA binds to A site

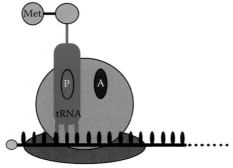

3. Transfer of Met from tRNA to form peptide bond
to second amino acid; movement of tRNA with
nascent peptide to P site

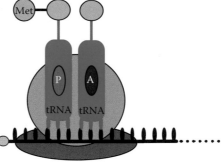

4. Next aminoacyl tRNA binds to A site;
steps 3 and 4 repeated until a STOP codon
is at the A site

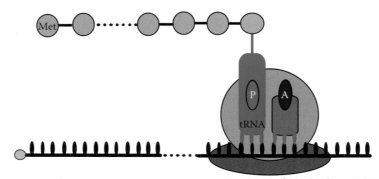

5. Termination factor binds to STOP codon at
A site; nascent peptide released and ribosome
disassembles, ready to translate another molecule
of mRNA

Figure 9.11 Ribosomal protein synthesis.

The first codon of mRNA to be translated (the initiator codon) is always AUG, the codon for methionine. This means that the amino terminal of all newly synthesised proteins is methionine, although this is often removed in post-translational modification of the protein (Section 9.2.3.4).

An initiator methionine-tRNA forms a complex with the small ribosomal subunit, then together with a variety of initiation factors (enzymes and other proteins) binds to the initiator codon of mRNA, then to a large ribosomal subunit, to form the complete ribosome. AUG is the only codon for methionine, and elsewhere in mRNA, it binds the normal methionine-tRNA. It is only adjacent to the 5′ cap that AUG binds the initiator methionine-tRNA.

After the ribosome has been assembled, with the initiator tRNA bound at the P site and occupying the AUG initiator codon, the next amino acyl tRNA binds to the A site of the ribosome, with its anti-codon bound to the next codon in the sequence.

The methionine is released from the initiator tRNA at the P site and forms a peptide bond to the amino group of the amino acyl tRNA at the A site of the ribosome. The initiator tRNA is then released from the P site, and the growing peptide chain, attached to its tRNA, moves from the A site to the P site. Since the peptide chain is attached to tRNA, which occupies a codon on the mRNA, this means that as the peptide chain moves from the A site to the P site, the whole assembly moves one codon along the mRNA.

As the growing peptide chain moves from the A site to the P site, and the ribosome moves along the mRNA chain, the next amino acyl tRNA occupies the A site, covering its codon. The growing peptide chain is transferred from the tRNA at the P site, forming a peptide bond to the amino acid at the A site. Again the free tRNA at the P site is released, and the growing peptide, attached to tRNA, moves from the A site to the P site, moving one codon along the mRNA as it does so.

The stop codons (UAA, UAG, and UGA) are not read by tRNA but by protein release factors. These occupy the A site of the ribosome and hydrolyse the peptide-tRNA bond. This releases the finished protein from the ribosome. As the protein leaves, the two subunits of the ribosome separate and leave the mRNA; they are now available to bind another initiator tRNA and begin the process of translation over again.

Just as several molecules of RNA polymerase can transcribe a gene at the same time, several ribosomes translate a molecule of mRNA at the same time. As the ribosomes travel along the ribosome, each has a longer growing peptide chain than the one before. Such assemblies of ribosomes on a molecule of mRNA are polysomes. Proteins that are to be exported from the cell have a sequence of hydrophobic amino acids at the amino terminal. This signal peptide draws the nascent polypeptide chain into the rough endoplasmic reticulum whilst it is being synthesised; thus, polysomes translating mRNA for proteins to be exported are attached to the rough endoplasmic reticulum.

Termination and release of the protein from the ribosome requires the presence of a stop codon and the protein release factors. However, protein synthesis will also come to a halt if there is not enough of one of the amino acids bound to tRNA. In this case, the growing peptide chain is not released from the ribosome, but remains, in arrested development, until the required amino acyl tRNA is available. This means that if the intake of one of the essential amino acids is inadequate, then once supplies are exhausted, protein synthesis will cease.

9.2.3.3   The energy cost of protein synthesis

Protein synthesis is an energy-expensive process. There is a cost of 4 mol of ATP equivalents per peptide bond synthesised (2.8 kJ/g of protein synthesised):

- Formation of the amino acyl tRNA requires the formation of amino acyl AMP, with the release of pyrophosphate; thus, for each amino acid attached to tRNA, there is a cost equivalent to 2 mol of ATP → ADP + phosphate.
- The binding of each amino acyl tRNA to the A site of the ribosome involves the hydrolysis of GTP → GDP + phosphate, which is equivalent to ATP → ADP + phosphate.
- Movement of the growing peptide chain from the A site of the ribosome to the P site again involves the hydrolysis of ATP → ADP + phosphate.

Allowing for active transport of amino acids into cells (Sections 3.2.2.3 and 4.4.3.2) increases this to 3.6 kJ/g of protein synthesised and allows for the nucleoside triphosphates required for mRNA synthesis gives a total cost of 4.2 kJ/g of protein synthesised.

In the fasting state, when the rate of protein synthesis is relatively low, about 9% of total energy expenditure (i.e., about 12% of the basal metabolic rate) is accounted for by protein synthesis. After a high carbohydrate meal, the rate of protein synthesis increases and accounts for 12% of energy expenditure. A high protein intake increases protein synthesis (and catabolism) further, and after a high protein meal, protein turnover accounts for almost 20% of energy expenditure.

9.2.3.4   Post-translational modification of proteins

The signal peptide of proteins that are exported from the cell is cleaved as part of the post-translational processing in the rough endoplasmic reticulum and Golgi apparatus. Many other proteins also lose short peptides from the amino or carboxyl terminal, and the initial (amino terminal) methionine is removed from most newly synthesised proteins.

Many proteins contain carbohydrates and lipids, which are covalently bound to amino acid side chains. Others contain covalently bound prosthetic groups, such as vitamins and their derivatives, metal ions or haem. The attachment of these non-amino acid parts of the protein is part of the process of post-translational modification to yield the active protein.

Some proteins contain unusual amino acids for which there is no codon and no tRNA. These are formed by modification of the protein after translation is complete. When the protein is catabolised, these modified amino acids cannot be re-utilised, but are either metabolised or excreted unchanged. Such amino acids include

- Methyl-histidine in the contractile proteins of muscle.
- Hydroxyproline and hydroxylysine in the connective tissue proteins formed via a reaction that requires vitamin C as a cofactor. This explains why wound healing, which requires new synthesis of connective tissue, is impaired in vitamin C deficiency (Section 11.14.3).
- Inter-chain links in collagen and elastin, formed by the oxidation of lysine residues. This reaction is catalysed by a copper-dependent enzyme, and copper deficiency leads fragility of bones and loss of the elasticity of connective tissues (Section 11.15.2.2). Measurement of urinary excretion of small peptides containing these cross-link compounds provides an index of bone turnover.
- γ-Carboxyglutamate in several of the blood clotting proteins and in osteocalcin in bone. The formation of γ-carboxyglutamate requires vitamin K (Section 11.5.2). Measurement of circulating the concentration of undercarboxylated prothrombin provides a sensitive index of vitamin K nutritional status.

9.3   The metabolism of amino acids

An adult has a requirement for a dietary intake of protein because there is continual oxidation of amino acids both as a source of metabolic fuel and, more importantly, for gluconeogenesis in the fasting state. In the fed state, amino acids in excess of immediate requirements for protein synthesis are oxidised and the carbon skeletons are used mainly for synthesis of fatty acids. Overall, for an adult in nitrogen balance, the total amount of amino acids being metabolised will be equal to the total absorption of amino acids from dietary proteins.

Amino acids are also required for the synthesis of a variety of metabolic products, including

- Purines (synthesised from glycine) and pyrimidines (synthesised from aspartate) for nucleic acid synthesis
- Haem, synthesised from glycine
- The catecholamine neurotransmitters, dopamine, noradrenaline, and adrenaline, synthesised from tyrosine
- The thyroid hormones thyroxine and tri-iodothyronine, synthesised from tyrosine (Section 11.15.3.3)
- Melanin, the pigment of skin and hair, synthesised from tyrosine
- The nicotinamide ring of the coenzymes NAD and NADP, synthesised from tryptophan (Section 11.8.2)
- The neurotransmitter serotonin (5-hydroxytryptamine), synthesised from tryptophan
- The neurotransmitter histamine, synthesised from histidine
- The neurotransmitter GABA (γ-aminobutyrate) synthesised from glutamate (Figure 5.19)
- Carnitine (Section 5.5.1), synthesised from lysine and methionine
- Creatine (Section 3.2.3.1), synthesised from arginine, glycine, and methionine
- The phospholipid bases ethanolamine and choline (Section 4.3.1.2), synthesised from serine and methionine. Acetyl choline is a neurotransmitter
- Taurine, synthesised from cysteine

In general, the amounts of amino acids required for synthesis of these products are small compared with the requirement for maintenance of nitrogen balance and protein turnover.

9.3.1   Metabolism of the amino nitrogen

The initial step in the metabolism of amino acids is the removal of the amino group ($-NH_3^+$), leaving the carbon skeleton of the amino acid. Chemically, these carbon skeletons are keto-acids (more correctly, they are oxo-acids). A keto-acid has a $- C = O$ group in place of the $HC-NH_3^+$ group of an amino acid; the metabolism of keto-acids is discussed in Section 9.3.2.

9.3.1.1   Deamination

Some amino acids can be directly oxidised to their corresponding keto-acids, releasing ammonia: the process of deamination (Figure 9.12). There is a general L-amino acid oxidase that catalyses the deamination of most amino acids, but it has a low activity and is relatively unimportant in amino acid metabolism.

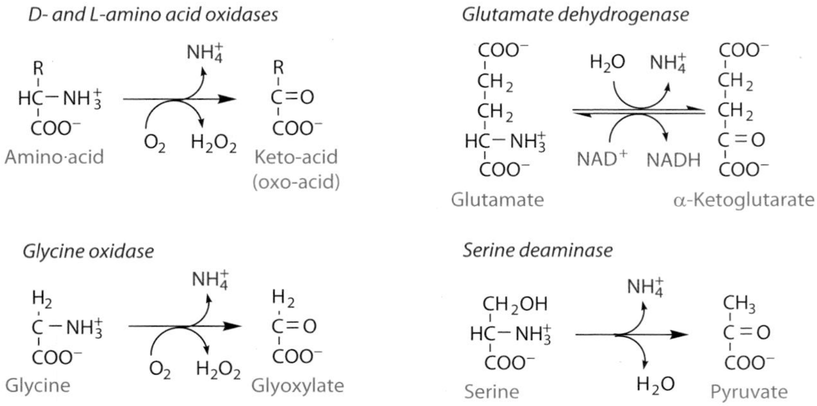

Figure 9.12 Deamination of amino acids.

Kidneys contain D-amino acid oxidase, which acts to deaminate, and hence detoxify, the small amounts of D-amino acids that arise from bacterial proteins. It also acts on D-serine, which has a neuromodulatory role in the central nervous system. The keto-acids resulting from the action of D-amino acid oxidase on D-amino acids can undergo transamination (Section 9.3.1.2) to yield the L-isomers. This means that, to a limited extent, D-amino acids can be isomerised and used for protein synthesis. Although there is evidence from experimental animals that D-isomers of (some of) the essential amino acids can be used to maintain nitrogen balance, there is little information on their utilisation in human beings.

Four amino acids are deaminated by specific enzymes:

1. Glycine is deaminated to glyoxylate and ammonium ions by glycine oxidase.
2. Glutamate is deaminated to α-ketoglutarate and ammonium ions by glutamate dehydrogenase.
3. Serine is deaminated and dehydrated to pyruvate by serine deaminase (sometimes called serine dehydratase).
4. Threonine is deaminated and dehydrated to oxo-butyrate by threonine deaminase.

9.3.1.2 Transamination

Most amino acids are not deaminated, but undergo transamination, in which the amino group is transferred onto the enzyme, leaving the keto-acid. In the second half of the reaction, the enzyme transfers the amino group onto an acceptor, which is a different keto-acid, thus, forming the amino acid corresponding to that keto-acid. This is a typical ping-pong reaction sequence (Section 2.3.3.2). The acceptor for the amino group at the active site of the enzyme is pyridoxal phosphate, the metabolically active coenzyme derived from vitamin B_6 (Section 11.9.2), forming pyridoxamine phosphate as an intermediate in the reaction. The reaction of transamination is shown in Figure 9.13, and the keto-acids corresponding to the amino acids in Table 9.9.

Transamination is a reversible reaction; thus, if the keto-acid can be synthesised in the body, so can the amino acid. The essential amino acids (Section 9.1.3) are those for which the only source of the keto-acid is the amino acid itself. Three of the keto-acids listed in Table 9.9 are common metabolic intermediates; they are the precursors of the three amino

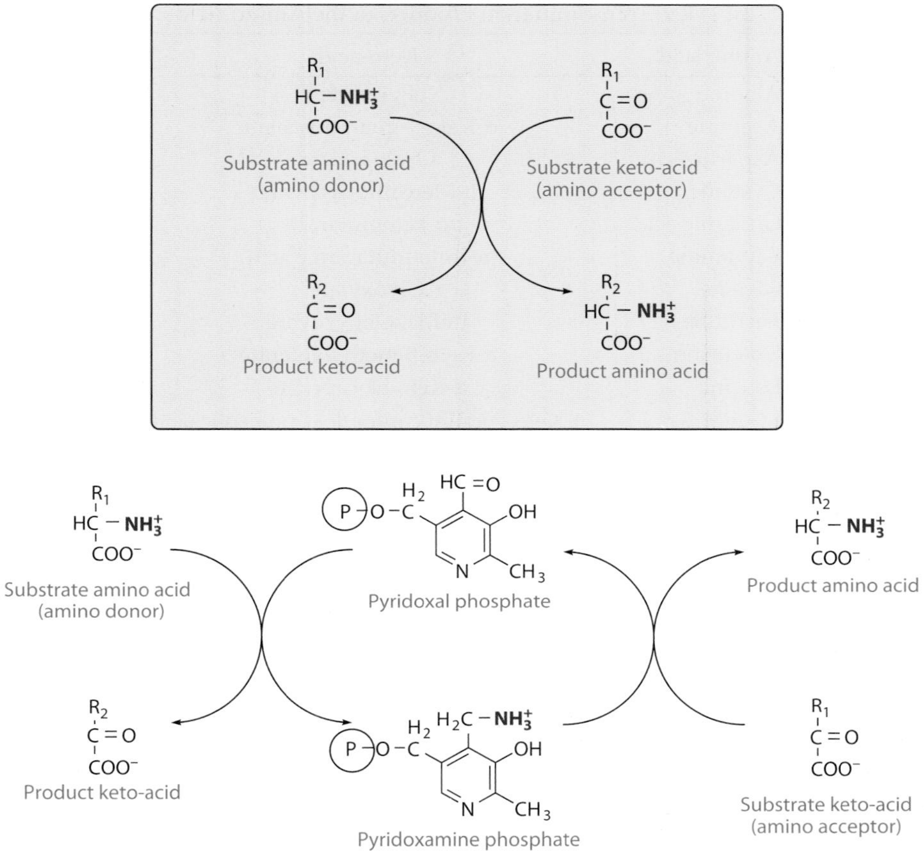

Figure 9.13 Transamination of amino acids. The overall reaction of transamination is shown in the yellow box; the role of pyridoxal phosphate as the intermediate amino acceptor is shown below.

acids that can be considered to be completely dispensable, in that there is no requirement for them in the diet:

1. Pyruvate—the keto-acid of alanine
2. α-Ketoglutarate—the keto-acid of glutamate
3. Oxaloacetate—the keto-acid of aspartate

The reversibility of transamination has been exploited in the treatment of patients in renal failure. The conventional treatment is to provide them with a very low protein diet to minimise the total amount of urea that has to be excreted (Section 9.3.1.4). However, they still have to be provided with the essential amino acids. If they are provided with the keto-acids corresponding to the essential amino acids, they can synthesise the amino acids by transamination, thus reducing yet further their nitrogen burden. The only amino acid for which this is not possible is lysine—the keto-acid corresponding to lysine undergoes rapid non-enzymic condensation to pipecolic acid, which cannot be metabolised further.

If the acceptor keto-acid in a transamination reaction is α-ketoglutarate, then glutamate is formed, and glutamate can readily be oxidised back to α-ketoglutarate and ammonium,

Table 9.9 Transamination Products of the Amino Acids

Amino acid	Keto-acid
Alanine	Pyruvate
Arginine	α-Keto-γ-guanidoacetate
Aspartic acid	Oxaloacetate
Cysteine	β-Mercaptopyruvate
Glutamic acid	α-ketoglutarate
Glutamine	α-Keto-glutaramic acid
Glycine	Glyoxylate
Histidine	Imidazolepyruvate
Isoleucine	α-Keto-β-methylvalerate
Leucine	α-Keto-isocaproate
Lysine[a]	α-Keto-ε-aminocaproate → pipecolic acid
Methionine	S-Methyl-β-thiol α-oxopropionate
Ornithine	Glutamic-γ-semialdehyde
Phenylalanine	Phenylpyruvate
Proline	γ-Hydroxypyruvate
Serine	Hydroxypyruvate
Threonine	α-Keto-β-hydroxybutyrate
Tryptophan	Indolepyruvate
Tyrosine	p-Hydroxyphenylpyruvate
Valine	α-Keto-isovalerate

[a] Lysine does not undergo reversible transamination because the keto-acid undergoes non-enzymic condensation to pipecolic acid.

catalysed by glutamate dehydrogenase. Similarly, if the acceptor keto-acid is glyoxylate, then the product is glycine, which can be oxidised back to glyoxylate and ammonium, catalysed by glycine oxidase. Thus, by means of a variety of transaminases and using the reactions of glutamate dehydrogenase and glycine oxidase, all of the amino acids can, indirectly, be converted to their keto-acids and ammonium (Figure 9.14). Aspartate can also act as an intermediate in the indirect deamination of a variety of amino acids (Figure 9.18).

9.3.1.3   *The metabolism of ammonia*

The deamination of amino acids (and a number of other reactions in the body, including oxidation to inactivate the amine neurotransmitters) results in the formation of ammonium ions. Ammonium is highly toxic. The normal plasma concentration is less than 50 μmol/L; an increase to 80–100 μmol/L (far too little to have any detectable effect on plasma pH) results in disturbance of consciousness, and in patients whose blood ammonium increases above approximately 200 μmol/L ammonia intoxication leads to coma and convulsions and may be fatal.

At any time, the total amount of ammonium being formed in various tissues that must be transported to the liver is greatly in excess of the toxic level. As it is formed in peripheral tissues, ammonium is metabolised to yield glutamine by the reactions of glutamate dehydrogenase and glutamine synthetase (Figure 9.15). Glutamine is transported in the bloodstream to the liver and kidneys.

It is the formation of glutamate from α-ketoglutarate that explains the neurotoxicity of ammonium; as ammonium concentrations in the nervous system increase, the reaction of

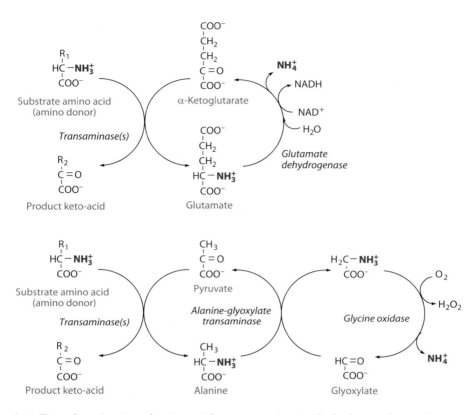

Figure 9.14 Transdeamination of amino acids—transamination linked to oxidative deamination.

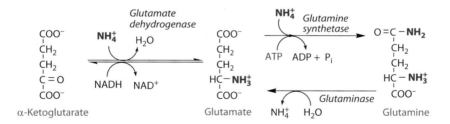

Figure 9.15 The synthesis of glutamate and glutamine from ammonium and hydrolysis of glutamine by glutaminase.

glutamate dehydrogenase depletes the mitochondrial pool of α-ketoglutarate, resulting in impairment of the activity of the citric acid cycle (Section 5.4.4), impairing energy-yielding metabolism and ATP formation.

   In the liver, glutamine may either be used directly as a source of nitrogen in a variety of pathways (including the synthesis of purines and pyrimidines) or may be hydrolysed by glutaminase to yield glutamate and ammonium, which is used as the nitrogen donor in other pathways. Glutaminase is also found in the kidneys, where it acts as a source of ammonium ions to neutralise excessively acidic urine.

9.3.1.4 *The synthesis of urea*

In the liver, ammonium arising from either the hydrolysis of glutamine or the reaction of adenosine deaminase (Figure 9.18) is the substrate for synthesis of urea, the main nitrogenous excretion product. The pathway for urea synthesis is shown in Figure 9.16. The key compound is ornithine, which acts as a carrier on which the molecule of urea is built up. At the end of the reaction sequence, urea is released by the hydrolysis of arginine, yielding ornithine to begin the cycle again. Although urea is an excretory end product of nitrogen

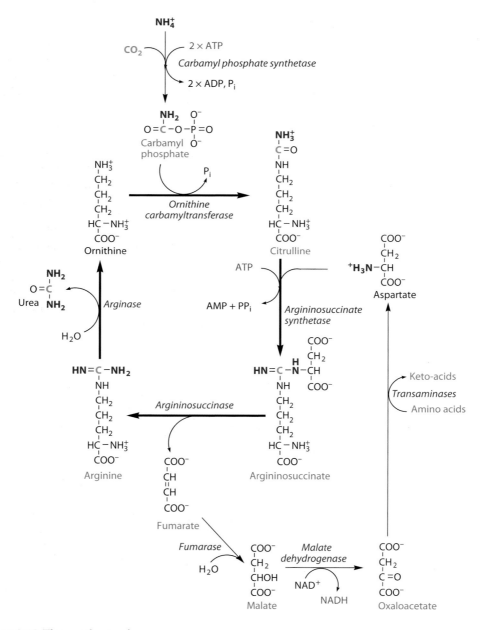

Figure 9.16 The synthesis of urea.

metabolism, it is reabsorbed in the distal renal tubules, where it maintains an osmotic gradient for the reabsorption of water.

The total amount of urea synthesised each day is several-fold higher than the amount that is excreted. Urea diffuses readily from the bloodstream into the large intestine, where it is hydrolysed by bacterial urease to carbon dioxide and ammonium. Much of the ammonium is reabsorbed and used in the liver for the synthesis of glutamate and glutamine, and then a variety of other nitrogenous compounds (Figure 9.17). Studies with ^{15}N urea show that a significant amount of label is found in essential amino acids. This may reflect intestinal bacterial synthesis of amino acids, or it may reflect the reversibility of the transamination of essential amino acids.

The urea synthesis cycle is also the pathway for the synthesis of the amino acid arginine. Ornithine is synthesised from glutamate, and then undergoes the reactions shown in Figure 9.16 to form arginine. Although the whole pathway of urea synthesis occurs only in the liver, the sequence of reactions leading to the formation of arginine also occurs in the kidneys, and the kidneys are the main source of arginine in the body.

Infants have relatively low activity of the urea synthesis cycle enzymes, which explains why at times of rapid growth arginine is an essential amino acid (Section 9.1.3). Young infants cannot be fed undiluted cows' milk because it provides more protein (as percentage of energy) than human milk and more than they can use for protein synthesis. The excess protein exceeds their capacity for urea synthesis, and they are at risk of hyperammonaemia. Infant formula is manufactured by diluting cows' milk to an appropriate protein concentration, then adding lactose to increase the energy yield to that of human milk.

The precursor for ornithine synthesis is *N*-acetyl glutamate, which is also an obligatory activator of carbamyl phosphate synthetase. This provides a regulatory mechanism—if *N*-acetyl glutamate is not available for ornithine synthesis (and hence there would be impaired activity of the urea synthesis cycle), then ammonium is not incorporated into carbamyl phosphate. This can be a cause of hyperammonaemia in a variety of metabolic disturbances that lead to either a lack of acetyl CoA for *N*-acetyl glutamate synthesis or an accumulation of propionyl CoA, which is a poor substrate for, and hence an inhibitor of, *N*-acetyl glutamate synthetase.

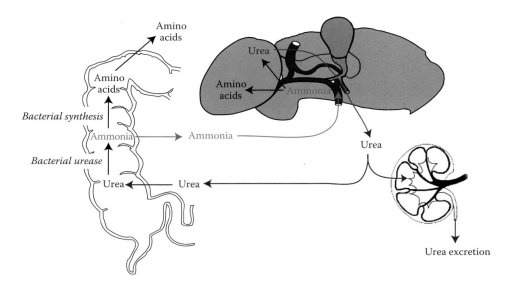

Figure 9.17 Enterohepatic cycling of urea.

9.3.1.5 Incorporation of nitrogen in biosynthesis

Amino acids are the only significant source of nitrogen for synthesis of nitrogenous compounds such as haem, purines, and pyrimidines. Three amino acids are especially important as nitrogen donors:

1. Glycine is incorporated intact into purines, haem, and other porphyrins, and creatine (Section 3.2.3.1).
2. Glutamine—the amide nitrogen is transferred in an ATP-dependent reaction, replacing an oxo-group in the acceptor with an amino group.
3. Aspartate undergoes an ATP- or GTP-dependent condensation reaction with an oxo-group, followed by cleavage to release fumarate.

Reactions in which aspartate acts as a nitrogen donor in this way result in a net gain of ATP, since the fumarate is hydrated to malate, then oxidised to oxaloacetate, which is then available to undergo transamination to aspartate (Figure 9.18). Adenosine deaminase converts adenosine monophosphate back to inosine monophosphate, liberating ammonia. This sequence of reactions thus provides a pathway for the deamination of a variety of amino acids, linked to transamination, similar to those shown in Figure 9.14 for transamination linked to glutamate dehydrogenase or glycine oxidase.

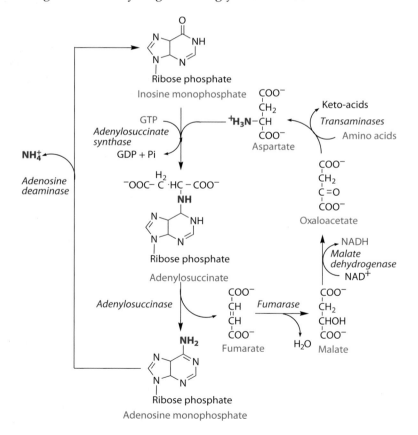

Figure 9.18 The role of aspartate as a nitrogen donor in synthetic reactions and of adenosine deaminase as a source of ammonium ions.

9.3.2 The metabolism of amino acid carbon skeletons

Acetyl CoA and acetoacetate arising from the carbon skeletons of amino acids may either be used for fatty acid synthesis (Section 5.6.1) or be oxidised as metabolic fuel, but cannot under any circumstances be utilised for the synthesis of glucose (gluconeogenesis, Section 5.7). Amino acids that yield acetyl CoA or acetoacetate are termed ketogenic. Those amino acids that yield intermediates that can be used for gluconeogenesis are termed glucogenic. Only two amino acids (leucine and lysine) are purely ketogenic; three others (tryptophan, isoleucine, and phenylalanine) yield both glucogenic and ketogenic fragments; the other amino acids are purely glucogenic (Table 9.10).

The principal substrate for gluconeogenesis is oxaloacetate, which undergoes the reaction catalysed by phospho-enolpyruvate carboxykinase to yield phospho-enolpyruvate (Figure 5.39). The onward metabolism of phospho-enolpyruvate to glucose is essentially the reverse of glycolysis (Figure 5.10).

The points of entry of amino acid carbon skeletons into central metabolic pathways are shown in Figure 5.20. Those that give rise to ketoglutarate, succinyl CoA, fumarate, or oxaloacetate can be regarded as directly increasing the tissue pool of citric acid cycle intermediates, and hence permitting the withdrawal of oxaloacetate for gluconeogenesis.

Those amino acids that give rise to pyruvate also increase the tissue pool of oxaloacetate because pyruvate can be carboxylated to oxaloacetate in the reaction catalysed by pyruvate carboxylase (Section 5.4.4.1).

Gluconeogenesis is an important fate of amino acid carbon skeletons in the fasting state, when the metabolic imperative is to maintain a supply of glucose for the central nervous system and red blood cells. However, in the fed state, the carbon skeletons of amino acids in excess of requirements for protein synthesis will mainly be used for formation of acetyl CoA for fatty acid synthesis and storage as adipose tissue triacylglycerol.

Table 9.10 Metabolic Fates of the Carbon Skeletons of Amino Acids (see also Figure 5.20)

	Glucogenic intermediates	Ketogenic intermediates
Alanine	Pyruvate	–
Glycine → serine	Pyruvate	–
Cysteine	Pyruvate	–
Tryptophan	Pyruvate	Acetyl CoA
Arginine → ornithine	α-Ketoglutarate	–
Glutamine → glutamate	α-Ketoglutarate	–
Proline → glutamate	α-Ketoglutarate	–
Histidine → glutamate	α-Ketoglutarate	–
Methionine	Propionyl CoA	–
Isoleucine	Propionyl CoA	Acetyl CoA
Valine	Succinyl CoA	–
Asparagine → aspartate	Oxaloacetate	–
Aspartate	Oxaloacetate or fumarate	–
Phenylalanine → tyrosine	Fumarate	Acetoacetate
Leucine	–	Acetoacetate and acetyl CoA
Lysine	–	Acetyl CoA

Key points

- Nitrogen balance is the difference between the dietary intake of nitrogenous compounds (mainly protein) and excretion of nitrogenous compounds. In an adult, the normal state is nitrogen equilibrium: intake = output.
- Positive nitrogen balance is normal in growth and pregnancy and after a period of protein loss from the body.
- Negative nitrogen balance occurs in response to trauma and when the intake of protein (or essential amino acids) is inadequate.
- There is continual catabolism of proteins and replacement synthesis. Different proteins turn over at different rates, and those that are regulatory enzymes have short half-lives.
- Protein requirements are estimated by determining the intake required to maintain nitrogen balance. For an adult, the average requirement is 0.66 g/kg body weight, equivalent to 8% of energy intake. Deficiency is unlikely in adults because most starchy dietary staples provide more than 8% of energy as protein.
- Nine amino acids cannot be synthesised in the body and are dietary essentials; of the remainder, two are synthesised from essential amino acids precursors, and under some circumstances, the demand for others may exceed the capacity to synthesise them. Only three amino acids, alanine, aspartate, and glutamate, can be considered to be completely dispensable, since they are synthesised from intermediates of carbohydrate metabolism.
- The nutritional value of a protein is determined by its content of essential amino acids compared with the amounts required for tissue protein synthesis. A deficit in one protein is complemented by a relative excess in others; thus, the protein quality of most diets is similar.
- DNA contains the information for synthesis of all tissue proteins; a copy of a gene is made by transcription to mRNA, and this is translated into the amino acid sequence during protein synthesis on the ribosome.
- Protein synthesis is energy expensive, accounting for about 8% of energy expenditure in the fasting state and up to 20% after a meal.
- Amino acids in excess of requirements for protein synthesis and those arising from protein catabolism in the fasting state are deaminated to keto-acids either directly or by deaminases linked to transaminases. Transamination is the process of transferring the amino group from an amino acid onto the keto-acid corresponding to another amino acid. The intermediate carrier of the amino group is the coenzyme pyridoxal phosphate, derived from vitamin B_6.
- Ammonium arising from deamination of amino acids is toxic; it is transported in the bloodstream as glutamine. Urea is synthesised in the liver as the main end product of nitrogen metabolism.
- Carbon skeletons of amino acids may be glucogenic or ketogenic.

Further resources on the CD

The nitrogen balance, peptide sequence, mutations in an exon and urea synthesis computer simulation exercises in the virtual laboratory on the CD.

Reference

American College of Sports Medicine and American Dietetic Association of Dietitians of Canada, 2009. *Nutrition and Athletic Performance*. Available from http://www.chap.uk.com/pdfs/Nutrition%20Athletic%20Performance.pdf.

chapter ten

The integration and control of metabolism

There is an obvious need to regulate metabolic pathways within individual cells to ensure that catabolic and biosynthetic pathways are not attempting to operate at the same time. There is also a need to integrate and coordinate metabolism throughout the body, to ensure a steady provision of metabolic fuels, and to control the extent to which different fuels are used by different tissues.

Objectives

After reading this chapter, you should be able to

- Explain what is meant by instantaneous, fast, and slow mechanisms of metabolic control.
- Explain what is meant by the terms hormone, and endocrine, paracrine and juxtacrine agents.
- Describe and explain allosteric regulation of enzyme activity.
- Describe and explain the regulation of glycolysis, explain what is meant by substrate cycling and why it is important.
- Describe and explain the hormonal control of glycogen synthesis and utilisation.
- Describe and explain the role of G-proteins and second messengers in signal transduction in response to fast-acting hormones, explain how there is amplification of the hormone signal and explain how there is desensitisation of the adrenoceptor in response to prolonged stimulation.
- Describe and explain the mechanisms involved in response to slow-acting hormones and explain how there is amplification of the hormone signal.
- Describe and explain the role of insulin and the insulin receptor substrate in short- and long-term metabolic control.
- Describe and explain hormonal control of the fed and fasting states and the hormonal control of adipose tissue and liver metabolism.
- Describe and explain the factors involved in the selection of fuels for muscle activity under different conditions.
- Describe and explain the biochemical basis of the metabolic derangements in diabetes mellitus and the metabolic syndrome.

10.1   Patterns of metabolic regulation

The rate at which different pathways operate is controlled by changes in the activity of key enzymes. In general, the first reaction unique to a given pathway or branch of a pathway will be most subject to regulation, although the activities of other enzymes are also regulated. The enzymes that exert the greatest control over flux (flow of metabolites) through a pathway are often those that catalyse essentially unidirectional reactions—i.e. those for which the substrates and products are far from thermodynamic equilibrium.

Within any one cell, the activities of regulatory enzymes may be controlled by two mechanisms that act instantaneously:

1. The availability of substrates
2. Inhibition or activation by accumulation of precursors, end products, or intermediates of a pathway

On a whole body basis, metabolic regulation is achieved by the actions of hormones. A hormone is released from the endocrine gland (Figure 10.1) in which it is synthesised in response to a stimulus such as the blood concentration of metabolic fuels, other hormones, or neuronal control. It circulates in the bloodstream and acts only on target cells that have receptors for the hormone, although all cells on the body are exposed to the hormone.

Paracrine agents are locally acting hormones that are secreted into the interstitial fluid (rather than the bloodstream) by cells that are close to the target cells. Juxtacrine agents are secreted into the intercellular space between the secreting cell and the target cell—neurotransmitters are juxtacrine agents. Some cells are targets for the hormones that they secrete—in this case, the hormone is an autocrine agent.

Some endocrine organs respond directly to changes in their immediate environment (e.g. the secretion of insulin by β-islet cells of the pancreas in response to an increasing concentration of glucose). Others are regulated by hormones released from the anterior pituitary gland. In turn, the secretion of hormones by the anterior pituitary is regulated by hormones secreted by the hypothalamus in response to various stimuli. The hormones secreted by the final target cells feed back on the hypothalamus and pituitary to inhibit the secretion of the stimulatory hormones, and so control their own secretion.

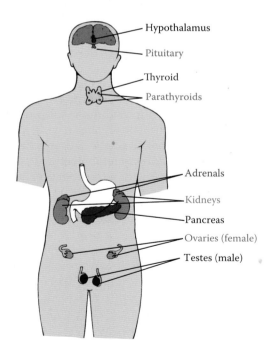

Figure 10.1 The major endocrine organs. In addition, adipose tissue and various regions of the gastrointestinal tract secrete hormones.

There are two types of response to hormones:

1. Fast responses due to changes in the activity of existing enzymes, as a result of covalent modification of the enzyme protein. Fast-acting hormones activate cell surface receptors, leading to the release of a second messenger inside the cell. The second messenger then acts directly or indirectly to activate an enzyme that catalyses the covalent modification of the target enzymes. This covalent modification may increase or decreased the activity of the target enzyme.
2. Slow responses due to changes in the rate of synthesis of enzymes. Slow-acting hormones activate intracellular receptors that bind to regulatory regions of DNA and increase or decrease the rate of transcription of one or more genes (Section 9.2.2.1).

Regardless of the mechanism by which a hormone acts, there are three key features of hormonal regulation:

1. Tissue selectivity, determined by whether or not the tissue contains receptors for the hormone
2. Amplification of the hormone signal
3. A mechanism to terminate or reverse the hormone action as its secretion decreases

10.2   Intracellular regulation of enzyme activity

As discussed in Section 2.3.3, the rate at which an enzyme catalyses a reaction increases with increasing concentration of substrate, until the enzyme is more or less saturated. This means that an enzyme that has a high K_m, relative to the usual concentration of its substrate, will be sensitive to changes in substrate availability. By contrast, an enzyme that has a low K_m, relative to the usual concentration of its substrate, will act at a more or less constant rate regardless of changes in substrate availability (Figure 2.9).

The availability of substrate may be regulated by uptake from the bloodstream—for example, muscle and adipose tissue only take up glucose to any significant extent in response to insulin. In the absence of insulin the glucose transporters are in intracellular vesicles; in response to insulin these vesicles migrate to the cell surface and fuse with the cell membrane, revealing active glucose transporters.

10.2.1   Allosteric modification of the activity of regulatory enzymes

Allosteric regulation of enzyme activity is due to reversible, non-covalent, binding of effectors to regulatory sites, leading to a change in the conformation of the active site. This may result in either increased catalytic activity (allosteric activation) or decreased catalytic activity (allosteric inhibition). Enzymes that are subject to allosteric regulation are usually multiple subunit proteins.

Many enzymes that are subject to allosteric regulation have two interconvertible conformations (Figure 10.2):

1. A tense (T) form, which binds substrates poorly and therefore has low catalytic activity. Allosteric inhibitors bind to and stabilise the less active T form of the enzyme.
2. A relaxed (R) form, which binds substrates well and therefore has high catalytic activity. Allosteric activators bind to and stabilise the active R form of the enzyme.

Allosteric inhibition
The inhibitor stabilises the T form of the enzyme, which binds substrate poorly

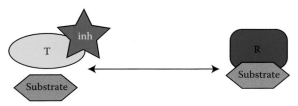

Allosteric activation
The activator stabilises the R form of the enzyme, which binds substrate well

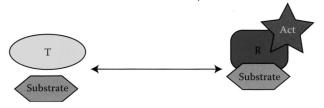

Figure 10.2 Allosteric inhibition and activation of enzymes.

Compounds that act as allosteric inhibitors are often end products of the pathway, and this type of inhibition is known as end product inhibition. The decreased rate of enzyme activity results in a lower rate of formation of a product that is present in adequate amounts.

Compounds that act as allosteric activators of enzymes are often precursors of the pathway; this is a mechanism for feed-forward activation, increasing the activity of a controlling enzyme in anticipation of increased availability of substrate.

Enzymes that consist of multiple subunits frequently display cooperativity between the subunits; binding of substrate to the active site of one subunit leads to conformational changes that enhance the binding of substrate to the other active sites of the complex (Section 2.3.3.3). This again is allosteric activation of the enzyme, in this case, by the substrate itself. The activity of such cooperative enzymes is more sharply dependent on the concentration of substrate than is the case for enzymes that do not show cooperativity.

As shown in Figure 10.3, an allosteric activator of an enzyme that shows substrate cooperativity acts by decreasing the cooperativity, so that the enzyme has a greater activity at a low concentration of the substrate than would otherwise be the case. Conversely, an allosteric inhibitor of a cooperative enzyme acts by increasing cooperativity, so that the enzyme has less activity at a low concentration of substrate than it would in the absence of the inhibitor.

10.2.2 *Control of glycolysis—the allosteric regulation of phosphofructokinase*

In glycolysis (Figure 5.10), most control is at the level of phosphofructokinase, which catalyses the (irreversible) phosphorylation of fructose 6-phosphate to fructose 1,6-bisphosphate. In gluconeogenesis, the hydrolysis of fructose 1,6-bisphosphate is catalysed by a separate enzyme, fructose bisphosphatase. Regulation of the activities of these two enzymes determines whether the overall metabolic flux is in the direction of glycolysis or gluconeogenesis.

Inhibition of phosphofructokinase leads to an accumulation of glucose 6-phosphate in the cell, and this results in inhibition of hexokinase, which has an inhibitory binding site

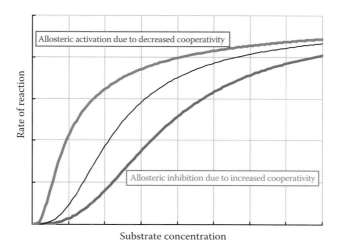

Figure 10.3 Allosteric inhibition and activation of an enzyme showing subunit cooperativity.

for its product. The result of this is a decreased rate of entry of glucose into glycolysis. In addition to hexokinase, the liver also contains glucokinase, which is not inhibited by glucose 6-phosphate (Section 5.3.1). This means that despite inhibition of utilisation of glucose as a metabolic fuel, the liver can take up glucose for glycogen synthesis (Section 5.6.3).

10.2.2.1 Feedback control of phosphofructokinase

ATP can be considered to be an end product of glycolysis, and phosphofructokinase is allosterically inhibited by ATP binding at a regulatory site that is distinct from the substrate-binding site for ATP. As shown in Figure 10.4, at physiological concentrations of ATP, phosphofructokinase has very low activity, and a more markedly sigmoid dependency on the concentration of its substrate. In the presence of a physiological concentration of

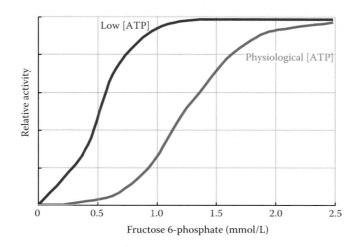

Figure 10.4 The substrate dependence of phosphofructokinase at low and physiological concentrations of ATP.

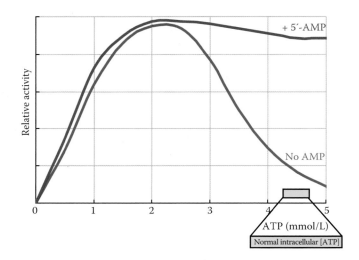

Figure 10.5 The inhibition of phosphofructokinase by ATP and relief of inhibition by 5'-AMP. The yellow bar shows the normal range of intracellular ATP.

ATP, the activity of phosphofructokinase at normal intracellular concentrations of fructose 6-phosphate is only about 10% of V_{max}.

When there is a requirement for increased glycolysis, and hence increased ATP production, the inhibition by ATP is relieved, and there may be a 100-fold or higher increase in glycolytic flux in response to increased demand for ATP. However, there is less than a 10% change in the intracellular concentration of ATP, which, as shown in Figure 10.5, would not have a significant effect on the activity of the enzyme. As the concentration of ADP begins to increase, adenylate kinase catalyses the reaction:

$$2 \times ADP \rightleftharpoons ATP + 5'\text{-}AMP$$

5'-AMP acts as a sensitive intracellular signal that energy reserves are low, and ATP formation must be increased. It binds to phosphofructokinase and both reverses the inhibition caused by ATP and also decreases the cooperativity between the subunits, so that the enzyme has greater affinity for fructose 6-phosphate. AMP also binds to fructose 1,6-bisphosphatase, reducing its activity.

In liver and adipose tissue, citrate in excess of requirements for citric acid cycle activity leaves mitochondria to provide a source of acetyl CoA for fatty acid synthesis (Section 5.6.1). As citrate accumulates in the cytosol in excess of the need for fatty acid synthesis, it inhibits phosphofructokinase, so reducing its own formation. In muscle, creatine phosphate (Section 3.2.3.1) has a similar effect.

Phosphoenolpyruvate is synthesised in the liver for gluconeogenesis (Section 5.7); under these conditions, there is obviously a need to inhibit glycolysis, and phosphoenolpyruvate inhibits phosphofructokinase.

10.2.2.2   *Feed-forward control of phosphofructokinase*

High intracellular concentrations of fructose 6-phosphate activate a second enzyme, phosphofructokinase-2, which catalyses the synthesis of fructose 2,6-bisphosphate from fructose 6-phosphate (Figure 10.6). Fructose 2,6-bisphosphate is an allosteric activator of

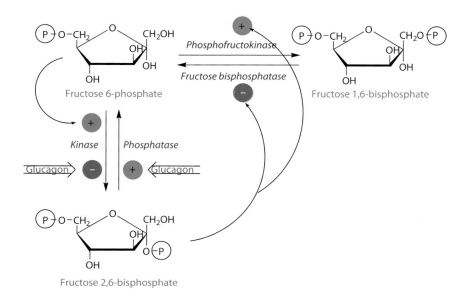

Figure 10.6 The role of 2,6-fructose bisphosphate in the regulation of phosphofructokinase.

phosphofructokinase and an allosteric inhibitor of fructose 1,6-bisphosphatase. It thus acts both to increase glycolysis and inhibit gluconeogenesis. This is feed-forward control— allosteric activation of phosphofructokinase because there is an increased concentration of substrate available.

Phosphofructokinase-2 is a bifunctional enzyme—a single protein with two catalytic sites. One site is the kinase that catalyses the phosphorylation of fructose 6-phosphate to fructose 2,6-bisphosphate, while the other is the phosphatase that catalyses hydrolysis of fructose 2,6-bisphosphate to fructose 6-phosphate and inorganic phosphate. A single regulatory site controls the activity of the two catalytic sites in opposite directions. In response to glucagon (which stimulates gluconeogenesis and inhibits glycolysis, Section 10.5), kinase activity is decreased and phosphatase activity increased. This results in a low concentration of fructose 2,6-bisphosphate, and hence decreased activity of phosphofructokinase and increased activity of fructose 1,6-bisphosphatase.

10.2.2.3   Substrate cycling

A priori, it would seem obvious that the activities of opposing enzymes such as phosphofructokinase and fructose 1,6-bisphosphatase should be regulated in such a way that one is active and the other inactive at any time. If both were active at the same time, then there would be cycling between fructose 6-phosphate and fructose 1,6-bisphosphate, with hydrolysis of ATP—an apparently futile cycle with no product formation. However, both enzymes are indeed active to some extent at the same time, although the activity of one is considerably greater than the other, so that there is a net metabolic flux. A relatively small change in the activity of both enzymes (in opposite directions) will lead to a very large change in the rate of flux through the pathway. This permits rapid and sensitive control.

Another function of substrate cycling is thermogenesis—deliberate hydrolysis of ATP for heat production. It is not known to what extent substrate cycling can be increased to enhance thermogenesis (which is normally mediated by uncoupling of electron transport and oxidative phosphorylation, Section 3.3.1.5). However, it is noteworthy that the honey-bee, which does not exhibit significant substrate cycling, cannot fly in cold weather, while the bumblebee, which has adaptive substrate cycling, can initiate thermogenesis and so fly in cold weather.

10.3 Responses to fast-acting hormones by covalent modification of enzyme proteins

A number of regulatory enzymes have a serine, tyrosine, or threonine residue at a regulatory site. This can undergo phosphorylation catalysed by a protein kinase (Figure 10.7). Phosphorylation increases the activity of some enzymes and reduces that of others. Later, often as the result of secretion and action of a counter-regulatory hormone, the phosphate group is removed from the enzyme by a phosphoprotein phosphatase, thus restoring the enzyme to its original state. These responses are not instantaneous, but they are rapid, with a maximum response developing within a few seconds of hormone stimulation.

The reduction in activity of pyruvate dehydrogenase in response to an increased concentration of acetyl CoA and NADH (Section 10.5.2) is the result of phosphorylation. This control of enzyme phosphorylation by substrates is unusual. In most cases, the activities

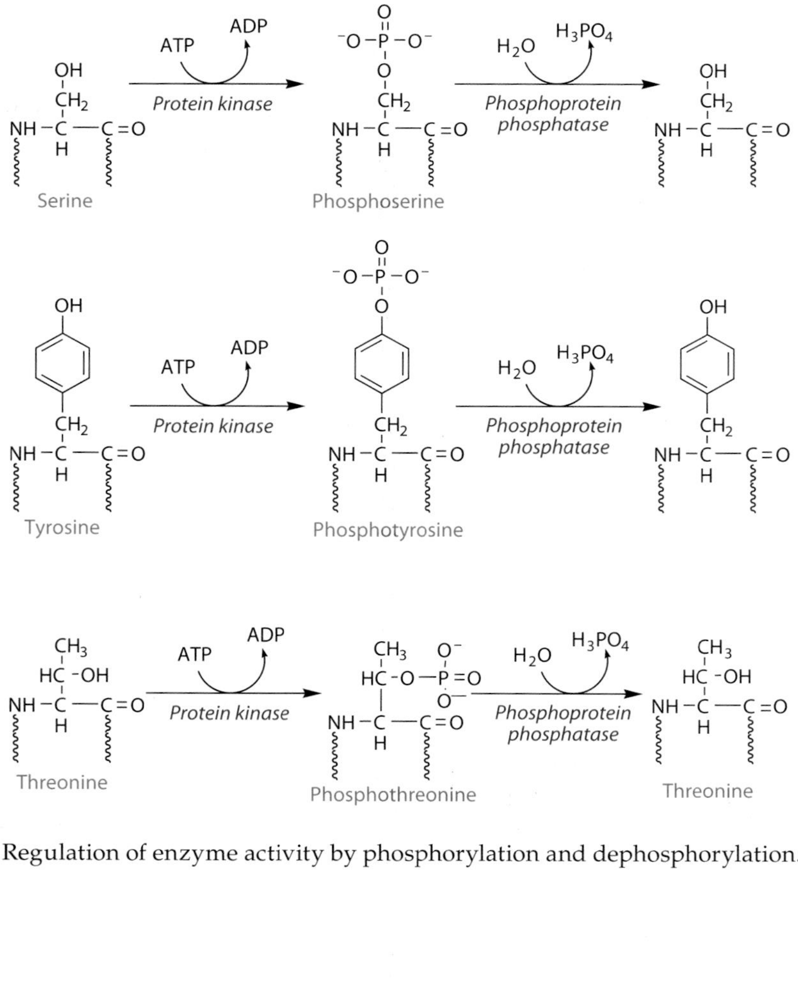

Figure 10.7 Regulation of enzyme activity by phosphorylation and dephosphorylation.

of protein kinases and phosphoprotein phosphatases are regulated by second messengers released intracellularly in response to fast-acting hormones binding to receptors at the cell surface. 5′-AMP, formed by the action of adenylate kinase (Section 10.2.2.1), also activates a protein kinase—in this case, it is acting as an intracellular messenger in response to changes in ATP availability, rather than in response to an external stimulus.

The hormonal regulation of glycogen synthesis and utilisation is one of the best understood of such mechanisms. Two enzymes are involved, and obviously it is not desirable that both enzymes should be active at the same time:

1. Glycogen synthase catalyses the synthesis of glycogen, adding glucose units from UDP-glucose (Section 5.6.3 and Figure 5.37).
2. Glycogen phosphorylase catalyses the removal of glucose units from glycogen, as glucose 1-phosphate (Section 5.6.3.1 and Figure 5.9).

In response to insulin (secreted in the fed state), there is increased synthesis of glycogen and inactivation of glycogen phosphorylase. In response to glucagon (secreted in the fasting state) or adrenaline (secreted in response to fear or fright), there is inactivation of glycogen synthase and activation of glycogen phosphorylase, permitting mobilisation of glucose from glycogen reserves. As shown in Figure 10.8, both effects are mediated by protein phosphorylation and dephosphorylation.

Protein kinase is activated in response to glucagon or adrenaline:

- Phosphorylation of glycogen synthase results in loss of activity.
- Phosphorylation of glycogen phosphorylase results in activation of the inactive enzyme.

Phosphoprotein phosphatase is activated in response to insulin:

- Dephosphorylation of phosphorylated glycogen synthase restores its activity.
- Dephosphorylation of phosphorylated glycogen phosphorylase results in loss of activity.

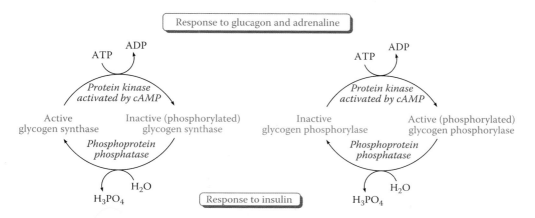

Figure 10.8 Hormonal regulation of glycogen synthase and glycogen phosphorylase: responses to glucagon or adrenaline and insulin.

There is a further measure of instantaneous control by intracellular metabolites that can override this hormonal regulation:

- Inactive glycogen synthase is allosterically activated by high concentrations of glucose 6-phosphate.
- Active glycogen phosphorylase is allosterically inhibited by ATP, glucose, and glucose 6-phosphate.

10.3.1   *Membrane receptors and G-proteins*

A cell responds to a fast-acting hormone if it has cell-surface receptors for the hormone. The receptors are transmembrane proteins; at the outer face of the membrane, they have a site that binds the hormone, in the same way as an enzyme binds its substrate, by non-covalent equilibrium binding. When the receptor binds the hormone, it undergoes a conformational change that permits it to interact with proteins at the inner face of the membrane. These are known as G-proteins because they bind guanine nucleotides (GDP or GTP). They function to transmit information from an occupied membrane receptor protein to an intracellular effector, which in turn leads to the release into the cytosol of a second messenger, ultimately resulting in the activation of protein kinases.

The G-proteins that are important in hormone responses consist of three subunits, α, β, and γ (Figure 10.9). In the resting state, the α-subunit is GDP bound and is separate from the $\beta\gamma$-dimer. When the receptor is occupied by the hormone, it undergoes a conformational change and recruits the subunits to form a (G-protein trimer)-receptor complex. The complex then binds GTP, which displaces the bound GDP. Once GTP has bound, the complex dissociates.

The α-subunit of the G-protein with GTP bound then binds to, and activates, the effector, which may be adenylyl cyclase (Section 10.3.2) or phospholipase C (Section 10.3.3), resulting in release of a second messenger.

The α-subunit has relatively slow GTPase activity that catalyses hydrolysis of the bound GTP to GDP. As this occurs, the α-subunit-effector complex dissociates, and the effector loses its activity. The G-protein subunits are then available to be recruited by another receptor that has been activated by binding the hormone.

There is an animation of the action of a G-protein-coupled receptor on the CD.

10.3.2   *Cyclic AMP and cyclic GMP as second messengers*

One of the intracellular effectors that is activated by the G-protein α-subunit-GTP complex is adenylyl cyclase. This is an integral membrane protein that catalyses the formation of cyclic AMP (cAMP) from ATP (Figure 10.10) as the second messenger in response to hormones such as glucagon and adrenaline. cAMP is an allosteric activator of protein kinases. It is also formed in the same way in response to a number of neurotransmitters.

Phosphodiesterase catalyses the hydrolysis of cAMP to yield 5′-AMP, thus providing a mechanism for termination of the intracellular response to the hormone. Under normal conditions, 5′-AMP is then phosphorylated to ADP by the reaction of adenylate kinase—it is only under conditions of relatively low ATP availability and relatively high ADP that adenylate kinase acts to form 5′-AMP as an intracellular signal of the energy state of the cell (Section 10.2.2.1).

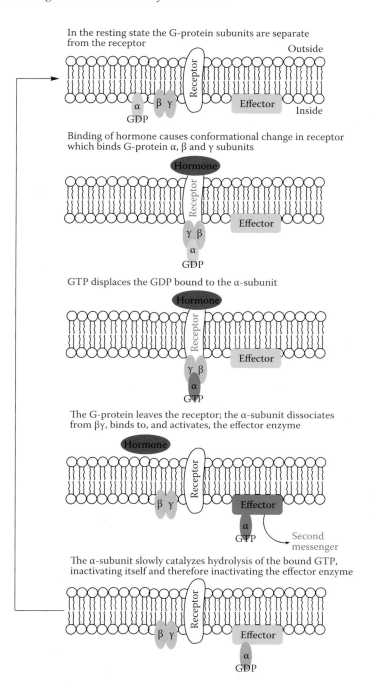

Figure 10.9 The role of G-proteins in the response to fast-acting (surface acting) hormones. See also the animation on the CD.

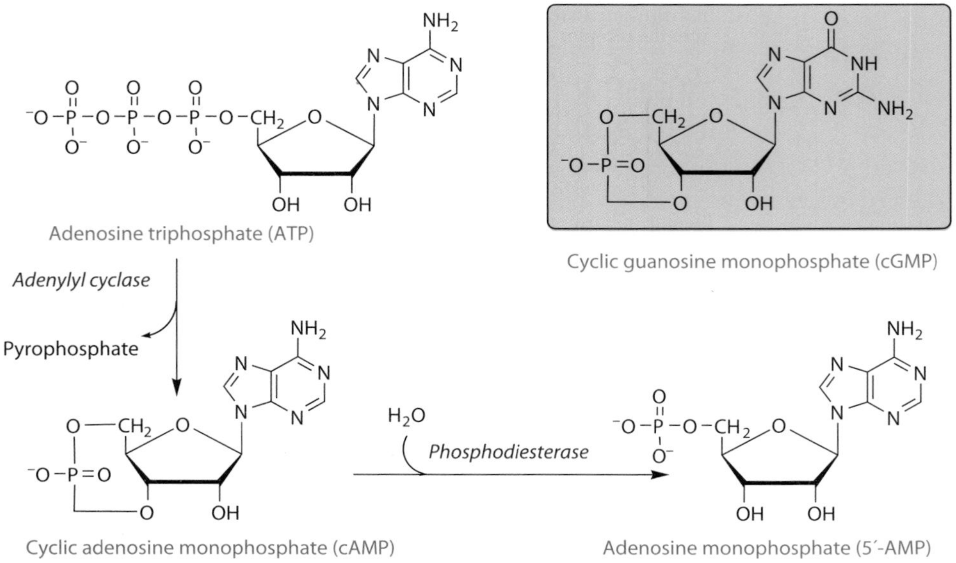

Figure 10.10 Adenylyl cyclase and the formation of cyclic AMP as an intracellular second messenger. (The structure of cyclic GMP is shown in the box.)

Phosphodiesterase is activated in response to insulin action (which thus acts to terminate the actions of glucagon and adrenaline) and is inhibited by drugs such as caffeine and theophylline, which therefore potentiate hormone and neurotransmitter action.

In the same way as cAMP is formed from ATP by adenylyl cyclase, the guanine analogue, cGMP can be formed from GTP by guanylyl cyclase. This may either be an integral membrane protein, like adenylyl cyclase, or a cytosolic protein. cGMP is produced in response to a number of neurotransmitters and also nitric oxide, the endothelium-derived relaxation factor that is important in vasodilatation.

10.3.2.1 Amplification of the hormone signal

In response to fear or fright, adrenaline is secreted by the adrenal glands; its plasma concentration is in the nanomolar range (10^{-9} mol/L). Within a few seconds, as a result of activation of glycogen phosphorylase in the liver, the blood concentration of glucose increases by several millimoles per litre—an approximately million-fold amplification of the hormone signal.

As shown in Figure 10.11, the active (G-protein α-subunit)–GTP released in response to binding of 1 mol of hormone to the surface receptor will activate adenylyl cyclase for as long as it contains GTP. The hydrolysis to yield inactive (G-protein α-subunit)-GDP occurs relatively slowly; a single molecule of (G-protein α-subunit)–GTP will lead to the production of about 40 mol of cAMP as second messenger.

There is an equilibrium between cAMP bound to protein kinase and that in free solution in the cytosol and therefore accessible to phosphodiesterase for inactivation. Each molecule of cAMP activates a molecule of protein kinase A for as long as it remains bound.

Phosphorylase kinase remains active until it is dephosphorylated in response to insulin or another counter-regulatory hormone, and so phosphorylates some 200 molecules

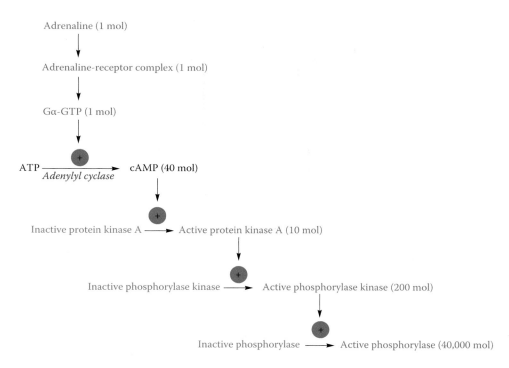

Figure 10.11 Amplification of the hormone signal through a phosphorylation cascade.

of glycogen phosphorylase. Similarly, glycogen phosphorylase remains active until it is dephosphorylated in response to a counter-regulatory hormone and will catalyse the release of several thousand molecules of glucose 6-phosphate per second.

10.3.2.2   Desensitisation of the adrenaline receptor

Continuous exposure to adrenaline leads to desensitisation. This may occur in two ways:

1. Desensitisation of multiple G-protein-coupled receptors—the process of heterologous desensitisation. Protein kinase A catalyses the phosphorylation of several serine and threonine residues in the cytosolic domain of all G-protein-coupled receptors; thus, the cell loses the ability to respond to multiple stimuli acting through different receptors but the same signalling pathway.
2. Specific desensitisation of the β-adrenoceptor—homologous desensitisation, in which the cell ceases to respond to adrenaline but continues to respond to other hormones acting via G-protein-coupled receptors. When adrenaline is bound to the receptor, the G-protein binds to the carboxy terminal and third intracellular loop of the receptor. In response to prolonged adrenergic stimulation, the receptor stimulates the β-adrenoceptor kinase (βARK), which catalyses phosphorylation of serine and threonine residues in the carboxy terminal and third intracellular loop of the receptor. This leads to a conformational change that permits the binding of β-arrestin to the receptor, and prevents binding of the G-protein. The receptor with β-arrestin bound undergoes endocytosis and is catabolised.

10.3.3   *Inositol trisphosphate and diacylglycerol as second messengers*

The other response to G-protein activation involves phosphatidylinositol, one of the phospholipids in cell membranes (Section 4.3.1.2). Phosphatidylinositol can undergo two phosphorylations, catalysed by phosphatidylinositol kinase, to yield phosphatidylinositol bisphosphate (PIP_2). PIP_2 is a substrate for phospholipase C inside the membrane, which is activated by the binding of a G-protein α-subunit with GTP bound. The products of phospholipase C action are inositol trisphosphate (IP_3) and diacylglycerol (Figure 10.12), both of which act as intracellular second messengers.

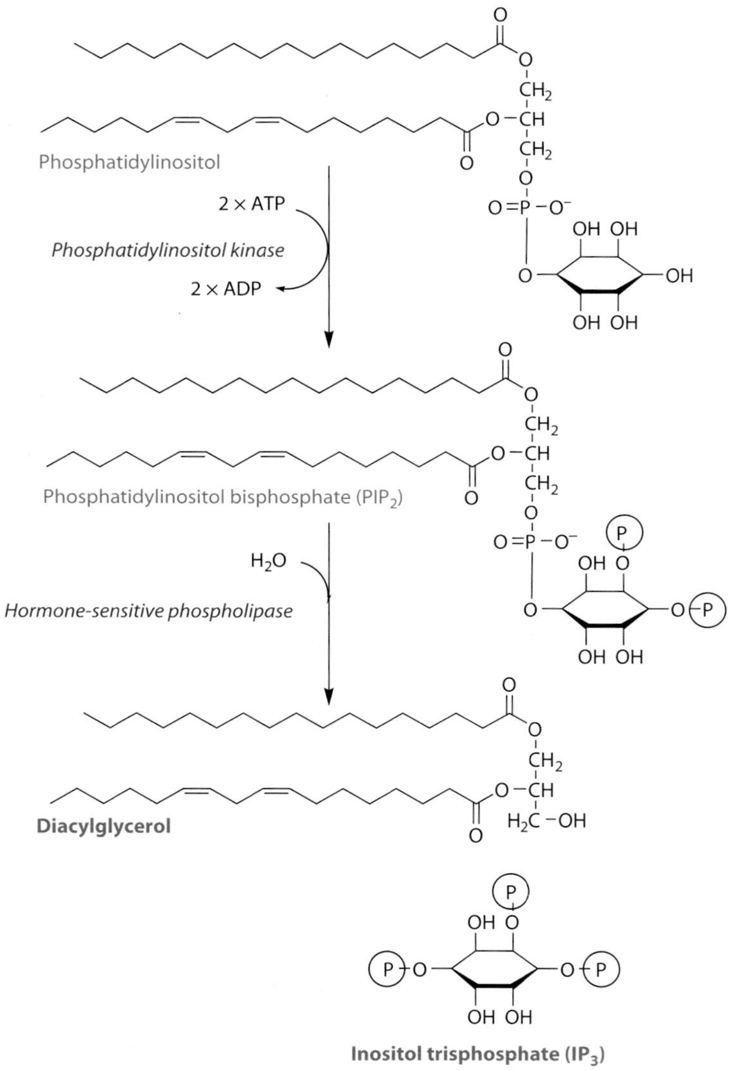

Figure 10.12 Hormone-sensitive phospholipase and the formation of inositol trisphosphate and diacylglycerol as intracellular messengers.

Inositol trisphosphate opens a calcium transport channel in the membrane of the endoplasmic reticulum. This leads to an influx of calcium from storage in the endoplasmic reticulum and a 10-fold increase in the cytosolic concentration of calcium ions. A number of enzymes are directly sensitive to this increased intracellular calcium, including protein kinase C, which phosphorylates target proteins in the same way as does protein kinase A activated by cAMP (Section 10.3.2).

Calmodulin is a small calcium binding protein found in all cells. Its affinity for calcium is such that at the resting concentration of calcium in the cytosol (of the order of 0.1 μmol/L), little or none is bound to calmodulin. When the cytosolic concentration of calcium increases to about 1 μmol/L in response to opening of the endoplasmic reticulum calcium transport channel, each molecule of calmodulin binds 4 mol of calcium. When this occurs, it undergoes a conformational change, and calcium–calmodulin binds to, and activates, cytosolic protein kinases, which, in turn phosphorylates target enzymes.

Some of the diacylglycerol released by phospholipase C action remains in the membrane, where it activates a membrane-bound protein kinase. Some diffuses into the cytosol, where it enhances the binding of calcium–calmodulin to cytosolic protein kinases.

Inositol trisphosphate is inactivated by further phosphorylation to inositol tetrakisphosphate (IP_4), and the diacylglycerol is inactivated by hydrolysis to glycerol and fatty acids.

10.3.3.1   *Amplification of the hormone signal*

The active (G-protein α-subunit)–GTP released in response to binding of 1 mol of hormone to the cell surface receptor will activate phospholipase C for as long as it contains GTP, and therefore, a single molecule of (G-protein α-subunit)–GTP complex will lead to the production of many moles of IP_3 and diacylglycerol as second messengers.

Each molecule of diacylglycerol will activate the membrane-bound protein kinase until it is hydrolysed (relatively slowly) by lipase, thus resulting in the phosphorylation of many molecules of target protein, each of which will catalyse the metabolism of many thousands of mol of substrate per second, until it is dephosphorylated by phosphoprotein phosphatase.

Similarly, each molecule of IP_3 will continue to keep the endoplasmic reticulum calcium channel open until it is phosphorylated to inactive inositol tetrakisphosphate, thus maintaining a flow of calcium ions into the cytosol. Each molecule of calcium–calmodulin will bind to, and activate, a molecule of protein kinase for as long as the cytosol calcium concentration remains high. It is only as the calcium is pumped back into the endoplasmic reticulum that the calcium concentration falls low enough for calmodulin to lose its bound calcium and be inactivated. Again, each molecule of phosphorylated enzyme will catalyse the metabolism of many thousands of mol of substrate per second until it is dephosphorylated by phosphoprotein phosphatase.

10.3.4   *The insulin receptor*

The insulin receptor consists of two α-subunits at the outer face of the membrane, which bind insulin and two β-subunits that span the membrane. In response to insulin binding to the α-subunit dimer, there is a conformational change in the receptor, leading to activation of the protein kinase activity of the cytosolic region of the β-subunits, and autophosphorylation of tyrosine residues on the β-subunits. The phosphorylated β-subunits then bind and phosphorylate the insulin receptor substrate protein (Figure 10.13).

The insulin receptor is a dimer of two α–β subunits linked by S-S bridges

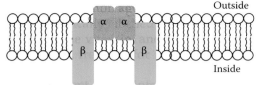

Binding of insulin causes a conformational change and activation of the tyrosine kinase activity of the β-subunits, which catalyse autophosphorylation

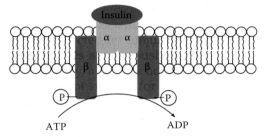

The phosphorylated receptor binds and phosphorylates insulin receptor substrate proteins

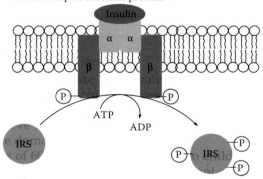

Phosphorylated insulin receptor substrate binds to and activates protein kinase B and mitogen-activated protein kinase

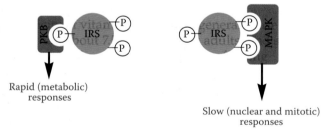

Figure 10.13 Signalling in response to stimulation of the insulin receptor.

Phosphorylated insulin receptor substrate can bind to either of two protein kinases:

1. Protein kinase B is responsible for initiating the cascade of actions leading to the rapid metabolic responses to insulin—stimulation of glucose transport, glycogen and fatty acid synthesis, inhibition of lipolysis and glycogenolysis, stimulation of protein synthesis by increasing translation.
2. The mitogen-activated protein kinases (MAP kinases) are responsible for initiating a cascade of actions leading to increased gene expression and cell division.

A number of growth factor receptors act in the same way as the insulin receptor to activate MAP kinases; a mutant of the epidermal growth factor (EGF) receptor is permanently activated, even when not occupied. This results in continuous signalling for cell division, and is one of the underlying mechanisms in many cancers.

10.4   Slow-acting hormones: changes in enzyme synthesis

There is continual turnover of proteins in the cell, and not all proteins are broken down and replaced at the same rate. Some are relatively stable, whilst others, and especially enzymes that are important in metabolic regulation, have short half-lives—of the order of minutes or hours (Table 9.2). This rapid turnover means that it is possible to control metabolic pathways by changing the rate at which a key regulatory enzyme is synthesised, so changing the total amount of that enzyme in the tissue. An increase in the rate of synthesis of an enzyme is induction, whilst the reverse, a decrease in the rate of synthesis of the enzyme by a metabolite, is repression. A number of key enzymes in metabolic pathways are induced by their substrates, and similarly many are repressed by high concentrations of the end products of the pathways they control.

Slow-acting hormones, including the steroid hormones such as cortisol and the sex steroids (androgens, oestrogens, and progesterone), retinoic acid derived from vitamin A (Section 11.2.3.2), calcitriol derived from vitamin D (Section 11.3.3), and the thyroid hormones (Section 11.15.3.3), act by changing the rate at which the genes for specific enzymes are expressed.

The responses are slower than for hormones that increase the activity of existing enzyme molecules because of the need for an adequate amount of new enzyme protein to be synthesised or the need for existing enzyme protein to be catabolised in the case of repression. The response is prolonged because, in the case of induction, after the hormone has ceased to act there is still an increased amount of enzyme protein in the cell, and the effect will only diminish as the newly synthesised enzyme is catabolised. In the case of repression, it will take time for there to be enough synthesis of new enzyme protein. The time scale of action of slow-acting hormones ranges between a few hours to several days.

Slow-acting hormones are commonly hydrophobic and circulate bound to proteins in the bloodstream. The hormone-binding protein complex enters the cell by endocytosis. The binding protein is then hydrolysed, liberating the hormone, which binds to an intracellular receptor protein. Binding of the hormone causes a conformational change in the receptor protein, and loss of a chaperone protein (heat shock protein) that is bound to the unoccupied receptor. Loss of the chaperone protein reveals a dimerisation site on the receptor. The hormone–receptor complex dimerises and undergoes phosphorylation that enables it to bind to a hormone response element on DNA (Figure 10.14). For induction of new protein synthesis, binding of the activated hormone-receptor complex to the

Hormone circulates in plasma bound to binding protein

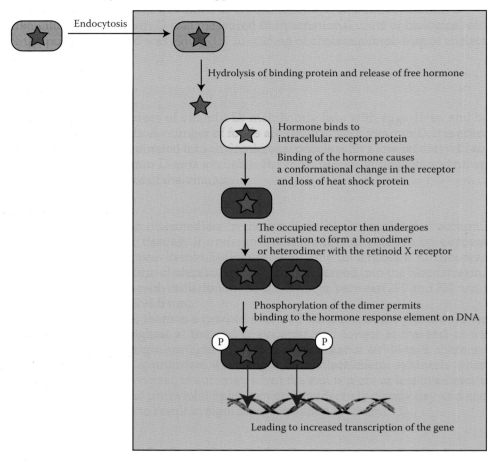

Figure 10.14 The action of steroid hormones.

hormone response element acts as a signal to recruit the various transcription factors required for transcription of the gene, leading to increased synthesis of mRNA (Section 9.2.2.1). Increased synthesis of mRNA results in increased synthesis of the protein (Section 9.2.3). For repression, binding of the activated hormone-receptor complex to the hormone response element blocks the access of transcription factors and so reduces transcription to mRNA.

Whilst some slow-acting hormone receptors form homodimers (two identical receptor proteins, each with hormone bound), others form heterodimers with the vitamin A RXR receptor that binds 9-*cis*-retinoic acid (Section 11.2.3.2). This means that vitamin A is important in the actions of a number of hormones. Vitamin A deficiency will lead to a lack of occupied RXR to form active heterodimers. However, RXR without 9-*cis*-retinoic acid bound can also form heterodimers with vitamin D and thyroid hormone receptors; these bind to, and block, rather than activate, hormone response elements. This means that in vitamin A deficiency, not only is there not the expected increase in transcription in response to vitamin D or thyroid hormone, but there is a reduction to below the basal rate of transcription. Conversely, excessive vitamin A may also impair hormone responses because the occupied RXR can form a homodimer, meaning that less is available to form heterodimers. There is some evidence that excessive intake of vitamin A impairs vitamin D responsiveness, and may be a factor in bone disease (Sections 11.3.3.1 and 11.3.4).

A cell will only respond to a slow-acting hormone if it synthesises the receptor protein. The response to the same hormone in different tissues, and at different stages in development, may well be different because only genes that are expressed in the cell will be induced. The control of gene expression by slow-acting hormones is not a matter of switching on or off a gene that is otherwise silent; the hormone increases or decreases the expression of a gene that is anyway being transcribed in the cell. Similarly, the secretion of steroid hormones is not a strictly an on/off affair, but a matter of changes in the amount being secreted.

Although there is a great deal of information about the molecular mechanisms involved in initiating the responses to nuclear-acting hormones, less is known about the termination of their action. Vitamin B_6 (Section 11.9.2) displaces hormone–receptor complexes from DNA binding, and there is evidence that the responsiveness of target tissues to slow-acting hormones is increased in vitamin B_6 deficiency.

10.4.1   Amplification of the hormone signal

The amplification of the hormone signal in response to a slow-acting hormone is the result of increased synthesis of mRNA—there is increased transcription for as long as the hormone-receptor complex remains bound to the hormone-response element on DNA. Each molecule of mRNA is translated many times over, leading to a considerable, albeit (relatively) slow, increase in the amount of enzyme protein in the cell. Each molecule of enzyme will then catalyse the metabolism of many thousands of mol of substrate per second until it is catabolised.

10.5   Hormonal control in the fed and fasting states

In the fed state (Figure 5.6), when there is an ample supply of metabolic fuels from the gut, the main processes occurring are synthesis of reserves of triacylglycerol and glycogen; glucose is in plentiful supply and is the main fuel for most tissues. At the same time, there is an increase in protein synthesis, to replace that lost in the fasting state (Section 9.2.3.3).

In the fasting state (Figure 5.7), the reserves of triacylglycerol and glycogen are mobilised for use; glucose, which is now scarce, must be spared for use by the brain and red blood cells, and protein synthesis slows down, so that there is net protein catabolism, releasing amino acids for gluconeogenesis (Section 5.7).

The principal hormones involved are insulin, in the fed state, and glucagon, in the fasting state. Adrenaline and noradrenaline share many of the actions of glucagon, and act to provide an increased supply of metabolic fuels from triacylglycerol and glycogen reserves in response to fear or fright, regardless of whether or not fuels are being absorbed from the gut.

In liver and muscle, insulin and glucagon act to regulate the synthesis and breakdown of glycogen, as shown in Figure 10.8. They also regulate glycolysis (stimulated by insulin and inhibited by glucagon) and gluconeogenesis (inhibited by insulin and stimulated by glucagon). The result of this is that in the fed state the liver takes up and utilises glucose, to form either glycogen, which is stored in the liver, or triacylglycerol, which is exported to other tissues in very-low-density lipoproteins. By contrast, in the fasting state the liver exports glucose arising from both the breakdown of glycogen and gluconeogenesis. It also oxidises fatty acids and exports ketone bodies for use by other tissues (Section 5.5.3).

10.5.1 Hormonal control of adipose tissue metabolism

Insulin has three actions in adipose tissue in the fed state (Figure 10.15):

1. *Stimulation of glucose uptake.* In the absence of insulin, glucose transporters in adipose tissue are in intracellular vesicles. An early response to insulin is migration of these vesicles to the cell surface, where they fuse with the cell membrane, exposing glucose transporters. This results in an increased rate of glucose uptake, and hence increased glycolysis (Section 5.4.1) and increased availability of acetyl CoA for fatty acid synthesis (Section 5.6.1). In the fasting state, when insulin secretion is low, little or no glucose is taken up into adipose tissue cells.

2. *Induction of lipoprotein lipase.* Lipoprotein lipase has a half life of about 1 h (Table 9.2). It is induced in response to insulin action, and the newly synthesised enzyme migrates to the surface of the blood vessel endothelial walls, where it binds chylomicrons or VLDL (Sections 5.6.2.1 and 5.6.2.2) and catalyses the hydrolysis of triacylglycerol. The non-esterified fatty acids are mainly taken up by adipose tissue and used for synthesis of triacylglycerol reserves.

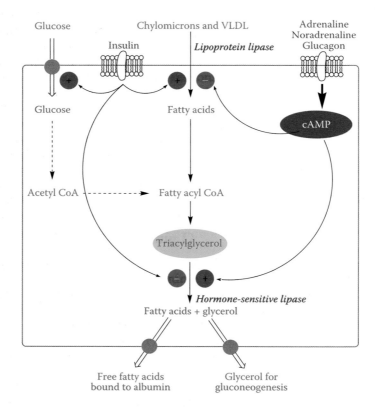

Figure 10.15 Hormonal control of the synthesis and hydrolysis of triacylglycerol in adipose tissue.

3. *Inhibition of intracellular lipase (hormone-sensitive lipase).* This reduces the hydrolysis of triacylglycerol reserves and halts the release of non-esterified fatty acids into the bloodstream.

cAMP, produced in response to adrenaline and noradrenaline, stimulates protein kinase, which activates intracellular hormone-sensitive lipase and represses the synthesis of lipoprotein lipase. Hormone-sensitive lipase catalyses the hydrolysis of the triacylglycerol stored in adipose tissue cells, leading to release into the bloodstream of free fatty acids, which are transported bound to albumin, and glycerol, which is a substrate for gluconeogenesis in the liver.

Even in the fed state, there is some release of non-esterified fatty acids into the bloodstream, as a result of the extracellular action of lipoprotein lipase—not all of the fatty acid released enters the adipocytes. In the fed state, most of this fatty acid is taken up by the liver, re-esterified to form triacylglycerol, and exported in VLDL (Section 5.6.2.2). This ATP-expensive cycling between lipolysis in adipose tissue and re-esterification in the liver provides a continual supply of non-esterified fatty acid for muscle. The extent to which muscle utilises fatty acids is determined more by the intensity of physical activity than by their availability (Section 10.6), and muscle has a requirement for fatty acids that is independent of the relative concentrations of insulin and glucagon.

10.5.2 Control of lipid metabolism in the liver

The liver synthesises fatty acids in the fed state and oxidises them in the fasting state. The direction of metabolic flux (lipogenesis or lipolysis) is controlled both in response to insulin and glucagon and also by the intracellular concentrations of substrates.

In the fed state, insulin stimulates glycolysis (and inhibits gluconeogenesis), leading to increased formation of pyruvate, which results in increased formation of acetyl CoA, and hence increased formation of citrate, which is exported to the cytosol for fatty acid synthesis (Section 5.6.1). Insulin also stimulates the activity of acetyl CoA carboxylase, leading to increased formation of malonyl CoA for fatty acid synthesis (Figure 5.29).

In the fasting state, glucagon has the opposite actions, decreasing glycolysis (and so reducing the availability of pyruvate, acetyl CoA, and hence citrate for fatty acid synthesis), increasing gluconeogenesis, and decreasing the activity of acetyl CoA carboxylase.

Pyruvate dehydrogenase is inhibited in response to increased acetyl CoA and also an increase in the $NADH/NAD^+$ ratio in the mitochondrion. The concentration of acetyl CoA will be high when β-oxidation of fatty acids is occurring, and there is no need to utilise pyruvate as a metabolic fuel. Similarly, the $NADH/NAD^+$ ratio will be high when there is an adequate amount of metabolic fuel being oxidised in the mitochondrion; again pyruvate is not required as a source of acetyl CoA. Under these conditions, pyruvate will mainly be carboxylated to oxaloacetate for gluconeogenesis (Section 5.7).

The regulation of pyruvate dehydrogenase is the result of phosphorylation of the enzyme (Figure 10.7). Pyruvate dehydrogenase kinase is allosterically activated by acetyl CoA and NADH and catalyses the phosphorylation of pyruvate dehydrogenase to an inactive form. Pyruvate dehydrogenase phosphatase acts constantly to dephosphorylate the inactive enzyme, thus restoring its activity and maintaining sensitivity to changes in the concentrations of acetyl CoA and NADH.

Citrate only leaves the mitochondria to provide a source of acetyl CoA for fatty acid synthesis when there is an adequate amount to maintain citric acid cycle activity. As citrate accumulates in the cytosol, it acts as a feed-forward activator of acetyl CoA carboxylase, increasing the formation of malonyl CoA. If citrate in the cytosol is not used as a source of acetyl CoA for fatty acid synthesis, it inhibits phosphofructokinase, thus inhibiting its own formation (Section 10.2.2.1).

Fatty acyl CoA in the cytosol implies a high rate of fatty acid uptake from the bloodstream; fatty acyl CoA inhibits acetyl CoA carboxylase, thus reducing the rate of malonyl CoA synthesis and fatty acid synthesis.

As well as being the substrate for fatty acid synthesis, malonyl CoA is important in controlling the β-oxidation of fatty acids. Malonyl CoA is a potent inhibitor of carnitine acyl transferase 1, the mitochondrial outer membrane enzyme that regulates uptake of fatty acyl CoA into the mitochondria (Section 5.5.1). This means that under conditions when fatty acids are being synthesised in the cytosol, they will not be taken up into the mitochondria for β-oxidation. (See also Section 10.6.2.1 for a discussion of the role of malonyl CoA in regulating muscle fuel selection.)

10.6   Selection of fuel for muscle activity

Muscle can use a variety of fuels:

- Plasma glucose
- Its own reserves of glycogen
- Triacylglycerol from plasma lipoproteins
- Plasma non-esterified fatty acids
- Plasma ketone bodies
- Triacylglycerol from adipose tissue reserves within the muscle

The selection of metabolic fuel depends on the intensity of work being performed, the duration of the exercise, and whether the individual is in the fed or fasting state.

10.6.1   The effect of work intensity on muscle fuel selection

Skeletal muscle contains two types of fibres:

1. Type I (red muscle) fibres. These are also known as slow-twitch muscle fibres. They are relatively rich in mitochondria and myoglobin (hence their colour) and have a high rate of citric acid cycle metabolism, with a low rate of glycolysis. They metabolise mainly fatty acids. These are the fibres used mainly in prolonged, relatively moderate, work.
2. Type II (white muscle) fibres. These are also known as fast-twitch fibres. They are relatively poor in mitochondria and myoglobin and have a high rate of glycolysis. Type IIA fibres also have a high rate of aerobic (citric acid cycle) metabolism, whilst type IIB have a low rate of citric acid cycle activity, and are mainly glycolytic. White muscle fibres are used mainly in high-intensity work of short duration (e.g., sprinting, weight-lifting).

Intense physical activity requires rapid production of ATP, usually for a relatively short time. Under these conditions, substrates and oxygen cannot enter the muscle at an adequate rate to meet the demand. While there will be as much aerobic metabolism as the available oxygen permits, muscle will depend to a considerable extent on anaerobic glycolysis of its glycogen reserves. This leads to the release of lactate into the bloodstream, which is used as a substrate for gluconeogenesis in the liver (Section 5.7 and Figure 5.13). Less intense physical activity is often referred to as aerobic exercise because it involves mainly red muscle fibres (and type IIA white fibres), and there is little accumulation of lactate.

Resting muscle is relatively poorly perfused with blood, and resting muscle tone is largely maintained by anaerobic glycolysis, producing lactate. In response to stimulation, blood flow through the muscle increases, and in moderate exercise there is mainly aerobic metabolism.

The increased rate of glycolysis for exercise is achieved in three ways:

1. As ADP begins to accumulate in muscle, it undergoes the reaction catalysed by adenylate kinase: $2 \times ADP \rightleftharpoons ATP + 5'\text{-}AMP$. $5'$-AMP is a potent activator of phosphofructokinase, reversing the inhibition of this key regulatory enzyme by ATP, and so increasing the rate of glycolysis (Section 10.2.2).
2. Nerve stimulation of muscle results in an increased cytosolic concentration of calcium ions, and hence activation of calmodulin (Section 10.3.3). Calcium–calmodulin activates glycogen phosphorylase, thus increasing the rate of formation of glucose 1-phosphate and providing an increased amount of substrate for glycolysis.
3. Adrenaline, released from the adrenal glands in response to fear or fright, acts on cell surface receptors, leading to the formation of cAMP, which leads to increased activity of protein kinase and glycogen phosphorylase (Figure 10.8).

In prolonged aerobic exercise at a relatively high intensity (e.g. cross-country or marathon running), muscle glycogen and endogenous triacylglycerol are the major fuels initially, with a modest contribution from plasma non-esterified fatty acids and glucose (Figure 10.16). As the exercise continues, and muscle glycogen and triacylglycerol begin to be depleted, plasma non-esterified fatty acids become more important.

At more moderate levels of exercise (e.g. gentle jogging or walking briskly), plasma non-esterified fatty acids provide the major fuel. This means that for weight reduction, where the aim is to reduce adipose tissue reserves, relatively prolonged exercise of moderate intensity is more desirable than shorter periods of more intense exercise. More importantly for overweight people, most of the non-esterified fatty acids that are metabolised in moderate exercise are derived from abdominal rather than subcutaneous adipose tissue (Section 7.2.2.1).

At rest, triacylglycerol from plasma lipoproteins is a significant fuel for muscle, providing 5%–10% of the fatty acids for oxidation, but non-esterified fatty acids are more important in exercise.

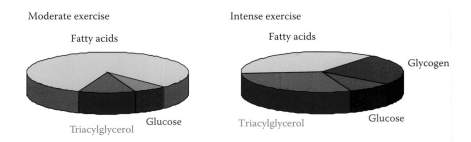

Figure 10.16 Utilisation of different metabolic fuels in muscle in moderate and intense exercise.

10.6.2   *Muscle fuel utilisation in the fed and fasting states*

Glucose is the main fuel for muscle in the fed state, but in the fasting state, glucose is spared for use by the brain and red blood cells; glycogen, fatty acids, and ketone bodies are now the main fuels for muscle.

There are five mechanisms involved in the control of glucose utilisation by muscle (Figure 10.17):

1. Glucose transport into muscle is dependent on insulin, as it is in adipose tissue (Section 10.5.1); thus, in the fasting state, when insulin secretion is low, there will be little uptake of glucose.
2. Hexokinase is inhibited by its product, glucose 6-phosphate, which may arise either as a result of the action of hexokinase on glucose or by isomerisation of glucose 1-phosphate from glycogen breakdown (Figure 5.9). Activation of glycogen phosphorylase leads to increased glucose 6-phosphate, which inhibits the utilisation of glucose that has entered the cell, and so further reduces the uptake of glucose.
3. The activity of pyruvate dehydrogenase is reduced in response to increasing concentrations of both NADH and acetyl CoA (Section 10.5.2). This means that the oxidation of fatty acids and ketone bodies will inhibit the decarboxylation of pyruvate. Under these conditions, the pyruvate that is formed from muscle glycogen by glycolysis will

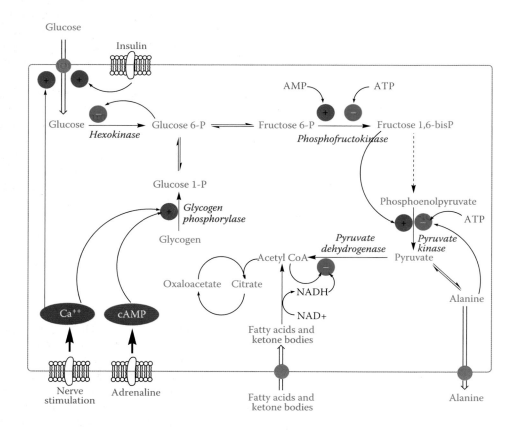

Figure 10.17 Control of the utilisation of metabolic fuels in muscle.

undergo transamination (Section 9.3.1.2) to form alanine. Alanine is exported from muscle and used for gluconeogenesis in the liver (Section 5.7 and Figure 5.38). Thus, although muscle cannot directly release glucose from its glycogen reserves (because it lacks glucose 6-phosphatase), muscle glycogen is an indirect source of blood glucose in the fasting state.

4. If alanine accumulates in muscle, it acts as an allosteric inhibitor of pyruvate kinase, thus reducing the rate at which pyruvate is formed. This end product inhibition of pyruvate kinase by alanine is over-ridden by high concentrations of fructose-bisphosphate, which acts as a feed-forward activator of pyruvate kinase.

5. ATP is an inhibitor of pyruvate kinase and phosphofructokinase (Section 10.2.2.1). This means that under conditions where the supply of ATP (which can be regarded as the end product of all energy-yielding metabolic pathways) is more than adequate to meet requirements, the metabolism of glucose is inhibited.

10.6.2.1   Regulation of fatty acid metabolism in muscle

β-Oxidation of fatty acids is controlled by the uptake of fatty acids into the mitochondria; in turn, this is controlled by the activity of carnitine acyl transferase on the outer mitochondrial membrane and the counter-transport of acyl-carnitine and free carnitine across the inner mitochondrial membrane (Section 5.5.1).

Carnitine acyl transferase activity is regulated by malonyl CoA. In liver and adipose tissue, this serves to inhibit mitochondrial uptake and β-oxidation of fatty acids when fatty acids are being synthesised in the cytosol. Muscle also has an active acetyl CoA carboxylase and synthesises malonyl CoA, although it does not synthesise fatty acids. Muscle carnitine acyl transferase is more sensitive to inhibition by malonyl CoA than is the enzyme in liver and adipose tissue.

Muscle also has malonyl CoA decarboxylase, which acts to decarboxylate malonyl CoA back to acetyl CoA. Acetyl CoA carboxylase and malonyl CoA decarboxylase are regulated in opposite directions by phosphorylation catalysed by a 5′-AMP-dependent protein kinase (which reflects the state of ATP reserves in the cell, Section 10.2.2.1). Phosphorylation in response to an increase in intracellular 5′-AMP results in inactivation of acetyl CoA carboxylase and activation of malonyl CoA decarboxylase. This results in a rapid fall in the concentration of malonyl CoA, thus relieving the inhibition of carnitine acyl transferase and permitting mitochondrial uptake and β-oxidation of fatty acids in response to a fall in ATP, signalling a need for increased energy-yielding metabolism.

In the fed state, there is decreased oxidation of fatty acids in muscle as a result of increased activity of acetyl CoA carboxylase in response to insulin action.

10.7   Diabetes mellitus—a failure of regulation of blood glucose concentration

Diabetes mellitus is an impaired ability to regulate the concentration of blood glucose, as a result of a failure of the normal control by insulin. Therefore, the plasma glucose concentration is considerably higher than normal, both in the fasting state and after a meal. When it increases above the capacity of the kidney to resorb it from the glomerular filtrate (the renal threshold, approximately 11 mmol/L), the result is glucosuria—excretion of glucose in the urine. As a result of glucosuria, there is increased excretion of urine because of osmotic diuresis; one of the common presenting signs of diabetes is frequent urination, accompanied by excessive thirst.

Diabetes mellitus is diagnosed by elevated fasting glucose, followed by measurement of plasma glucose after an oral dose of 1 g per kg body weight—an oral glucose tolerance test. The normal response is a modest increase in plasma glucose, followed by a return to the initial level as it is taken up into liver, muscle, and adipose tissue for synthesis of glycogen and fatty acids (Sections 5.6.3 and 5.6.1). In a diabetic person, fasting plasma glucose is higher than normal, and in response to the test dose, it increases considerably higher (possibly to above the renal threshold), and remains elevated for a considerable time (Figure 10.18).

There are two main types of diabetes mellitus:

1. Type I diabetes (insulin-dependent diabetes mellitus, IDDM) is due to a failure to secrete insulin, as a result of damage to the β-cells of the pancreatic islets resulting from viral infection or autoimmune disease. There is a genetic susceptibility; the concordance of IDDM in monozygotic (identical) twins is about 50%. Type I diabetes commonly develops in childhood, and is sometimes known as juvenile-onset diabetes. Injection of insulin and strict control of carbohydrate intake are essential for control of blood glucose—this explains why it is sometimes called insulin-dependent diabetes.
2. Type II diabetes (non-insulin-dependent diabetes mellitus, NIDDM) is due to failure of responsiveness to insulin (insulin resistance), as a result of decreased sensitivity of insulin receptors (Section 7.2.3.1). There is a genetic susceptibility to type II diabetes, which usually develops in middle age, with a gradual onset, and is sometimes known as maturity-onset diabetes, although it is increasingly common in obese young adults and adolescents.

Initially, insulin secretion, in response to glucose, is normal or higher than normal in people with insulin resistance, and they can maintain adequate glycaemic control, although they have an impaired response to a glucose tolerance test. When the demand for insulin exceeds the synthetic capacity of the β-islet cells of the pancreas, overt diabetes is the result.

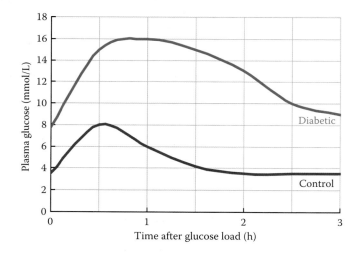

Figure 10.18 The oral glucose tolerance test in control and diabetic subjects.

Type II diabetes is more common in obese people, and especially those with abdominal, rather than subcutaneous, obesity. Significant weight loss can often restore normal glycaemic control without the need for any other treatment. The metabolic syndrome (Section 7.2.3) is the simultaneous development of insulin resistance, hypertension, and hypertriglyceridaemia, all associated with (abdominal) obesity.

At least in the early stages of type II diabetes, control of glucose metabolism can be achieved using oral hypoglycaemic agents, which both stimulate increased insulin secretion and also enhance insulin receptor function. Increasingly, as biosynthetic human insulin has become widely available, treatment of type II diabetes includes insulin injection to maintain better glycaemic control.

10.7.1   Adverse effects of poor glycaemic control

Acutely, diabetics are liable to coma as a result of hypoglycaemia or hyperglycaemia. Hypoglycaemic coma occurs if the plasma concentration of glucose falls below about 2 mmol/L, as a result of administration of insulin or oral hypoglycaemic agents without an adequate intake of carbohydrate. Strenuous exercise without additional food intake can also cause hypoglycaemia. In such cases, oral or intravenous glucose is required.

Hyperglycaemic coma develops in people with type I diabetes because, despite an abnormally high plasma concentration of glucose, tissues are unable to utilise it in the absence of insulin. The high plasma concentration of glucose leads to elevated plasma osmolarity, which results in coma. Because glucose cannot be utilised, ketone bodies are synthesised in the liver (Section 5.5.3). However, when the metabolism of glucose is impaired, there is little pyruvate available for synthesis of oxaloacetate to maintain citric acid cycle activity (Section 5.4.4). The result is ketoacidosis together with a very high plasma concentration of glucose. In such cases, insulin injection is required as well as intravenous bicarbonate if the acidosis is severe.

In the long term, failure of glycaemic control and a persistently high plasma glucose concentration result in damage to capillary blood vessels (especially in the retina, leading to a risk of blindness), kidneys, and peripheral nerves (leading to loss of sensation), and the development of cataracts in the lens of the eye and abnormal metabolism of plasma lipoproteins (which increases the risks of atherosclerosis and ischaemic heart disease). At high concentrations, glucose can be reduced to sorbitol by aldose reductase. In tissues such as the lens of the eye and nerves, which cannot metabolise sorbitol, it accumulates, causing osmotic damage.

Glucose can react non-enzymically with free amino groups on proteins, resulting in glycation of the proteins (Figure 10.19). Glycated proteins include

- Collagen, leading to the thickening of basement membranes in blood capillaries, resulting in kidney damage and retinopathy. Glycated collagen in joints also explains the increased risk of osteoarthritis.
- Apolipoprotein B, leading to increased risk of atherosclerosis and ischemic heart disease.
- α-Crystallin in the lens, leading to the development of cataracts.
- Haemoglobin A, leading to reduced oxygen carrying capacity of the blood.

Glycation of haemoglobin A (with the formation of what can be measured as haemoglobin A_{1c}) provides a sensitive means of assessing glycaemic control over the preceding 4–6

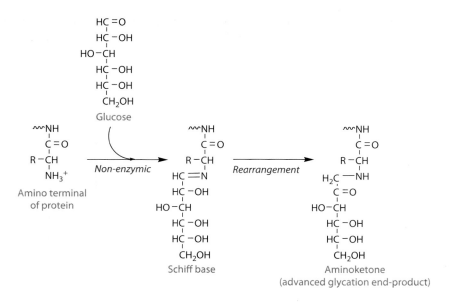

Figure 10.19 Non-enzymic glycation of proteins by high concentrations of glucose in poorly controlled diabetes mellitus.

weeks. It provides a better index of compliance with dietary restriction and maintenance of glycaemic control than a simple spot test of plasma glucose.

Key points

- Within any one cell, metabolism can be regulated instantaneously in response to changes in concentrations of substrates as well as in response to precursors and end products that act as allosteric regulators of key enzymes.
- Phosphofructokinase is a key regulatory enzyme of glycolysis and is inhibited by ATP and citrate. The inhibition by physiological concentrations of ATP is relieved by 5′-AMP, which acts as a signal of the energy state of the cell.
- Substrate cycling permits rapid and sensitive control over pathways and may also be important in thermogenesis.
- Fast-acting hormones act by changing the activity of existing enzyme protein by covalent modification. They bind to cell surface receptors, activating G-proteins that lead to the synthesis of intracellular second messengers. These initiate cascades of intracellular responses, resulting in considerable amplification of the hormone signal.
- Prolonged stimulation of the β-adrenoceptor leads to desensitisation of either responses to multiple different hormones or specifically to adrenaline.
- Slow-acting hormones act by changing the rate of gene expression. They bind to, and activate, intracellular receptors that bind to hormone response elements on DNA.
- In adipose tissue and liver, lipolysis and lipogenesis are controlled in opposite directions in response to insulin, glucagon, and adrenaline.
- Muscle can use a variety of fuels; the selection of fuel to be metabolised depends on the intensity and duration of exercise and whether the subject is in the fed or fasting state.

- Diabetes mellitus is impaired ability to regulate the concentration of blood glucose; it may be due to failure of insulin synthesis and secretion (type I diabetes) or loss of insulin receptor sensitivity (type II diabetes).

Further resources on the CD

The radio-immunoassay program in the virtual laboratory on the CD.

chapter eleven

Micronutrients
The vitamins and minerals

In addition to an adequate source of metabolic fuels (carbohydrates, fats, and proteins, Chapter 5) and protein (Chapter 9), there is a requirement for very much smaller amounts of other nutrients: the vitamins and minerals. Collectively, these are referred to as micronutrients because of the small amounts that are required.

Vitamins are organic compounds that are required for the maintenance of normal health and metabolic integrity. They cannot be synthesised in the body but must be provided in the diet. They are required in very small amounts, of the order of mg or µg/day, and thus can be distinguished from the essential fatty acids (Sections 5.6.1.1 and 6.3.2.1) and the essential amino acids (Section 9.1.3), which are required in amounts of grams/day.

The essential minerals are those inorganic elements that have a physiological function in the body. Obviously, since they are elements, they must be provided in the diet because elements cannot be interconverted. The amounts required vary from grams/day for sodium and calcium, through mg/day (e.g. iron) to µg/day for the trace elements (so called because they are required in such small amounts).

Objectives

After reading this chapter, you should be able to

- Describe and explain the way in which micronutrient requirements are determined and how reference intakes are calculated; explain how it is that different national and international authorities have different reference intakes for some nutrients.
- Describe and explain the chemistry, metabolic functions, and deficiency signs associated with each of the vitamins and important minerals.
- Describe the whole body maintenance of calcium homeostasis.
- Describe and explain the various micronutrient deficiencies that can lead to the development of anaemia.

11.1   The determination of requirements and reference intakes

For any nutrient, there is a range of intakes between that which is clearly inadequate, leading to clinical deficiency disease, and that which is so much in excess of the body's metabolic capacity that there may be signs of toxicity. Between these two extremes is a level of intake that is adequate for normal health and the maintenance of metabolic integrity, and a series of more precisely definable levels of intake that are adequate to meet specific criteria, and may be used to determine requirements and appropriate levels of intake:

- Clinical deficiency disease, with clear anatomical and functional lesions, and severe metabolic disturbances, possibly proving fatal. Prevention of deficiency disease is a minimal goal in determining requirements.

- Covert deficiency, where there are no signs of deficiency under normal conditions, but any trauma or stress reveals the precarious state of the body reserves and may precipitate clinical signs. For example, an intake of 10 mg of vitamin C/day is adequate to prevent clinical deficiency, but at least 20 mg/day is required for healing of wounds (Section 11.14.4).
- Metabolic abnormalities under normal conditions, such as impaired carbohydrate metabolism in thiamin deficiency (Section 11.6.3) or excretion of methylmalonic acid in vitamin B_{12} deficiency (Section 11.10.4).
- Abnormal response to a metabolic load, such as the inability to metabolise a test dose of histidine in folate deficiency (Section 11.11.6.1) or tryptophan in vitamin B_6 deficiency (Section 11.9.5.1), although at normal levels of intake there may be no metabolic impairment.
- Inadequate saturation of enzymes with (vitamin-derived) coenzymes (Section 2.7.3). This can be tested for three vitamins, using red blood cell enzymes: thiamin (Section 11.6.4), riboflavin (Section 11.7.4), and vitamin B_6 (Section 11.9.4).
- Low plasma concentration of the nutrient, indicating that there is an inadequate amount in tissue reserves to permit normal transport between tissues. For some nutrients, this may reflect failure to synthesise a transport protein rather than primary deficiency of the nutrient itself.
- Low urinary excretion of the nutrient, reflecting low intake and changes in metabolic turnover.
- Incomplete saturation of body reserves.
- Adequate body reserves and normal metabolic integrity.
- Possibly beneficial effects of intakes more than adequate to met requirements—the promotion of optimum health and life expectancy.
- Pharmacological (drug-like) actions at very high levels of intake.
- Abnormal accumulation in tissues and overloading of normal metabolic pathways, leading to signs of toxicity and possibly irreversible lesions. Iron (Sections 4.5.3.1 and 11.15.2.3), selenium (Section 11.15.2.5), niacin (Section 11.8.5.1), and vitamins A (Section 11.2.5.2), D (Section 11.3.5.1), and B_6 (Section 11.9.6.1) are all known to be toxic in excess.

Having decided on an appropriate criterion of adequacy, requirements are determined by feeding volunteers an otherwise adequate diet, but lacking the nutrient under investigation, until there is a detectable metabolic or other abnormality. They are then repleted with graded intakes of the nutrient until the abnormality is just corrected.

Problems arise in interpreting the results, and therefore defining requirements, when different markers of adequacy respond to different levels of intake. This explains the difference in the tables of reference intakes published by different national and international authorities (see Tables 11.1 through 11.3).

11.1.1 *Dietary reference values*

Individuals do not all have the same requirement for nutrients, even when calculated on the basis of body size or energy expenditure. There is a range of individual requirements of up to 25% around the average. Therefore, to set population goals and assess the adequacy of diets, it is necessary to set a reference level of intake that is high enough to ensure that no one will either suffer from deficiency or be at risk of toxicity.

Table 11.1 Reference Nutrient Intakes of Vitamins and Minerals, UK, 1991

Age	Vitamins									Minerals							
	B$_1$ (mg)	B$_2$ (mg)	Niacin (mg)	B$_6$ (mg)	B$_{12}$ (µg)	Folate (µg)	C (mg)	A (µg)	D (µg)	Ca (mg)	P (mg)	Mg (mg)	Fe (mg)	Zn (mg)	Cu (mg)	Se (µg)	I (µg)
0–3 months	0.2	0.4	3	0.2	0.3	50	25	350	8.5	525	400	55	1.7	4.0	0.2	10	50
4–6 months	0.2	0.4	3	0.2	0.3	50	25	350	8.5	525	400	60	4.3	4.0	0.3	13	60
7–9 months	0.2	0.4	4	0.3	0.4	50	25	350	7	525	400	75	7.8	5.0	0.3	10	60
10–12 months	0.3	0.4	5	0.4	0.4	50	25	350	7	525	400	80	7.8	5.0	0.3	10	60
1–3 years	0.5	0.6	8	0.7	0.5	70	30	400	7	350	270	85	6.9	5.0	0.4	15	70
4–6 years	0.7	0.8	11	0.9	0.8	100	30	500	–	450	350	120	6.1	6.5	0.6	20	100
7–10 years	0.7	1.0	12	1.0	1.0	150	30	500	–	550	450	200	8.7	7.0	0.7	30	110
Males																	
11–14 years	0.9	1.2	15	1.2	1.2	200	35	600	–	1000	775	280	11.3	9.0	0.8	45	130
15–18 years	1.1	1.3	18	1.5	1.5	200	40	700	–	1000	775	300	11.3	9.5	1.0	70	140
19–50 years	1.0	1.3	17	1.4	1.5	200	40	700	–	700	550	300	8.7	9.5	1.2	75	140
50+ years	0.9	1.3	16	1.4	1.5	200	40	700	10	700	550	300	8.7	9.5	1.2	75	140
Females																	
11–14 years	0.7	1.1	12	1.0	1.2	200	35	600	–	800	625	280	14.8	9.0	0.8	45	130
15–18 years	0.8	1.1	14	1.2	1.5	200	40	600	–	800	6254	300	14.8	7.0	1.0	60	140
19–50 years	0.8	1.1	13	1.2	1.5	200	40	600	–	700	550	270	14.8	7.0	1.2	60	140
50+ years	0.8	1.1	12	1.2	1.5	200	40	600	10	700	550	270	8.7	7.0	1.2	60	140
Pregnant	+0.1	+0.3	–	–	–	+100	+10	+100	10	–	–	–	–	–	–	–	–
Lactating	+0.1	+0.5	+2	–	+0.5	+60	+30	+350	10	+550	+440	+50	–	+6.0	+0.3	+15	–

Source: Department of Health. *Dietary Reference Values for Food Energy and Nutrients for the United Kingdom.* HMSO, London, 1991.

Table 11.2 Population Reference Intakes of Vitamins and Minerals, European Union, 1993

Age	Vitamins								Minerals						
	A (µg)	B$_1$ (mg)	B$_2$ (mg)	Niacin (mg)	B$_6$ (mg)	Folate (µg)	B$_{12}$ (µg)	C (mg)	Ca (mg)	P (mg)	Fe (mg)	Zn (mg)	Cu (mg)	Se (µg)	I (µg)
6–12 months	350	0.3	0.4	5	0.4	50	0.5	20	400	300	6	4	0.3	8	50
1–3 years	400	0.5	0.8	9	0.7	100	0.7	25	400	300	4	4	0.4	10	70
4–6 years	400	0.7	1.0	11	0.9	130	0.9	25	450	350	4	6	0.6	15	90
7–10 years	500	0.8	1.2	13	1.1	150	1.0	30	550	450	6	7	0.7	25	100
Males															
11–14 years	600	1.0	1.4	15	1.3	180	1.3	35	1000	775	10	9	0.8	35	120
15–17 years	700	1.2	1.6	18	1.5	200	1.4	40	1000	775	13	9	1.0	45	130
18+ years	700	1.1	1.6	18	1.5	200	1.4	45	700	550	9	9.5	1.1	55	130
Females															
11–14 years	600	0.9	1.2	14	1.1	180	1.3	35	800	625	18	9	0.8	35	120
15–17 years	600	0.9	1.3	14	1.1	200	1.4	40	800	625	17	7	1.0	45	130
18+ years	600	0.9	1.3	14	1.1	200	1.4	45	700	550	16[1]	7	1.1	55	130
Pregnant	700	1.0	1.6	14	1.3	400	1.6	55	700	550	1	7	1.1	55	130
Lactating	950	1.1	1.7	16	1.4	350	1.9	70	1200	950	16	12	1.4	70	160

Source: Scientific Committee for Food. *Nutrient and energy intakes for the European Community.* Commission of the European Communities, Luxembourg, 1993.

Table 11.3 Recommended Dietary Allowances and Acceptable Intakes for Vitamins and Minerals, United States and Canada, 1997–2011

Age	A (µg)	D (µg)	E (mg)	K (µg)	B₁ (mg)	B₂ (mg)	Niacin (mg)	B₆ (mg)	Folate (µg)	B₁₂ (µg)	Vit C (mg)	Ca (mg)	P (mg)	Fe (mg)	Zn (mg)	Cu (mg)	Se (µg)	I (µg)
0–6 months	400	10	4	2.0	0.2	0.3	2	0.1	65	0.4	40	200	100	–	2.0	200	15	110
7–12 months	500	10	5	2.5	0.3	0.4	4	0.3	80	0.5	50	260	275	11	3	220	20	130
1–3 years	300	15	6	30	0.5	0.5	6	0.5	150	0.9	15	700	460	7	3	340	20	90
4–8 years	400	15	7	55	0.5	0.6	8	0.6	200	1.2	25	1000	500	10	5	440	30	90
Males																		
9–13 years	600	15	11	60	0.9	0.9	12	1.0	300	1.8	45	1300	1250	8	8	700	40	120
14–18 years	900	15	15	75	1.2	1.3	16	1.3	400	2.4	75	1300	1250	11	11	890	55	150
19–30 years	900	15	15	120	1.2	1.3	16	1.3	400	2.4	90	1000	700	8	11	900	55	150
31–50 years	900	15	15	120	1.2	1.3	16	1.3	400	2.4	90	1000	700	8	11	900	55	150
51–70 years	900	15	15	120	1.2	1.3	16	1.7	400	2.4	90	1200	700	8	11	900	55	150
>70 years	900	20	15	120	1.2	1.3	16	1.7	400	2.4	90	1200	700	8	11	900	55	150
Females																		
9–13 years	600	15	11	60	0.9	0.9	12	1.0	300	1.8	45	1300	1250	8	8	700	40	120
14–18 years	700	15	15	75	1.0	1.0	14	1.2	400	2.4	65	1300	1250	15	9	890	55	150
19–30 years	700	15	15	90	1.1	1.1	14	1.3	400	2.4	75	1000	700	18	8	900	55	150
31–50 years	700	15	15	90	1.1	1.1	14	1.3	400	2.4	75	1000	700	18	8	900	55	150
51–70 years	700	15	15	90	1.1	1.1	14	1.5	400	2.4	75	1200	700	8	8	900	55	150
>70 years	700	20	15	90	1.1	1.1	14	1.5	400	2.4	75	1200	700	8	8	900	55	150
Pregnant	770	15	15	90	1.4	1.4	18	1.9	600	2.6	85	1000	700	27	11	1000	60	220
Lactating	900	15	16	90	1.4	1.6	17	2.0	500	2.8	120	1000	700	9	12	1300	70	290

Source: Standing Committee on the Scientific Evaluation of Dietary Reference Intakes, Food and Nutrition Board, Institute of Medicine. *Dietary Reference Intakes for Calcium, Phosphorus, Magnesium, Vitamin D, and Fluoride*, 1997; *Dietary Reference Intakes for Thiamin, Riboflavin, Niacin, Vitamin B₆, Folate, Vitamin B₁₂, Pantothenic Acid, Biotin, and Choline*, 1998; *Dietary Reference Intakes for Vitamin C, Vitamin E, Selenium, and Carotenoids*, 2000; *Dietary Reference Intakes for Vitamin A, Vitamin K, Arsenic, Boron, Chromium, Copper, Iodine, Iron, Manganese, Molybdenum, Nickel, Silicon, Vanadium, and Zinc*, 2001; *Dietary Reference Intakes for Calcium and Vitamin D*, 2011; National Academy Press, Washington, DC.

Note: Figures for infants younger than 12 months are adequate intakes, based on the observed mean intake of infants fed principally on breast milk; for nutrients other than vitamin K figures are RDA, based on estimated average requirement + 2 sᴅ; figures for vitamin K are adequate intakes, based on observed average intakes.

Table 11.4 Recommended Nutrient Intakes for Vitamins, FAO, 2001

Age	Vitamin A (µg)	Vitamin D (µg)	Vitamin K (µg)	Vitamin B$_1$ (mg)	Vit B$_2$ (mg)	Niacin (mg)	Vitamin B$_6$ (mg)	Folate (µg)	Vitamin B$_{12}$ (µg)	Vitamin C (mg)	Pantothenic acid (mg)	Biotin (µg)
0–6 months	375	5	5	0.2	0.3	2	0.1	80	0.4	25	1.7	5
7–12 months	400	5	10	0.3	0.4	4	0.3	80	0.5	30	1.8	6
1–3 years	400	5	15	0.5	0.5	6	0.5	160	0.9	30	2.0	8
4–6 years	450	5	20	0.6	0.6	8	0.6	200	1.2	30	3.0	12
7–9 years	500	5	25	0.9	0.9	12	1.0	300	1.8	35	4.0	20
Males												
10–18 years	600	5	35–55	1.2	1.3	16	1.3	400	2.4	40	5.0	30
19–50 years	600	5	65	1.2	1.3	16	1.3	400	2.4	45	5.0	30
50–65 years	600	10	65	1.2	1.3	16	1.7	400	2.4	45	5.0	30
>65 years	600	15	65	1.2	1.3	16	1.7	400	2.4	45	5.0	30
Females												
10–18 years	600	5	35–55	1.1	1.0	16	1.2	400	2.4	40	5.0	25
19–50 years	600	5	55	1.1	1.1	14	1.3	400	2.4	45	5.0	30
50–65 years	600	10	55	1.1	1.1	14	1.5	400	2.4	45	5.0	30
> 65 years	600	15	55	1.1	1.1	14	1.5	400	2.4	45	5.0	30
Pregnant	800	5	55	1.4	1.4	18	1.9	600	2.6	55	6.0	30
Lactating	850	5	55	1.5	1.6	17	2.0	500	2.8	70	7.0	35

Source: Food and Agriculture Organization of the United Nations and World Health Organization, *Human Vitamin and Mineral Requirements*, FAO, Rome, 2001.

As shown in the upper graph in Figure 11.1, if it is assumed that individual requirements are normally distributed around the observed mean requirement, then a range of ± 2 × the standard deviation (SD) around the mean will include the requirements of 95% of the population. This 95% range is conventionally used as the 'normal' or reference range (e.g. in clinical chemistry to assess the normality or otherwise of a test result) and is used to define three levels of nutrient intake:

1. The Estimated Average Requirement (EAR). This is the observed mean requirement to meet the chosen criterion of adequacy in experimental studies.
2. The Reference Nutrient Intake (RNI). This is 2 × SD above the observed mean requirement, and is therefore more than adequate to meet the individual requirements of 97.5% of the population. This is the goal for planning diets, e.g. in institutional feeding, and the standard against which the intake of a population can be assessed. In the European Union tables (Table 11.2), this is called the Population Reference Intake

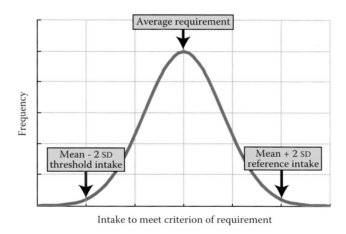

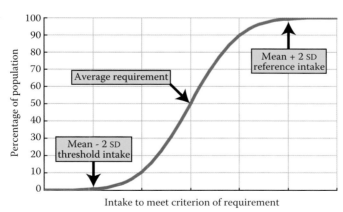

Figure 11.1 The derivation of reference intakes of nutrients from the distribution around the observed mean requirement; plotted below as a cumulative distribution curve, permitting estimation of the probability that a given level of intake is adequate to meet an individual's requirement.

(PRI); in the United States, it is called the Recommended Dietary Allowance (RDA, Table 11.3).

3. The Lower Reference Nutrient Intake (LNRI). This is 2 × sd below the observed mean requirement, and is therefore adequate to meet the requirements of only 2.5% of the population. In the European Union tables, this is called the Lower Threshold Intake, to stress that it is a level of intake at or below which it is extremely unlikely that normal metabolic integrity could be maintained.

The reference intake is greater than the requirement of almost all members of the population; thus, there is no cause for concern if an individual has an intake below the reference intake. Indeed, if a population survey shows that the average intake is below the reference intake, there is still no cause for concern. It is only when the average intake is below the average requirement that deficiency is likely to be a problem. The lower graph in Figure 11.1 shows the distribution of requirements plotted as the cumulative percentage of the population whose requirements have been met at each level of intake. This can therefore be used to estimate the probability that a given level of intake is adequate to meet an individual's requirements.

For some nutrients, deficiency is unknown except under experimental conditions, and there are no estimates of average requirements, and therefore no reference intakes. Since deficiency does not occur, it is obvious that average levels of intake are more than adequate to meet requirements, and for these nutrients there is a range of intakes that is defined as safe and adequate, based on the observed range of intakes.

The reference intakes of vitamins and minerals shown in Tables 11.1 through 11.4 are age- and gender-specific. Apart from foods for infants and children, the highest requirement for any population group is used to provide the basis for nutritional labelling of foods (Section 6.3).

11.1.1.1 Supplements and safe levels of intake

In general, the amounts of micronutrients in foods pose no health hazards, although liver may contain high levels of vitamin A that pose a risk to pregnant women (Section 11.2.5.2). However, the amounts that may be consumed in supplements may be hazardous. Table 11.5 shows the tolerable upper levels of habitual intake for those nutrients where there is adequate evidence to set a level of intake at or below which there is no evidence of any hazard.

11.1.2 The vitamins

Vitamins are organic compounds that are required in small amounts for the maintenance of normal health and metabolic integrity. Deficiency causes a specific disease, which is cured or prevented only by restoring the vitamin to the diet. This is important—it is not enough just to show that a compound has effects, since these may be pharmacological actions, not related to the maintenance of normal health and metabolic integrity.

As can be seen from Table 11.6, the vitamins are named in a curious way. This is a historical accident, and results from the way in which they were discovered. Studies at the beginning of the 20th century showed that there was something in milk that was essential, in very small amounts, for the growth of animals fed on a diet consisting of purified fat, carbohydrate, protein, and mineral salts. Two factors were found to be essential: one was found in the cream and the other in the watery part of milk. Logically, they were called Factor A (fat-soluble, in the cream) and Factor B (water-soluble, in the watery part of the

Table 11.5 Tolerable Upper Levels of Vitamin and Mineral Intake for Adults

	Tolerable upper intake level	
	U.S. Institute of Medicine	European Food Safety Authority
Vitamin A (μg)	3000	3000
Vitamin D (μg)	100	100
Vitamin E (mg)	100	300
Niacin (mg)	900	Nicotinic acid 10 Nicotinamide 900
Vitamin B_6 (mg)	100	25
Folate (μg)	1000	1000
Vitamin C (mg)	2000	Not determined
Choline (mg)	3500	100
Boron (mg)	20	10
Calcium (mg)	2000	2500
Copper (mg)	10	5
Fluoride (mg)	10	7
Iodine (μg)	1100	600
Iron (mg)	45	Not determined
Magnesium (mg)	350	250
Manganese (mg)	11	Not determined
Molybdenum (μg)	2000	500
Nickel (mg)	1	Not determined
Phosphorus (mg)	4000	Not determined
Selenium (μg)	400	300
Vanadium (mg)	1800	Not determined
Zinc (mg)	40	25
Sodium (mg)	2300	Not determined
Chloride (mg)	3600	Not determined

Source: Institute of Medicine. *Dietary Reference Intakes: The Essential Guide to Nutrient Requirements,* 2006; *Dietary Reference Intakes for Calcium and Vitamin D,* 2011, Washington, DC, National Academies Press; European Food Safety Authority, *Tolerable Upper Intake Levels for Vitamins and Minerals,* Scientific Committee on Food, Scientific Panel on Dietetic Products, Nutrition, and Allergies, EFSA 2012.

milk). Factor B was identified chemically as an amine, and in 1913, the name 'vitamin' was coined for these 'vital amines'.

Further studies showed that 'vitamin B' was a mixture of a number of compounds, only one of which was chemically an amine. These different compounds of 'vitamin B' have different functions, and they were given numbers as well: vitamin B_1, vitamin B_2, and so on. There are gaps in the numerical order of the B vitamins. When what might have been called vitamin B_3 was discovered, it was found to be a chemical compound that was already known, nicotinic acid. It was therefore not given a number. Other gaps are because compounds that were believed to be vitamins were later shown either not to be dietary essentials or to be vitamins that had already been described by other workers and given other names.

As the chemistry of the vitamins was elucidated, they were given names as well. When only one chemical compound has the biological activity of the vitamin, this is quite easy. Thus, vitamin B_1 is thiamin, vitamin B_2 is riboflavin, etc. With several vitamins, a number of chemically related compounds found in foods can be interconverted in the body, and all

Table 11.6 The Vitamins

Vitamin		Functions	Deficiency disease
A	Retinol β-Carotene	Visual pigments in the retina; regulation of gene expression and cell differentiation β-carotene is an antioxidant	Night blindness, xerophthalmia; keratinisation of skin
D	Calciferol	Maintenance of calcium balance; enhances intestinal absorption of Ca^{2+} and mobilises bone mineral	Rickets = poor mineralisation of bone Osteomalacia = bone demineralisation
E	Tocopherols Tocotrienols	Antioxidant, especially in cell membranes	Extremely rare—serious neurological dysfunction
K	Phylloquinone Menaquinones	Coenzyme in formation of γ-carboxy-glutamate in proteins of blood clotting and bone matrix	Impaired blood clotting, haemorrhagic disease
B_1	Thiamin	Coenzyme in pyruvate and α-ketoglutarate dehydrogenases and transketolase; role in nerve conduction	Peripheral nerve damage (beriberi) or central nervous system lesions (Wernicke–Korsakoff syndrome)
B_2	Riboflavin	Coenzyme in oxidation and reduction reactions; prosthetic group of flavoproteins	Lesions of corner of mouth, lips, and tongue, seborrhoeic dermatitis
Niacin	Nicotinic acid Nicotinamide	Coenzyme in oxidation and reduction reactions, functional part of NAD and NADP	Pellagra—photosensitive dermatitis, depressive psychosis
B_6	Pyridoxine Pyridoxal Pyridoxamine	Coenzyme in transamination and decarboxylation of amino acids and glycogen phosphorylase; role in steroid hormone action	Disorders of amino acid metabolism, convulsions
	Folic acid	Coenzyme in transfer of one-carbon fragments	Megaloblastic anaemia
B_{12}	Cobalamin	Coenzyme in transfer of one-carbon fragments and metabolism of folate	Pernicious anaemia = megaloblastic anaemia with degeneration of the spinal cord
	Pantothenic acid	Functional part of CoA and acyl carrier protein fatty acid synthesis and metabolism	Peripheral nerve damage (burning foot syndrome)
H	Biotin	Coenzyme in carboxylation reactions in gluconeogenesis and fatty acid synthesis	Impaired fat and carbohydrate metabolism, dermatitis
C	Ascorbic acid	Coenzyme in hydroxylation of proline and lysine in collagen synthesis; antioxidant; enhances absorption of iron	Scurvy—impaired wound healing, loss of dental cement, subcutaneous haemorrhage

show the same biological activity. Such chemically related compounds are called vitamers, and a generic descriptor is used to include all compounds that display the same biological activity. Thus, niacin is the generic descriptor for two compounds, nicotinic acid and nicotinamide, which have the same biological activity. Vitamin B_6 is used to describe the six compounds that have vitamin B_6 activity.

Correctly, for a compound to be classified as a vitamin, it should be a dietary essential that cannot be synthesised in the body. By this strict definition, two vitamins should not really be included since they can be made in the body. However, both were discovered as a result of investigations of deficiency diseases, and they are usually considered as vitamins:

1. Vitamin D is made in the skin after exposure to sunlight (Section 11.3.2.1) and should really be regarded as a steroid hormone rather than a vitamin. It is only when sunlight exposure is inadequate that a dietary source is required.
2. Niacin can be formed from the essential amino acid tryptophan (Section 11.8.2). Indeed, synthesis from tryptophan is probably more important than a dietary intake of preformed niacin.

11.2   Vitamin A

Vitamin A was the first vitamin to be discovered, initially as an essential dietary factor for growth. It has roles in vision (where retinaldehyde provides the prosthetic group of the light-sensitive proteins in the retina) and in the regulation of gene expression and tissue differentiation (where it is retinoic acid that is important). Deficiency is a major problem of public health in large areas of the world, and the commonest cause of preventable blindness worldwide. Together with iron (Section 11.15.2.3) and iodine (Section 11.15.3.3), elimination of vitamin A deficiency is one of the three key micronutrient targets of the World Health Organisation. Golden rice is a strain of rice that has been genetically engineered to produce β-carotene (a precursor of vitamin A, Sections 11.2.1 and 11.2.2.1) in relatively large amounts—an example of biofortification of a staple food that promises to have a significant impact on vitamin A deficiency.

11.2.1   Vitamin A vitamers and international units

Two groups of compounds (Figure 11.2) have vitamin A activity: retinol, retinaldehyde, and retinoic acid (preformed vitamin A); and a variety of carotenes and related compounds (collectively known as carotenoids), which can be cleaved oxidatively to yield retinaldehyde, and hence retinol and retinoic acid. Those carotenoids that can be cleaved to yield retinaldehyde are known as pro-vitamin A carotenoids.

Retinol and retinoic acids are found only in foods of animal origin, and a small number of bacteria, mainly as the ester retinyl palmitate. The oxidation of retinaldehyde to retinoic acid is irreversible; retinoic acid cannot be converted to retinol *in vivo*, and does not support either vision or fertility in deficient animals.

Some 50 or more dietary carotenoids are potential sources of vitamin A: α-, β-, and γ-carotenes and cryptoxanthin are quantitatively the most important. Although it would appear from its structure that one molecule of β-carotene will yield two of retinol, this is not so in practice (Section 11.2.2.1); 6 μg of β-carotene is equivalent to 1 μg of preformed retinol. For other carotenes with vitamin A activity, 12 μg is equivalent to 1 μg of preformed retinol.

The total amount of vitamin A in foods is expressed as μg retinol equivalents, calculated from the sum of μg preformed vitamin A + 1/6 × μg β-carotene + 1/12 × μg other provitamin A carotenoids.

Before pure vitamin A was available for chemical analysis, the vitamin A content of foods was determined by biological assay, and the results expressed in international units

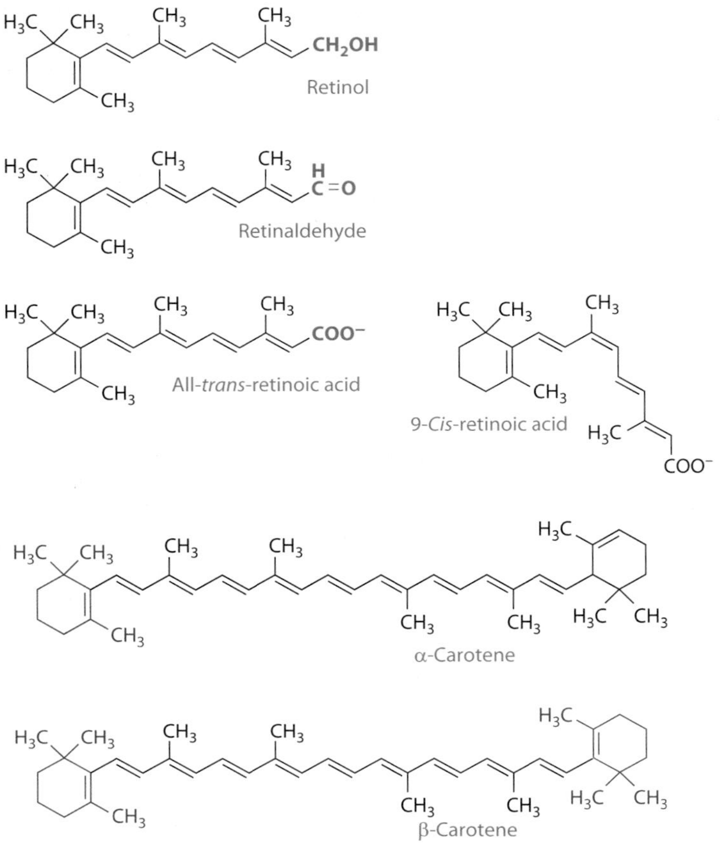

Figure 11.2 Vitamin A: retinoids and major pro-vitamin A carotenoids.

(iu): 1 iu = 0.3 μg retinol, or 1 μg of retinol = 3.33 iu. Although obsolete, iu are sometimes still used in food labelling.

11.2.2 *Metabolism of vitamin A and pro-vitamin A carotenoids*

Retinol and carotene are absorbed from the small intestine dissolved in lipid; with diets providing less than about 10% of energy from fat, absorption is impaired, and very low fat diets are associated with vitamin A deficiency. About 70%–90% of dietary retinol is normally absorbed, and even at high levels of intake this falls only slightly. Between 5% and 60% of dietary carotene is absorbed, depending on the nature of the food, whether it is cooked or raw and how much fat was present in the meal. A number of interventions in developing counties to improve vitamin A nutritional status by persuading people to consume carotene-rich leafy vegetables have been disappointing because there was inadequate fat in the diet to permit useful absorption of carotene.

Retinyl esters formed in the intestinal mucosa enter the lymphatic circulation, in chylomicrons (Sections 4.3.2.2 and 5.6.2.1) together with dietary lipid and carotenoids. Tissues can take up retinyl esters from chylomicrons, but most remains in the chylomicron remnants that are taken up by the liver. Here the esters are hydrolysed, and the vitamin may either be secreted from the liver bound to retinol binding protein (RBP), or be transferred to stellate cells in the liver, where it is stored as esters in intracellular lipid droplets.

At normal levels of intake, most retinol is catabolised by oxidation to retinoic acid and excreted in the bile as retinoyl glucuronide. As the liver concentration of retinol increases above 70 μmol/kg, microsomal cytochrome P_{450}-dependent oxidation occurs, leading to polar metabolites that are excreted in urine and bile. At high intakes, this pathway becomes saturated and excess retinol is toxic because there is no further capacity for its catabolism and excretion.

11.2.2.1   *Carotene dioxygenase and the formation of retinol from carotenes*

As shown in Figure 11.3, β-carotene and other provitamin A carotenoids are cleaved in the intestinal mucosa by carotene dioxygenase, yielding retinaldehyde, which is reduced to retinol, esterified, and secreted in chylomicrons together with esters formed from dietary retinol.

Only a proportion of carotene is oxidised in the intestinal mucosa, and a significant amount enters the circulation in chylomicrons (Sections 4.3.2.2 and 5.6.2.1). Carotene in the chylomicron remnants is cleared by the liver, where some is cleaved by hepatic carotene dioxygenase, and the remainder is secreted in very-low-density lipoprotein.

Central oxidative cleavage of β-carotene, as shown in Figure 11.3 should yield two molecules of retinaldehyde, which can be reduced to retinol. However, the biological activity

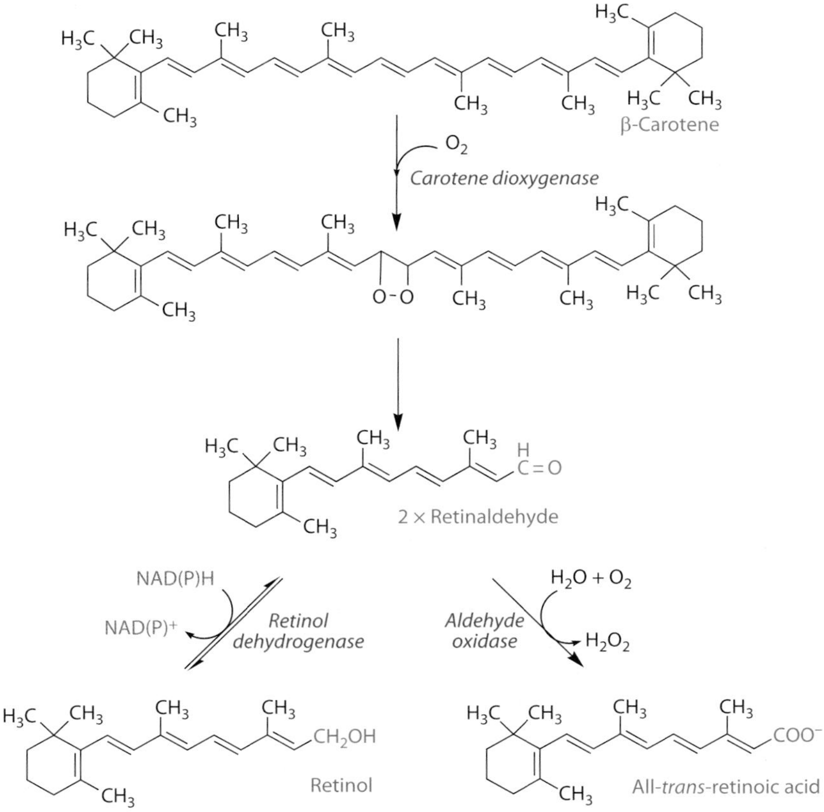

Figure 11.3 The reaction of carotene dioxygenase.

of β-carotene, on a molar basis, is considerably lower than that of retinol, not two-fold higher as might be expected. In addition to the relatively poor absorption of carotene from the diet, three factors may account for this:

1. The intestinal activity of carotene dioxygenase is relatively low; thus, a significant proportion of ingested β-carotene may appear in the circulation unchanged.
2. Other carotenoids in the diet that are not substrates may inhibit carotene dioxygenase and reduce the proportion that is converted to retinol.
3. There are two isoenzymes of carotene dioxygenase. One catalyses central cleavage, as shown in Figure 11.3. The other catalyses asymmetric cleavage, which leads to the formation of 8′-, 10′-, and 12′-apo-carotenals, which are oxidised to retinoic acid but cannot be precursors of retinol or retinaldehyde because the reaction of aldehyde oxidase to form retinoic acid is irreversible.

11.2.2.2   *Plasma retinol binding protein*

Retinol is released from the liver bound to an α-globulin, RBP; this serves to maintain the vitamin in aqueous solution, protects it against oxidation, and also delivers the vitamin to target tissues. The synthesis of RBP is reduced very considerably in protein-energy malnutrition, and in severely undernourished people, there may be functional vitamin A deficiency despite apparently adequate liver reserves, as a result of lack of RBP.

RBP is secreted from the liver as a 1:1 complex with the thyroxine-binding pre-albumin, transthyretin (Section 11.15.3.3). This is important to prevent urinary loss of retinol, since RBP alone is small enough to be filtered by the kidney, with a considerable loss of vitamin A from the body. Cell surface receptors on target tissues take up retinol from the RBP-transthyretin complex. The cell surface receptors also remove the carboxy terminal arginine residue from RBP, thus, inactivating it by reducing its affinity for both transthyretin and retinol. The apo-protein is not recycled; it is filtered at the glomerulus, reabsorbed in the proximal renal tubules, and then hydrolysed.

11.2.3   *Metabolic functions of vitamin A*

Vitamin A has two major functions: as retinaldehyde in vision and as retinoic acids in regulation of gene expression and tissue differentiation. In addition to their role as vitamin A precursors, carotenes can act as radical trapping antioxidants, although they may also have pro-oxidant actions (Section 6.5.3.3).

11.2.3.1   *Vitamin A in vision*

In the retina, retinaldehyde functions as the prosthetic group of the light-sensitive opsin proteins, forming rhodopsin (in rods) and iodopsin (in cones). Any one cone cell contains only one type of opsin and is sensitive to only one colour of light. Colour blindness results from loss or mutation of one or other of the cone opsins.

In the pigment epithelium of the retina, all-*trans*-retinol is isomerised to 11-*cis*-retinol and oxidised to 11-*cis*-retinaldehyde. This reacts with a lysine residue in opsin, forming the holo-protein rhodopsin (sometimes called visual purple because of its colour). Opsins are cell-type specific; they shift the absorption of 11-*cis*-retinaldehyde from the UV into what we call, in consequence, the visible range—either a relatively broad spectrum of sensitivity for vision in dim light (in the rods) or more defined spectral peaks for differentiation of colours in bright light (in the cones).

As shown in Figure 11.4, the absorption of light by rhodopsin causes isomerisation of the retinaldehyde bound to opsin from 11-*cis* to all-*trans* and a series of conformational changes in opsin. This results in the release of retinaldehyde from the protein and the initiation of a nerve impulse. The overall process is known as bleaching since it results in the loss of the purple colour of rhodopsin.

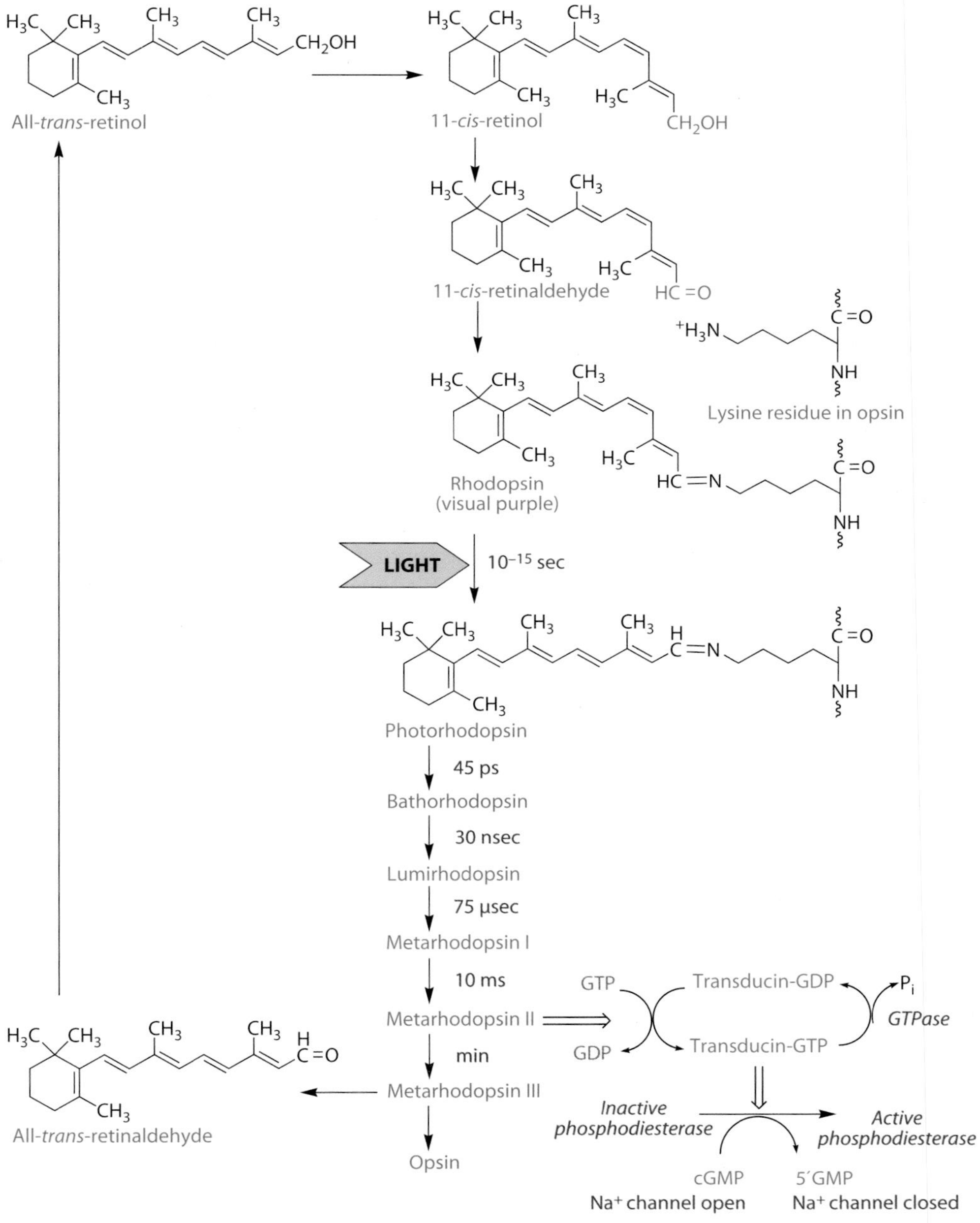

Figure 11.4 The role of retinaldehyde in the visual cycle.

The all-*trans*-retinaldehyde released from rhodopsin is reduced to all-*trans*-retinol and joins the pool of retinol in the pigment epithelium for isomerisation to 11-*cis*-retinol and regeneration of rhodopsin. The key to initiation of the visual cycle is the availability of 11-*cis*-retinaldehyde, and hence vitamin A. In deficiency, both the time taken to adapt to darkness and the ability to see in poor light are impaired.

The formation of the initial excited form of rhodopsin, bathorhodopsin, occurs within picoseconds of illumination and is the only light dependent step in the visual cycle. Thereafter there is a series of conformational changes leading to the formation of metarhodopsin II. The conversion of metarhodopsin II to metarhodopsin III is relatively slow, with a time-course of minutes. The final step is hydrolysis to release all-*trans*-retinaldehyde and opsin.

Metarhodopsin II is the excited form of rhodopsin that initiates a G-protein cascade (Section 10.3.1) leading to a nerve impulse.

11.2.3.2   *Retinoic acid and the regulation of gene expression*

The most important function of vitamin A is in the control of cell differentiation and turnover. All-*trans*-retinoic acid and 9-*cis*-retinoic acid (Figure 11.5) act in the regulation of growth, development and tissue differentiation; they have different actions in different tissues. Like the steroid hormones (Section 10.4) and vitamin D (Section 11.3.3), retinoic acid binds to nuclear receptors that bind to response elements (control regions) of DNA and regulate the transcription of specific genes.

There are two families of nuclear retinoid receptors: the retinoic acid receptors (RAR) bind all-*trans*-retinoic acid or 9-*cis*-retinoic acid and the retinoid X receptors (RXR) bind

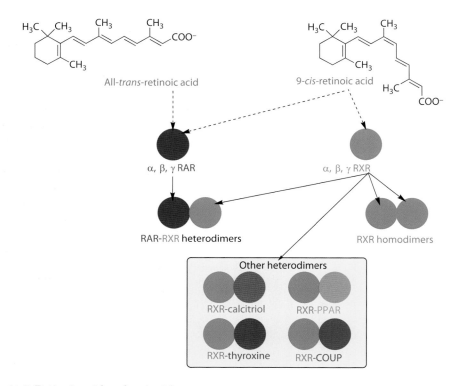

Figure 11.5 Retinoic acid and retinoid receptors.

9-*cis*-retinoic acid. (The RXR is so called because when it was discovered, its physiological ligand was unknown.) Retinoic acid is involved in the regulation of a wide variety of genes; there are three types of activated retinoid receptor dimers that bind to different response elements on DNA:

1. RXR can form homodimers (i.e., RXR-RXR dimers).
2. RAR and RXR can form RAR-RXR heterodimers.
3. RXR can form heterodimers with a wide variety of other nuclear acting receptors, including those for vitamin D (Section 11.3.3), thyroid hormone (Section 11.15.3.3), long-chain polyunsaturated fatty acid derivatives (the PPAR receptors), and one for which the physiological ligand has not yet been identified (the COUP receptor).

Either deficiency or excess of vitamin A can impair the function of vitamin D, thyroid hormone, PPAR, and COUP receptors.

- In vitamin A deficiency, there is insufficient 9-*cis*-retinoic acid to form occupied RXR. Unoccupied RXR can still form heterodimers, but not only do these not activate gene transcription, they act as repressors. Not only is there not the expected increase in gene expression in response to vitamin D or thyroid hormone, there is a reduction to below the basal level of expression.
- In vitamin A excess, there is increased availability of 9-*cis*-retinoic acid and increased formation of RXR homodimers, leaving less RXR available to form heterodimers.

11.2.4 *Vitamin A deficiency—night blindness and xerophthalmia*

Worldwide, vitamin A deficiency is a major public health problem, and the most important preventable cause of blindness. The earliest signs of deficiency are connected with vision. Initially, there is a loss of sensitivity to green light. This is followed by impairment of dark adaptation—the ability to adapt when moving from normal light into dim light. As the deficiency progresses, there is night blindness—the inability to see at all in dim light. More prolonged or severe deficiency leads to the condition called xerophthalmia: keratinisation of the cornea, followed by ulceration—irreversible damage to the eye that causes blindness. At the same time, there are changes in the skin, again with excessive keratinisation.

Vitamin A also has an important role in the differentiation of immune system cells and mild deficiency, not severe enough to cause any disturbance of vision, that leads to increased susceptibility to infectious diseases. At the same time, the synthesis of RBP is reduced in response to infection (it is a negative acute phase protein), so that there is a reduction in the circulating concentration of the vitamin, and further impairment of immune responses.

Signs of vitamin A deficiency also occur in protein-energy malnutrition (Section 8.2), even when the intake of vitamin A is adequate, because of reduced synthesis of plasma RBP. In this case, there is severely impaired immunity to infection, as a result of both the functional vitamin A deficiency and also the impairment of immune responses associated with undernutrition.

11.2.5 *Vitamin A requirements and reference intakes*

There have been relatively few studies of vitamin A requirements in which subjects have been depleted of the vitamin for long enough to permit the development of clear deficiency signs. Current estimates of requirements are based on the intakes required to maintain a concentration of 70 μmol retinol/kg in the liver, as determined by measurement of the rate of metabolism of isotopically labelled vitamin A. This is adequate to maintain normal plasma concentrations of the vitamin, and people with this level of liver reserves can be maintained on a vitamin A free diet for many months before they develop any signs of deficiency.

The average requirement to maintain a concentration of 70 μmol/kg of liver is 6.7 μg retinol equivalents/kg body weight, and this is the basis for calculation of reference intakes.

11.2.5.1   *Assessment of vitamin A status*

In field surveys, to identify those suffering from vitamin A deficiency, the earliest signs of corneal damage are detected by conjunctival impression cytology; abnormalities only develop when liver reserves are seriously depleted. The ability to adapt to dim light is impaired early in deficiency, and dark adaptation time is sometimes used to assess vitamin A status. The test is not suitable for use on children (the group most at risk of deficiency), and the apparatus is not suited to use in the field.

The plasma concentration of vitamin A only falls when then liver reserves are nearly depleted. In deficiency there is accumulation of apo-RBP in the liver, which can only be secreted when vitamin A is available. This provides the basis for the relative dose response test for vitamin A status—the ability of a dose of retinol to raise the plasma concentration several hours later, after chylomicrons have been cleared from the circulation.

11.2.5.2   *Toxicity of vitamin A*

Although there is an increase in the rate of metabolism and excretion of retinol as the concentration in the liver increases above 70 μmol/kg, there is only a limited capacity to metabolise the vitamin. Excessively high intakes lead to accumulation in the liver and other tissues, above the capacity of binding proteins; free, unbound vitamin A is present, leading to tissue damage.

Single doses of 60 mg of retinol are given to children in developing countries as prophylaxis against vitamin A deficiency—an amount adequate to meet the child's needs for 4–6 months. About 1% of children so treated show transient signs of toxicity, but this is considered an acceptable risk in view of the high prevalence and devastating effects of deficiency.

The chronic toxicity of vitamin A is a more general cause for concern; prolonged habitual intake of more than about 7.5–9 mg/day by adults (and significantly less for children, Table 11.7) causes signs and symptoms of toxicity affecting

- The central nervous system: headache, nausea, ataxia, and anorexia, all associated with increased cerebrospinal fluid pressure.
- The liver: hepatomegaly with histological changes in the liver, increased collagen formation, and hyperlipidaemia.
- Bones: joint pains, thickening of the long bones, hypercalcaemia, and calcification of soft tissues.
- The skin: excessive dryness, scaling, and chapping of the skin, desquamation, and alopecia (hair loss).

Table 11.7 Tolerable Upper Levels of Habitual Intake of Preformed Retinol

	Tolerable upper limit (µg/day)	Reference intake (µg/day)	Ratio
Infants	900	350	2.6
1–3 years	1800	400	4.5
4–6 years	3000	500	6.0
6–12 years	4500	500	9.0
13–20 years	6000	600–700	8.6–10
Adult men	9000	700	12.9
Adult women	7500	600	12.5
Pregnant women	3000	700	4.3

The synthetic vitamin A analogs 13-*cis*-retinoic acid and etretinate that are used to treat dermatological problems are highly teratogenic, causing a variety of fetal abnormalities. After women have been treated with them, it is recommended that contraceptive precautions be continued for 12 months because of their retention in the body. By extrapolation, it has been assumed that retinol is also teratogenic, and pregnant women are advised not to consume more than 3000 µg of preformed vitamin A per day.

High intakes of carotene intake are not known to have any adverse effects, apart from giving an orange-yellow colour to the skin. However, in two intervention studies in the 1990s with supplements of β-carotene there was increased mortality from lung cancer in those receiving the supplements. Under conditions of high oxygen availability, β-carotene (and presumably also other carotenoids) has a pro-oxidant rather than an antioxidant action (Section 6.5.3.3).

11.3   *Vitamin D*

Vitamin D is not strictly a vitamin, since it can be synthesised in the skin, and indeed under most conditions, endogenous synthesis is the major source of the vitamin—it is only when sunlight exposure is inadequate that a dietary source is required. It is important in the regulation of calcium absorption and homeostasis, and has a wide range of other actions mediated by nuclear receptors that regulate gene expression and cell differentiation. Deficiency, leading to rickets in children and osteomalacia in adults, continues to be a problem in northern latitudes, where sunlight exposure is poor, and there is increasing evidence that higher levels of intake, or increased sunlight exposure, may provide protection against a number of chronic non-communicable diseases.

11.3.1   *Vitamers and international units*

The normal dietary form of vitamin D is cholecalciferol (also known as calciol). This is also the compound that is formed in the skin by ultraviolet irradiation of 7-dehydrocholesterol. Some foods are enriched with the synthetic compound ergocalciferol, which is synthesised by ultraviolet irradiation of the steroid ergosterol. Ergocalciferol is metabolised in the same way as cholecalciferol and has the same biological activity. Early studies assigned the name vitamin D_1 to an impure mixture of products derived from the irradiation of ergosterol; when ergocalciferol was identified, it was called vitamin D_2, and when the physiological compound was identified as cholecalciferol, it was called vitamin D_3.

Like vitamin A, vitamin D was measured in international units of biological activity before the pure compound was isolated: 1 iu = 25 ng of cholecalciferol; 1 µg of cholecalciferol = 40 iu.

11.3.2   *Absorption and metabolism of vitamin D*

There are few dietary sources of vitamin D: mainly oily fish, with eggs, liver, and butter providing modest amounts. A number of foods are fortified with vitamin D. It is absorbed in lipid micelles and incorporated into chylomicrons; people with a low-fat diet will absorb little of such dietary vitamin D as is available. For most people, endogenous synthesis in the skin is the major source of the vitamin.

11.3.2.1   *Synthesis of vitamin D in the skin*

7-Dehydrocholesterol is an intermediate in the synthesis of cholesterol that accumulates in the skin (but not other tissues). It undergoes a non-enzymic reaction on exposure to ultraviolet light, yielding previtamin D (Figure 11.6). This undergoes a further reaction over a period of hours to form cholecalciferol, which is absorbed into the bloodstream. The photolytic reaction occurs with radiation in the UV-B range, between 290 and 310 nm, with a relatively sharp peak at 296.5 nm.

In temperate climates, there is a marked seasonal variation in the plasma concentration of vitamin D; it is highest at the end of summer, and lowest at the end of winter. Although there may be bright sunlight in winter, beyond about 40° N or S, there is very little UV radiation of the appropriate wavelength for cholecalciferol synthesis when the sun is low in the sky. By contrast, in summer, when the sun is more or less overhead, there is a considerable amount of ultraviolet light even on a moderately cloudy day and enough can penetrate thin clothes to result in significant formation of vitamin D.

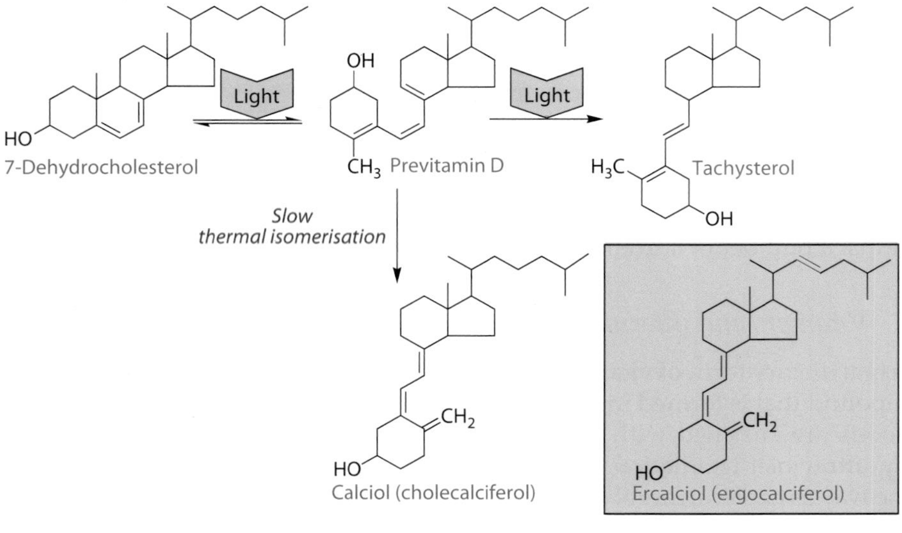

Figure 11.6 The synthesis of vitamin D in the skin. The structure of ergocalciferol (vitamin D_2) is shown in the yellow box.

11.3.2.2   *Metabolism to the active metabolite, calcitriol*

Cholecalciferol, either synthesised in the skin or taken in from foods, undergoes two hydroxylations to yield the active metabolite, 1,25-dihydroxyvitamin D or calcitriol (Figure 11.7). Ergocalciferol from fortified foods undergoes similar hydroxylation to yield ercalcitriol. The nomenclature of the vitamin D metabolites is shown in Table 11.8.

The first hydroxylation occurs in the liver, to form calcidiol (25-hydroxy-vitamin D). This is released into the circulation bound to a vitamin D binding globulin. There is no tissue storage of vitamin D; plasma calcidiol is the main reserve of the vitamin, and it is plasma calcidiol that shows the most significant seasonal variation in temperate climates.

The second hydroxylation occurs in the kidney, where calcidiol undergoes either 1-hydroxylation to yield the active metabolite 1,25-dihydroxy-vitamin D (calcitriol) or 24-hydroxylation to yield an apparently inactive metabolite, 24,25-dihydroxyvitamin D (24-hydroxycalcidiol). The plasma concentration of calcitriol is maintained within the normal range until that of calcidiol has fallen to very low levels.

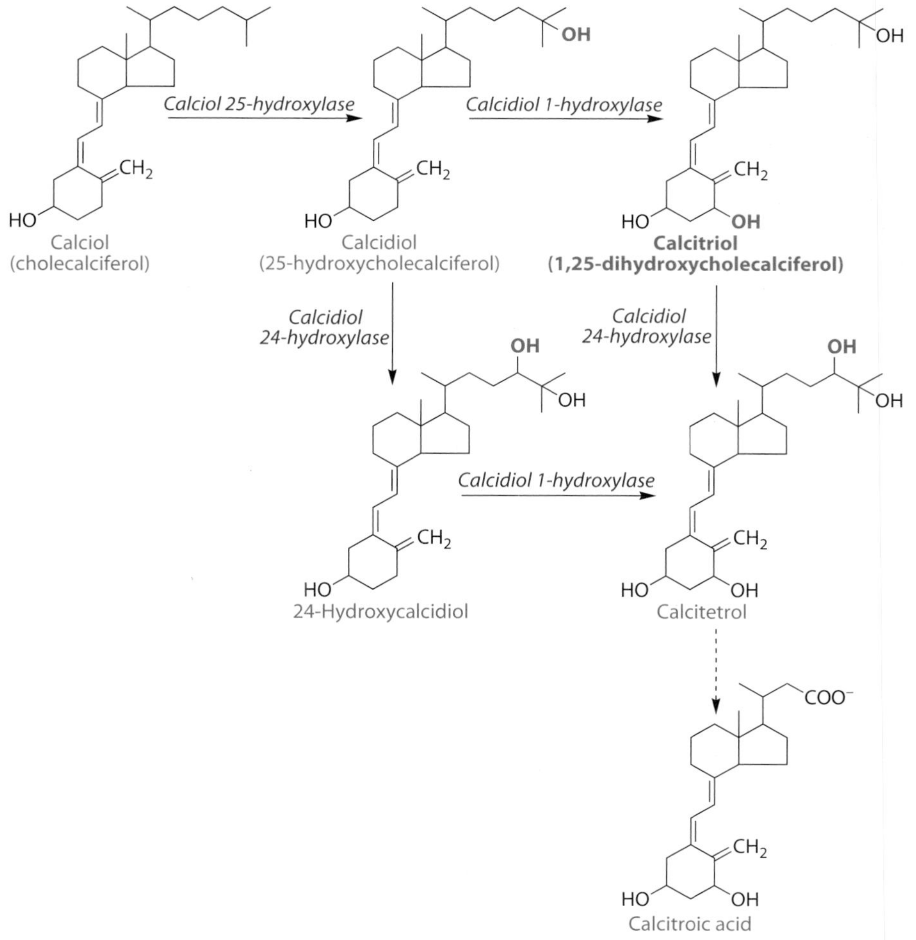

Figure 11.7 The metabolism of vitamin D to yield the active metabolite calcitriol, and its inactivation.

Table 11.8 Nomenclature of Vitamin D Metabolites

Trivial name	Recommended name	Abbreviation
Vitamin D_3		
Cholecalciferol	Calciol	–
25-Hydroxycholecalciferol	Calcidiol	$25(OH)D_3$
1α-Hydroxycholecalciferol	1(S)-Hydroxycalciol	$1α(OH)D_3$
24,25-Dihydroxycholecalciferol	24(R)-Hydroxycalcidiol	$24,25(OH)_2D_3$
1,25-Dihydroxycholecalciferol	Calcitriol	$1,25(OH)_2D_3$
1,24,25-Trihydroxycholecalciferol	Calcitetrol	$1,24,25(OH)_3D_3$
Vitamin D_2		
Ergocalciferol	Ercalciol	–
25-Hydroxyergocalciferol	Ercalcidiol	$25(OH)D_2$
24,25-Dihydroxyergocalciferol	24(R)-Hydroxyercalcidiol	$24,25(OH)_2D_2$
1,25-Dihydroxyergocalciferol	Ercalcitriol	$1,25(OH)_2 D_2$
1,24,25-Trihydroxyergocalciferol	Ercalcitetrol	$1,24,25(OH)_3D_2$

Note: The abbreviations shown in column 3 are not recommended but are frequently used in the literature.

The main function of vitamin D is in the control of calcium homeostasis (Section 11.15.1.1), and in turn, vitamin D metabolism is regulated, at the level of 1- or 24-hydroxylation, by factors that respond to plasma concentrations of calcium and phosphate:

- Calcitriol acts to reduce its own synthesis. It induces the 24-hydroxylase and represses the synthesis of 1-hydroxylase in the kidney, acting on gene expression through calcitriol receptors.
- Parathyroid hormone is secreted in response to a fall in plasma calcium. In the kidney, it acts to increase the activity of calcidiol 1-hydroxylase and decrease that of the 24-hydroxylase. This is not an effect on protein synthesis, but the result of changes in the activity of existing enzyme protein, mediated by cAMP (Section 10.3.2). In turn, both calcitriol and high blood concentrations of calcium repress the synthesis of parathyroid hormone.
- Calcium exerts its main effect on the synthesis and secretion of parathyroid hormone. However, calcium ions also have a direct effect in the kidney, reducing the activity of calcidiol 1-hydroxylase (but with no effect on the activity of 24-hydroxylase).

11.3.3 Metabolic functions of vitamin D

Calcitriol acts like a steroid hormone, binding to a nuclear receptor protein (Section 10.4), and forming a heterodimer with the vitamin A (RXR) receptor (Section 11.2.3.2). The active receptor complex binds to the enhancer site of the gene coding for a calcium binding protein, increasing its transcription, and so increasing the amount of calcium binding protein in the cell.

The principal function of vitamin D is to maintain the plasma concentration of calcium; calcitriol achieves this in three ways:

1. Increased intestinal absorption of calcium (Section 11.15.1)
2. Reduced excretion of calcium (by stimulating reabsorption in the distal renal tubules)
3. Mobilisation of bone mineral (Section 11.3.3.1)

In addition, calcitriol has a variety of permissive or modulatory effects; it is a necessary, but not a sufficient factor in

- Insulin secretion
- Synthesis and secretion of parathyroid and thyroid hormones
- Inhibition of production of interleukin by activated T-lymphocytes and of immunoglobulin by activated B-lymphocytes
- Differentiation of monocyte precursor cells in the immune system
- Modulation of cell proliferation

The best studied actions of vitamin D are in the intestinal mucosa, where the intracellular calcium binding protein is essential for the absorption of calcium from the diet. Here the vitamin has another action as well, to increase the transport of calcium across the mucosal membrane. The increase in calcium transport is seen immediately after feeding vitamin D, whereas the increase in absorption is slower, since it depends on new synthesis of the binding protein. The rapid response to vitamin D does not involve new protein synthesis, but reflects an effect on preformed calcium transport proteins in the cell membrane.

The effects of vitamin D other than on calcium homeostasis and bone metabolism are mainly the result of tissue uptake of calcidiol and hydroxylation to calcitriol within the target cells. These actions are therefore more sensitive to moderate vitamin D deficiency because the plasma concentration of calcitriol is maintained until circulating calcidiol has fallen to very low levels.

11.3.3.1   The role of calcitriol in bone metabolism

The maintenance of bone structure is due to balanced activity of osteoclasts, which erode existing bone mineral and organic matrix, and osteoblasts, which synthesise and secrete the proteins of bone matrix. Mineralisation of the organic matrix is largely controlled by the availability of calcium and phosphate.

Calcitriol raises plasma calcium by activating osteoblasts to secrete osteoclast stimulating factors. The activated osteoclasts then erode bone to mobilise calcium. Calcitriol acts later to stimulate the laying down of new bone to replace the loss, by stimulating the differentiation and recruitment of osteoblast cells.

11.3.4   Vitamin D deficiency: rickets and osteomalacia

Historically, rickets is a disease of toddlers, especially in northern industrial cities. Their bones are undermineralised as a result of poor absorption of calcium in the absence of adequate amounts of calcitriol. When the child begins to walk, the long bones of the legs are deformed, leading to bow-legs or knock-knees. More seriously, rickets can also lead to collapse of the rib-cage, and deformities of the bones of the pelvis. Similar problems may also occur in adolescents who are deficient in vitamin D during the adolescent growth spurt, when there is again a high demand for calcium for new bone formation.

Whilst florid rickets leading to bone deformities is now rare, there is still a significant problem of subclinical rickets, identified by elevated plasma alkaline phosphatase activity. A number of studies have shown that up to 10% of toddlers in northern cities have subclinical rickets, and it is also a problem amongst adolescents. There has been a resurgence of subclinical rickets amongst adolescents in northern countries as a result of reduced sunlight exposure, associated with an increase in indoor leisure activities at the expense of outdoor activities.

Osteomalacia is the adult equivalent of rickets. It results from the demineralisation of bone, rather than the failure to mineralise it in the first place, as is the case with rickets. Women who have little exposure to sunlight are especially at risk from osteomalacia after several pregnancies because of the strain that pregnancy places on their marginal reserve of calcium. Osteomalacia also occurs in the elderly. Here again, the problem may be inadequate exposure to sunlight, but there is also evidence that the capacity to form 7-dehydrocholesterol in the skin decreases with advancing age; thus, the elderly are more reliant on the few dietary sources of vitamin D.

11.3.5   Vitamin D requirements and reference intakes

It is difficult to determine requirements for dietary vitamin D, since the major source is synthesis in the skin. The main criterion of adequacy is the plasma concentration of calcidiol. In elderly subjects with little sunlight exposure, a dietary intake of 10 µg of vitamin D/day results in a plasma calcidiol concentration of 20 nmol/L, the lower end of the reference range for younger adults at the end of winter. Therefore, the UK reference intake for the elderly is 10 µg/day; the same figure is used for younger adults in the United States, with an RDA of 15 µg/day for older people. Average intakes of vitamin D are less than 4 µg/day; thus, to achieve an intake of 10–15 µg/day will almost certainly require either fortification of foods or the use of vitamin D supplements.

There is a great deal of evidence that the functions of vitamin D in the regulation of gene expression and cell differentiation are optimal at higher levels of vitamin D intake than current reference intakes. In addition to protecting bone health, higher intakes of vitamin D are likely to be protective against a number of cancers as well as type II diabetes and the metabolic syndrome (Sections 7.2.3 and 10.7). These desirable levels of intake cannot be achieved from unfortified foods, but would be achievable by increased sunlight exposure. The problem is that excessive sunlight exposure is associated with increased risk of skin cancer.

11.3.5.1   Vitamin D toxicity

During the 1950s, rickets was more or less totally eradicated in Britain and other temperate countries. This was due to enrichment of a large number of infant foods with vitamin D. However, a number of infants suffered from vitamin D poisoning, the most serious effect of which is hypercalcaemia—an elevated plasma concentration of calcium. This can lead to contraction of blood vessels, and hence dangerously high blood pressure, and calcinosis—the calcification of soft tissues, including the kidney, heart, lungs, and blood vessel walls.

Some infants are sensitive to intakes of vitamin D as low as 25–50 µg/day. To avoid the serious problem of vitamin D poisoning in these susceptible infants, the fortification of infant foods with vitamin D was reduced considerably. Reduction of intakes to below the level at which any infant shows signs of toxicity meant that about 10% were undersupplied with vitamin D, explaining the current prevalence of subclinical rickets in northern cities. A small number of children have been identified who show hypercalcaemia at normal levels of vitamin D intake. They have mutations affecting the activity of calcidiol 24-hydroxylase, the enzyme that inactivates calcidiol (Figure 11.7). It remains to be seen whether there are other mutations affecting this enzyme that might explain the hypercalcaemia seen in infants exposed to higher intakes of vitamin D.

The toxic threshold in adults is not known, but patients suffering from vitamin D intoxication who have been investigated were taking more than 250 µg of vitamin D/day.

Although excess dietary vitamin D is toxic, excessive exposure to sunlight does not lead to vitamin D poisoning. There is a limited capacity to form the precursor,

7-dehydrocholesterol, in the skin, and a limited capacity to take up cholecalciferol from the skin. Furthermore, prolonged exposure of previtamin D to UV light results in reversal of the reaction from 7-dehydrocholesterol as well as onward isomerisation of previtamin D to inactive tachysterol (Figure 7.6).

11.4   Vitamin E

Although vitamin E was identified as a dietary essential for animals in the 1920s, it was not until 1983 that it was clearly demonstrated to be a dietary essential for human beings. Vitamin E acts as a lipid-soluble antioxidant in cell membranes and plasma lipoproteins and has a number of other membrane-specific functions, including roles in cell signalling and platelet aggregation. There is epidemiological evidence that high intakes of vitamin E are associated with lower incidence of cardiovascular disease, although intervention trials have been disappointing (Section 6.5.3.5).

11.4.1   Vitamers and units of activity

Vitamin E is the generic descriptor for two families of compounds, the tocopherols and the tocotrienols (Figure 11.8). The different vitamers have different biological potency, as shown in Table 11.9. The most active is α-tocopherol, and it is usual to express vitamin E intake in terms of mg α-tocopherol equivalents. This is the sum of mg α-tocopherol + 0.5 × mg β-tocopherol + 0.1 × mg γ-tocopherol + 0.3 × mg α-tocotrienol. The other vitamers either occur in negligible amounts in foods or have negligible vitamin activity.

The obsolete international unit of vitamin E activity is still sometimes used: 1 iu = 0.67 mg α-tocopherol equivalent; 1 mg α-tocopherol = 1.49 iu.

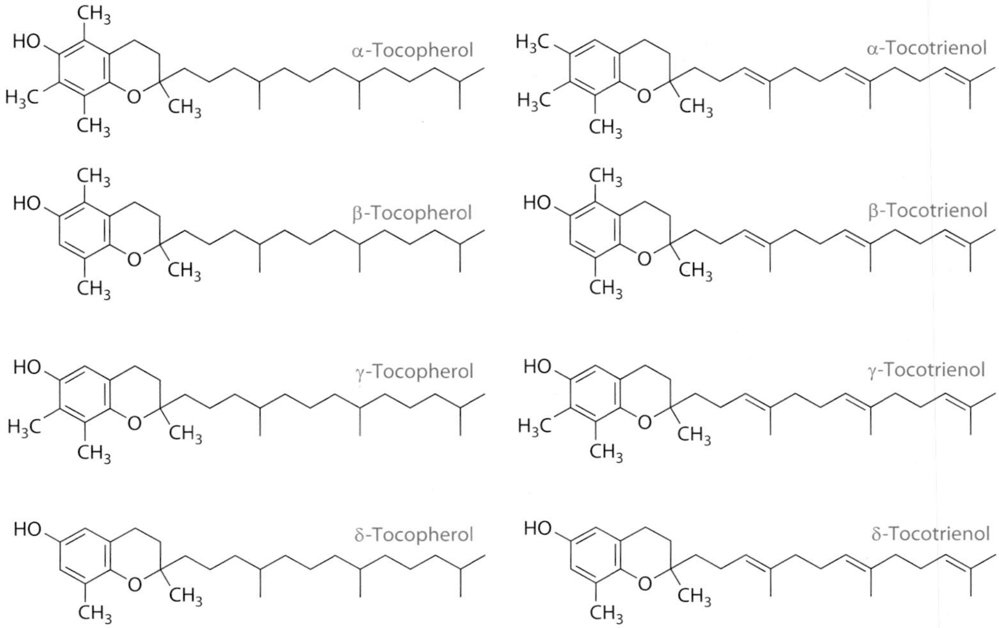

Figure 11.8 Vitamin E vitamers.

Table 11.9 Relative Biological Activity of the Vitamin E Vitamers

	iu/mg	Relative activity
D-α-Tocopherol (*RRR*)	1.49	1.0
D-β-Tocopherol (*RRR*)	0.75	0.49
D-γ-Tocopherol (*RRR*)	0.15	0.10
D-δ-Tocopherol (*RRR*)	0.05	0.03
D-α-Tocotrienol	0.45	0.29
D-β-Tocotrienol	0.08	0.05
D-γ-Tocotrienol	–	–
D-δ-Tocotrienol	–	–
L-α-Tocopherol (SRR)	0.46	0.31
RRS-α-Tocopherol	1.34	0.90
SRS-α-Tocopherol	0.55	0.37
RSS-α-Tocopherol	1.09	0.73
SSR-α-Tocopherol	0.31	0.21
RSR-α-Tocopherol	0.85	0.57
SSS-α-Tocopherol	1.10	0.74

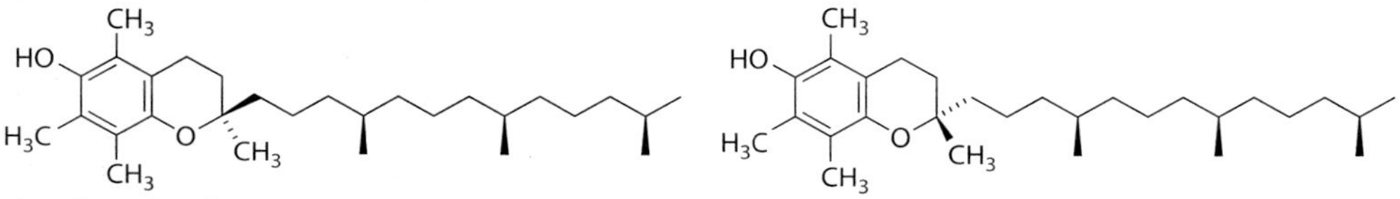

D-α-Tocopherol
2′R, 4′R, 8′R (*RRR* or all-*R*) α-tocopherol

L-α-Tocopherol
2′R, 4′R, 8′R (*SSR*) α-tocopherol

Figure 11.9 Asymmetric centres in α-tocopherol.

Synthetic α-tocopherol does not have the same biological potency as the naturally occurring compound because the side chain of tocopherol has three centres of asymmetry (Figure 11.9), and when it is synthesised chemically, the product is a mixture of the various isomers. In the naturally occurring compound all three centres of asymmetry have the *R*-configuration and naturally occurring α-tocopherol is all-*R*, or *RRR*-α-tocopherol.

11.4.2 Absorption and metabolism of vitamin E

Tocopherols and tocotrienols are absorbed in lipid micelles, and incorporated into chylomicrons (Sections 4.3.2.2 and 5.6.2.1), then secreted by the liver in VLDL (Section 5.6.2.2). The major route of excretion is in the bile, as a variety of metabolites. There may also be significant excretion of the vitamin through the skin.

There are two mechanisms for tissue uptake of vitamin E. Lipoprotein lipase releases the vitamin by hydrolysing the triacylglycerol in chylomicrons and VLDL, whilst separately there is uptake of LDL-bound vitamin E by means of LDL receptors. Retention within tissues depends on intracellular binding proteins, and the differences in biological activity of the vitamers are due to differential protein binding. γ-Tocopherol and α-tocotrienol bind relatively poorly, whilst *SRR*-α-tocopherol and *RRR*-α-tocopherol acetate do not bind to liver tocopherol binding protein to any significant extent.

11.4.3   Metabolic functions of vitamin E

The main function of vitamin E is as a radical trapping antioxidant in cell membranes and plasma lipoproteins. It is especially important in limiting radical damage resulting from oxidation of polyunsaturated fatty acids, by reacting with the lipid peroxide radicals before they can establish a chain reaction (Section 6.5.3.5). The radical formed from vitamin E is relatively unreactive, and persists long enough to undergo reaction to yield non-radical products. Commonly, the vitamin E radical in a membrane or lipoprotein is reduced back to tocopherol by reaction with vitamin C in plasma (Figure 6.15). The resultant monodehydroascorbate radical then undergoes enzymic or non-enzymic reaction to yield ascorbate and dehydroascorbate (Figure 6.16), neither of which is a radical.

The antioxidant function of vitamin E is dependent on the stability of the tocopheroxyl radical, which means that it survives long enough to undergo reaction to yield non-radical products. However, this stability also means that the tocopheroxyl radical can also penetrate further into cells or deeper into plasma lipoproteins, and potentially propagate a chain reaction. Therefore, although it is regarded as an antioxidant, vitamin E may, like other antioxidants, also have pro-oxidant actions, especially at high concentrations. This may explain why, although epidemiological studies have shown a clear association between high blood concentrations of vitamin E and lower incidence of atherosclerosis, the results of intervention studies with relatively high doses of vitamin E have generally been disappointing, with increased mortality amongst those taking vitamin E supplements (Section 6.5.3.5).

There is a considerable overlap between the functions of vitamin E and selenium (Section 11.15.2.5). Vitamin E reduces lipid peroxides to unreactive fatty acids (Figure 6.15); the selenium dependent enzyme glutathione peroxidase reduces hydrogen peroxide to water (Section 6.5.3.2), thus lowering the intracellular concentration of potentially lipid damaging peroxide. Glutathione peroxidase will also reduce the tocopheroxyl radical back to tocopherol. Thus, vitamin E acts to remove the products of lipid peroxidation, whilst selenium acts both to remove the cause of lipid peroxidation and also to recycle vitamin E. In vitamin E-deficient animals, selenium will prevent many of the signs of deficiency, but not central nervous system necrosis (Section 11.4.4).

11.4.3.1   Hypocholesterolaemic actions of tocotrienols

Tocotrienols have lower biological activity than tocopherols, and indeed it is conventional to consider only γ-tocotrienol as a significant part of vitamin E intake (Section 11.4.1). However, the tocotrienols have a hypocholesterolaemic action not shared by the tocopherols. In plants, tocotrienols are synthesised from hydroxymethylglutaryl CoA (HMG CoA), which is also the precursor for cholesterol synthesis. High levels of tocotrienols repress the synthesis of HMG CoA reductase, the rate-limiting enzyme in the pathway for synthesis of both cholesterol and (in plants) tocotrienols (Figure 6.25).

11.4.4   Vitamin E deficiency

In experimental animals, vitamin E deficiency results in a number of different conditions:

- Deficient female animals suffer the death and resorption of the fetuses. This provided the basis of the original biological assay of vitamin E.
- Deficient male animals suffer testicular atrophy and degeneration of the germinal epithelium of the seminiferous tubules.

- Both skeletal and cardiac muscle are affected in deficiency. This is sometimes called nutritional muscular dystrophy; an unfortunate term, since there is no evidence that human muscular dystrophy is related to vitamin E deficiency, and the condition is better called necrotising myopathy.
- The integrity of blood vessel walls is affected, with leakage of blood plasma into subcutaneous tissues, and accumulation under the skin of a green-coloured fluid—exudative diathesis.
- The nervous system is affected, with the development of central nervous system necrosis and axonal dystrophy. This is exacerbated by feeding diets rich in polyunsaturated fatty acids.

Dietary deficiency of vitamin E in human beings is unknown, although patients with severe fat malabsorption, cystic fibrosis, some forms of chronic liver disease or (very rare) congenital lack of plasma β-lipoprotein or intracellular vitamin E binding proteins, suffer deficiency because they are unable to absorb the vitamin or transport it around the body. They suffer from severe damage to nerve and muscle membranes.

Premature infants are at risk of vitamin E deficiency, since they are often born with inadequate reserves of the vitamin. The red blood cell membranes of deficient infants are abnormally fragile, as a result of unchecked oxidative radical attack. This may lead to haemolytic anaemia (Section 11.16) if they are not given supplements of the vitamin.

Experimental animals that are depleted of vitamin E become sterile. However, there is no evidence that vitamin E nutritional status is in any way associated with human fertility, and there is certainly no evidence that vitamin E supplements increase sexual potency, prowess, or vigor.

11.4.5   Vitamin E requirements

It is difficult to establish vitamin E requirements, partly because deficiency is more or less unknown and also because the requirement depends on the intake of polyunsaturated fatty acids. It is generally accepted that an acceptable intake of vitamin E is 0.4 mg α-tocopherol equivalent/g dietary polyunsaturated fatty acid. The plant oils that are rich sources of polyunsaturated fatty acids are also rich sources of vitamin E.

11.4.5.1   Indices of vitamin E status

Erythrocytes are incapable of *de novo* lipid synthesis; thus, peroxidative damage resulting from oxygen stress has a serious effect, shortening red cell life and possibly precipitating haemolytic anaemia (Section 11.16) in vitamin E deficiency. This can be used as a method of assessing status (although unrelated factors affect the results) by measuring the haemolysis of red cells induced by dilute hydrogen peroxide.

An alternative method of assessing functional antioxidant status, again one that is affected by both vitamin E and other antioxidants, is by measuring the exhalation of pentane arising from the metabolism of the peroxides ω6 polyunsaturated fatty acids or ethane from peroxides of ω3 polyunsaturated fatty acids.

11.5   Vitamin K

Vitamin K was discovered as a result of investigations into the cause of a bleeding disorder (haemorrhagic disease) of cattle fed on silage made from sweet clover and of chickens fed on a fat-free diet. The missing factor in the diet of the chickens was identified as vitamin K,

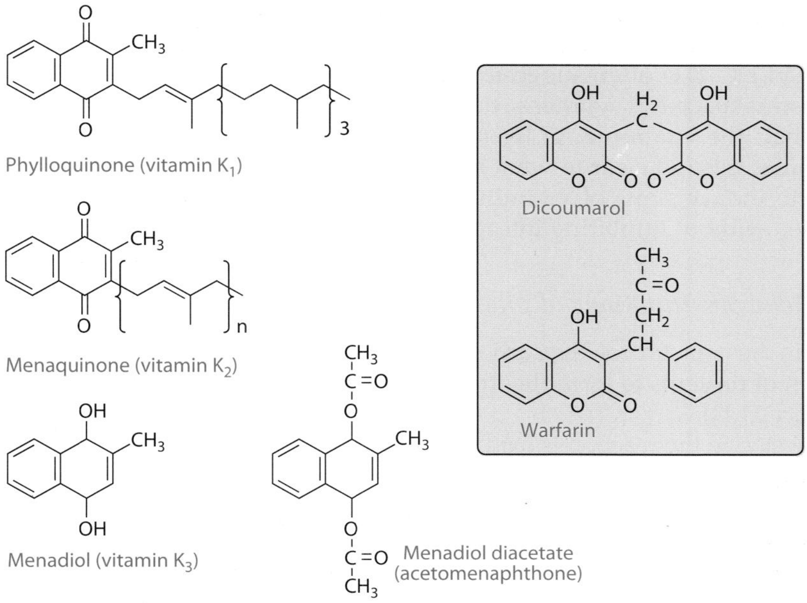

Figure 11.10 Vitamin K vitamers; the vitamin K antagonists dicoumarol and warfarin are shown in the yellow box. Menadione and menadiol diacetate are synthetic compounds that are converted to menaquinone in the liver.

whilst the problem in the cattle was that the feed contained dicoumarol (Figure 11.10), an antagonist of the vitamin. Because of its importance in blood coagulation, it was called the *koagulations-vitamine* (vitamin K) when the original results were reported (in German).

Since the effect an excessive intake of dicoumarol was severely impaired blood clotting, it was isolated and tested in low doses as an anticoagulant for use in patients at risk of thrombosis. Although it was effective, it had unwanted side effects, and synthetic vitamin K antagonists were developed for clinical use as anticoagulants. The most commonly used of these is warfarin (Figure 11.10), which is also used, in larger amounts, to kill rodents.

11.5.1 Vitamers of vitamin K

Three compounds have the biological activity of vitamin K (Figure 11.10):

1. Phylloquinone, the normal dietary source, found in green leafy vegetables.
2. Menaquinones, a family of related compounds synthesised by intestinal bacteria, with differing lengths of side chain.
3. Menadione and menadiol diacetate, synthetic compounds that can be metabolised to phylloquinone.

Phylloquinone is found in all green leafy vegetables; the richest sources are spring (collard) greens, spinach, and Brussels sprouts. In addition, soybean, rapeseed, cottonseed, and olive oils are relatively rich in vitamin K, although other oils are not.

About 80% of dietary phylloquinone is normally absorbed into the lymphatic system in chylomicrons and is then taken up by the liver from chylomicron remnants and released into the circulation in very-low-density lipoprotein.

Intestinal bacteria synthesise a variety of menaquinones, which are absorbed to a limited extent from the large intestine into the lymphatic system, cleared by the liver and released in VLDL. It is often suggested that about half the requirement for vitamin K is met by intestinal bacterial synthesis, but there is little evidence for this, other than the fact that about half the vitamin K in liver is phylloquinone, and the remainder a variety of menaquinones. It is not clear to what extent the menaquinones are biologically active—it is possible to induce signs of vitamin K deficiency simply be feeding a phylloquinone-deficient diet, without inhibiting intestinal bacterial action.

11.5.2   Metabolic functions of vitamin K

Vitamin K is the cofactor for the carboxylation of glutamate residues in the postsynthetic modification of proteins to form the unusual amino acid γ-carboxyglutamate, abbreviated to Gla (Figure 11.11).

The first step in the reaction is oxidation of vitamin K hydroquinone to the epoxide. This epoxide then activates a glutamate residue in the protein substrate to a carbanion that reacts with carbon dioxide to form γ-carboxyglutamate. Vitamin K epoxide is then reduced to the quinone by a warfarin-sensitive reductase and the quinone is reduced to the active hydroquinone by either the same warfarin-sensitive reductase or a warfarin-insensitive quinone reductase.

In the presence of warfarin, vitamin K epoxide cannot be reduced back to the active hydroquinone, but accumulates, and is conjugated and excreted. If enough vitamin K is provided in the diet, the quinone can be reduced to the active hydroquinone by the warfarin-insensitive enzyme, and carboxylation can continue, with stoichiometric utilisation of vitamin K and excretion of the epoxide. High doses of vitamin K are used to treat patients who have received an overdose of warfarin, and at least part of the resistance of some populations of rats to the action of warfarin is due to a high consumption of vitamin K

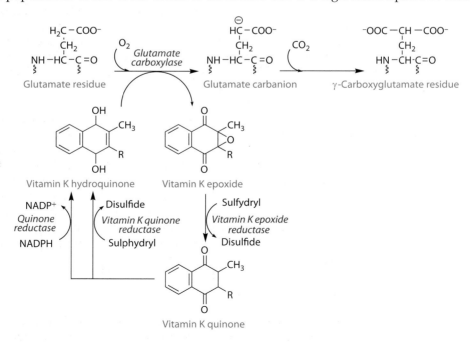

Figure 11.11 The role of vitamin K in γ-carboxyglutamate synthesis.

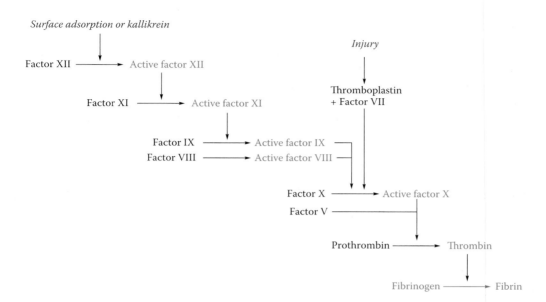

Figure 11.12 The intrinsic and extrinsic blood clotting cascades.

from maram grass, although there are also genetically resistant populations of rodents that have a warfarin-insensitive reductase.

Prothrombin and several other proteins of the blood clotting system (Factors VII, IX, and X, and proteins C and S, Figure 11.12) each contain between 4 and 6 γ-carboxyglutamate residues per mol. γ-Carboxyglutamate chelates calcium ions, and so permits the binding of the blood clotting proteins to membranes. In vitamin K deficiency, or in the presence of an antagonist such as warfarin, an abnormal precursor of prothrombin (preprothrombin) containing little or no γ-carboxyglutamate is released into the circulation. Preprothrombin cannot chelate calcium or bind to phospholipid membranes and so is unable to initiate blood clotting. Preprothrombin is sometimes known as PIVKA—the protein induced by vitamin K absence.

11.5.2.1   *Bone vitamin K dependent proteins*

Treatment of pregnant women with warfarin can lead to bone abnormalities in the child—the fetal warfarin syndrome. Two proteins in bone matrix contain γ-carboxyglutamate: osteocalcin and bone matrix Gla protein. Osteocalcin is interesting in that as well as γ-carboxyglutamate, it also contains hydroxyproline; thus, its synthesis is dependent not only on vitamin K but also on vitamin C (Section 11.14.2.1); in addition, its synthesis is induced by vitamin D, and the release into the circulation of osteocalcin provides a sensitive index of vitamin D action (Section 11.3.3.1). Osteocalcin comprises some 1%–2% of total bone protein, and it functions as a calcium-binding protein, modifying the crystallisation of bone mineral. The matrix Gla protein is found in a variety of tissues, where it functions to maintain calcium in solution and prevent mineralisation.

11.5.3   *Vitamin K deficiency and requirements*

Apart from experimental depletion, vitamin K deficiency is unknown, and determination of requirements is complicated by a lack of data on the importance of menaquinones synthesised by intestinal bacteria (Section 11.5.1).

The main way of determining vitamin K status, and monitoring the efficacy of anti-coagulant therapy, is by measuring the time required for the formation of a fibrin clot in citrated blood plasma after the addition of calcium ions and thromboplastin—the pro-thrombin time. To standardise the results, they are normally expressed as the international normalised ratio (INR)—the ratio of the patient's prothrombin time/that of a control sample, raised to the power of a sensitivity factor for the batch of thromboplastin used.

A more sensitive index of vitamin K status is provided by direct measurement of preprothrombin in plasma, most commonly by immunoassay using antisera against pre-prothrombin that do not react with prothrombin. Such studies suggest that an intake of 1 µg/kg body weight/day is adequate, leading reference intakes between 65 and 80 µg/day for adults.

A small number of newborn infants have very low reserves of vitamin K, and are at risk of potentially fatal haemorrhagic disease. It is therefore generally recommended that all neonates should be given a single prophylactic dose of vitamin K.

11.6   Vitamin B$_1$ (thiamin)

Historically, thiamin deficiency affecting the peripheral nervous system (beriberi) was a major public health problem in Southeast Asia following the introduction of the steam-powered mill that made highly polished (thiamin depleted) rice widely available. There are still sporadic outbreaks of deficiency amongst people whose diet is rich in carbohydrate and poor in thiamin. More commonly, thiamin deficiency affecting the heart and central nervous system is a problem in people with an excessive consumption of alcohol.

The structures of thiamin and the coenzyme thiamin diphosphate are shown in Figure 11.13. Thiamin is unstable to light, and although bread and flour contain significant amounts of thiamin, much or all of this can be lost when baked goods are exposed to sunlight in a shop window.

Thiamin is also destroyed by sulphites, and in potato products that have been blanched by immersion in sulphite solution, there is little or no thiamin remaining. Polyphenols, including tannic acid in tea and betel nuts, also destroy thiamin, and have been associated with thiamin deficiency. Fermented raw fish is also devoid of thiamin because of the action of thiaminases that cleave the vitamin.

11.6.1   Absorption and metabolism of thiamin

Most dietary thiamin is present as phosphates, which are readily hydrolysed by intestinal phosphatases, and free thiamin is readily absorbed in the duodenum and proximal jejunum, and then transferred to the portal circulation as free thiamin or thiamin monophosphate. The export of thiamin from the mucosal cells is by active transport (Section 3.2.2.3) and is inhibited by alcohol, which explains why alcoholics are especially susceptible to thiamin deficiency.

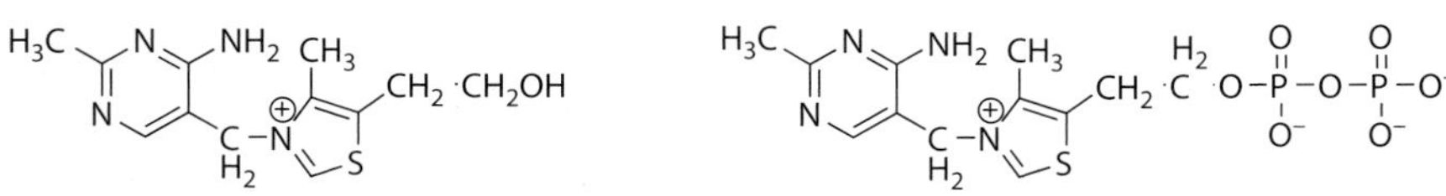

Figure 11.13 Thiamin (vitamin B$_1$) and the coenzyme thiamin diphosphate.

Tissues take up both free thiamin and thiamin monophosphate, then phosphorylate them further to yield thiamin diphosphate (the active coenzyme) and thiamin triphosphate. Some free thiamin is excreted in the urine, increasing with diuresis, and a significant amount may also be lost in sweat. Most urinary excretion is as thiochrome, the result of non-enzymic cyclisation, as well as a variety of products of side chain oxidation and ring cleavage.

There is little storage of thiamin in the body, and biochemical signs of deficiency can be observed within a few days of initiating a thiamin-free diet.

11.6.2   Metabolic functions of thiamin

Thiamin has a central role in energy-yielding metabolism and especially the metabolism of carbohydrates. Thiamin diphosphate (also known as thiamin pyrophosphate, Figure 11.13) is the coenzyme for three multi-enzyme complexes that catalyse oxidative decarboxylation of the substrate linked to reduction of enzyme-bound lipoamide and eventually reduction of NAD^+ to NADH:

- Pyruvate dehydrogenase in carbohydrate metabolism (Section 5.4.3.1 and Figure 5.16).
- α-Ketoglutarate dehydrogenase in the citric acid cycle (Section 5.4.4).
- The branched-chain keto-acid dehydrogenase involved in the metabolism of leucine, isoleucine, and valine.

Thiamin diphosphate is also the coenzyme for transketolase, in the pentose phosphate pathway of carbohydrate metabolism (Section 5.4.2). Thiamin triphosphate has a role in nerve conduction, as the phosphate donor for phosphorylation of a nerve membrane sodium transport channel.

11.6.3   Thiamin deficiency

Thiamin deficiency can result in three distinct syndromes:

1. A chronic peripheral neuritis, beriberi, which may or may not be associated with heart failure and oedema (Sections 11.6.3.1 and 11.6.3.2).
2. Acute pernicious (fulminating) beriberi (shoshin beriberi), in which heart failure and metabolic abnormalities predominate, with little evidence of peripheral neuritis (Section 11.6.3.3).
3. Wernicke's encephalopathy with Korsakoff's psychosis, a thiamin-responsive condition associated especially with alcohol and narcotic abuse (Section 11.6.3.4).

In general, a relatively acute deficiency is involved in the central nervous system lesions of the Wernicke–Korsakoff syndrome, and a high-energy intake, as in alcoholics, is also a predisposing factor. Dry beriberi (neuritis without oedema) is associated with a more prolonged, less severe, deficiency, with a generally low food intake, whilst higher carbohydrate intake and physical activity predispose to oedema and wet beriberi.

The role of thiamin diphosphate in pyruvate dehydrogenase means that in deficiency there is impaired conversion of pyruvate to acetyl CoA, and hence impaired entry of pyruvate into the citric acid cycle (Section 5.4.3.1). Especially in subjects on a relatively high carbohydrate diet, this results in increased plasma concentrations of lactate and pyruvate, which may lead to life-threatening lactic acidosis.

11.6.3.1   Dry beriberi

Chronic deficiency of thiamin, especially associated with a high carbohydrate diet, results in beriberi, which is a symmetrical ascending peripheral neuritis. Initially, the patient complains of weakness, stiffness, and cramps in the legs and is unable to walk more than a short distance. There may be numbness of the feet and ankles, and vibration sense may be diminished. As the disease progresses, the ankle jerk reflex is lost, and the muscular weakness spreads upward, involving first the extensor muscles of the foot, then the muscles of the calf, and finally the extensors and flexors of the thigh. At this stage, there is pronounced toe and foot drop—the patient is unable to keep either the toe or the whole foot extended off the ground. When the arms are affected there is a similar inability to keep the hand extended—wrist drop.

The affected muscles become tender, numb, and hyperaesthetic. The hyperaesthesia extends in the form of a band around the limb, the so-called stocking and glove distribution, and is followed by anesthesia. There is deep muscle pain, and in the terminal stages, when the patient is bed-ridden, even slight pressure, as from bed clothes, causes considerable pain.

11.6.3.2   Wet beriberi

The heart may also be affected in beriberi, with dilatation of arterioles, rapid blood flow and increased pulse rate and pressure, and increased jugular venous pressure leading to right-sided heart failure, and oedema—so-called wet beriberi. The signs of chronic heart failure may be seen without peripheral neuritis. The arteriolar dilatation, and possibly also the oedema, probably result from high circulating concentrations of lactate and pyruvate as a result of impaired activity of pyruvate dehydrogenase.

11.6.3.3   Acute pernicious (fulminating) beriberi—shoshin beriberi

Heart failure without increased cardiac output, and no peripheral oedema, may also occur acutely, associated with severe lactic acidosis. This was a common presentation of deficiency in Japan, where it was called shoshin (=acute) beriberi; in the 1920s, some 26,000 deaths a year were recorded.

With improved knowledge of the cause, and improved nutritional status, the disease has become more or less unknown, although in the 1980s, it reappeared amongst Japanese adolescents consuming a diet based largely on high-carbohydrate, low-nutrient foods such as sweet carbonated drinks, 'instant' noodles, and polished rice. It also occurs amongst alcoholics, when the lactic acidosis may be life threatening, without clear signs of heart failure. Acute beriberi has also been reported when previously starved subjects are given intravenous glucose.

11.6.3.4   The Wernicke–Korsakoff syndrome

While peripheral neuritis and acute cardiac beriberi with lactic acidosis occur in thiamin deficiency associated with alcohol abuse, the more usual presentation is the Wernicke–Korsakoff syndrome, due to central nervous system lesions. Initially, there is a confused state, Korsakoff's psychosis, which is characterised by confabulation and loss of recent memory, although memory for past events may be unimpaired. Later, neurological signs develop, Wernicke's encephalopathy, characterised by nystagmus and extra-ocular palsy. *Post mortem* examination shows characteristic brain lesions.

Like shoshin beriberi, Wernicke's encephalopathy can develop acutely, without the more gradual development of Korsakoff's psychosis, amongst previously starved patients given intravenous glucose and seriously ill patients given parenteral hyperalimentation.

11.6.4   Thiamin requirements

Because thiamin has a central role in energy-yielding, and especially carbohydrate, metabolism, requirements depend mainly on carbohydrate intake and have been related to non-fat energy intake. In practice, requirements and reference intakes are calculated on the basis of total energy intake, assuming that the average diet provides 40% of energy from fat. For diets that are lower in fat content, and hence higher in carbohydrate and protein, thiamin requirements may be somewhat higher.

The activation of apo-transketolase in erythrocyte lysate by thiamin diphosphate added *in vitro* has become the most widely used and accepted index of thiamin nutritional status (Sections 2.7.3 and 5.4.2). An activation coefficient >1.25 is indicative of deficiency, and <1.15 is considered to reflect adequate thiamin nutrition. The reference intake of 100 μg/MJ (0.5 mg/1000 kcal) is based on the amount to maintain a normal transketolase activation—with a minimum intake for people with a low energy intake of 0.8–1.0 mg/day to allow for metabolism of endogenous substrates.

11.7   Vitamin B₂ (riboflavin)

Riboflavin deficiency is a significant public health problem in many areas of the world. The vitamin has a central role as a coenzyme in energy-yielding metabolism, yet deficiency is rarely, if ever, fatal because there is very efficient conservation and recycling of riboflavin in deficiency. The structures of riboflavin and the riboflavin-derived coenzymes (also known as flavin coenzymes) are shown in Figures 2.18 and 2.19.

The main dietary sources of riboflavin are milk and dairy products, providing 25% or more of the total intake in most diets, and to a considerable extent, average riboflavin status in different countries reflects milk consumption. In addition, because of its intense yellow colour, riboflavin is widely used as a food colour.

Photolysis of riboflavin leads to the formation of lumiflavin (in alkaline solution), and lumichrome (in acidic or neutral solution), both of which are biologically inactive. Exposure of milk in clear glass bottles to sunlight or fluorescent light (with a peak wavelength of 400–550 nm) can result in the loss of nutritionally important amounts of riboflavin. Lumiflavin and lumichrome catalyse oxidation of lipids (to peroxides) and methionine (to methional), resulting in the development of an unpleasant flavour—the so-called 'sunlight' flavour. Light of 400–550 nm can penetrate both clear glass bottles and cardboard cartons; cartons for milk include a protective lining that is opaque at this wavelength.

11.7.1   Absorption and metabolism of riboflavin

Apart from milk and eggs, which contain relatively large amounts of free riboflavin, most of the vitamin in foods is as flavin coenzymes bound to enzymes, which are released when the protein is hydrolysed. Intestinal phosphatases then hydrolyse the coenzymes to riboflavin, which is absorbed in the upper small intestine. Much of the absorbed riboflavin is phosphorylated in the intestinal mucosa by flavokinase and enters the bloodstream as riboflavin phosphate.

Tissues contain very little free riboflavin; most is present as FAD and riboflavin phosphate bound to enzymes. Uptake into tissues is by passive carrier-mediated transport of free riboflavin, followed by metabolic trapping (Section 3.2.2.2) by phosphorylation to riboflavin phosphate, then onward metabolism to FAD.

FAD that is not protein bound is rapidly hydrolysed to riboflavin phosphate by nucleo-tide pyrophosphatase; unbound riboflavin phosphate is hydrolysed to riboflavin by non-specific phosphatases, and free riboflavin diffuses out of tissues into the bloodstream.

Riboflavin and riboflavin phosphate that are not bound to plasma proteins are filtered at the glomerulus. Renal tubular reabsorption of riboflavin is saturated at normal plasma concentrations. There is also active tubular secretion of the vitamin; urinary excretion of riboflavin after high doses can be twofold to threefold greater than the glomerular filtra-tion rate.

There is no significant storage of riboflavin; any surplus intake is excreted rapidly; thus, once metabolic requirements have been met, urinary excretion of riboflavin and its metabolites reflects intake until intestinal absorption is saturated. In depleted animals, the maximum growth response is achieved with intakes that give about 75% saturation of tissues, and the intake to achieve tissue saturation is that at which there is quantitative excretion of the vitamin.

There is very efficient conservation of tissue riboflavin in deficiency, with only a four-fold difference between the minimum liver concentration of flavins in deficiency and the level at which saturation occurs. In deficiency, almost the only loss of riboflavin from tis-sues will be the small amount that is covalently bound to enzymes; the non-covalently bound coenzymes are recycled when proteins are catabolised.

11.7.2   Metabolic functions of the flavin coenzymes

The metabolic function of the flavin coenzymes is as electron carriers in a wide variety of oxidation and reduction reactions central to all metabolic processes (Figure 2.19), includ-ing the mitochondrial electron transport chain (Section 3.3.3.1.2), and key enzymes in fatty acid (Section 5.5.2) and amino acid (Section 9.3.1.1) oxidation, and the citric acid cycle (Section 5.4.4.1). Flavin coenzymes remain bound to the enzyme throughout the catalytic cycle. The majority of flavoproteins have FAD as the prosthetic group; some have both FAD and riboflavin phosphate, and some have other prosthetic groups as well.

Reoxidation of the reduced flavin in oxygenases and mixed-function oxidases pro-ceeds by way of formation of the flavin radical and flavin hydroperoxide, with the interme-diate generation of superoxide and perhydroxyl radicals and hydrogen peroxide. Because of this, flavin oxidases make a significant contribution to the total oxidative stress in the body (Section 6.5.2.1).

11.7.3   Riboflavin deficiency

Although riboflavin is involved in all areas of metabolism and deficiency is widespread on a global scale, deficiency is not fatal. There seem to be two reasons for this:

1. Although deficiency is common, the vitamin is widespread in foods, and most diets will provide minimally adequate amounts to permit maintenance of central meta-bolic pathways.
2. There is efficient re-utilisation of the riboflavin that is released by the turnover of flavoproteins; a very small amount is catabolised or excreted.

Riboflavin deficiency is characterised by lesions of the margin of the lips (cheilosis) and corners of the mouth (angular stomatitis), a painful desquamation of the tongue, making it red, dry, and atrophic (magenta tongue), and a sebhorreic dermatitis, with filiform excrescences.

The main metabolic effect of riboflavin deficiency is on lipid metabolism. Riboflavin deficient animals have a lower metabolic rate than controls, and require a 15%–20% higher food intake to maintain body weight. Feeding a high fat diet leads to more marked impairment of growth, and a higher requirement for riboflavin to restore growth.

11.7.3.1 Resistance to malaria in riboflavin deficiency

A number of studies have noted that in areas where malaria is endemic, riboflavin deficient people are relatively resistant and have a lower parasite burden than adequately nourished people. The biochemical basis of this resistance to malaria in riboflavin deficiency is not known, but two possible mechanisms have been proposed:

1. Malarial parasites may have a particularly high requirement for riboflavin—a number of flavin analogues have anti-malarial action.
2. As a result of impaired antioxidant activity in erythrocytes, there may be increased fragility of erythrocyte membranes. As in sickle cell trait, which also protects against malaria, this may result in exposure of the parasites to the host's immune system at a vulnerable stage in their development, resulting in the production of protective antibodies.

11.7.4 Riboflavin requirements

Glutathione reductase is especially sensitive to riboflavin depletion, and the usual way of assessing riboflavin status is by measurement of the activation of red blood cell glutathione reductase by FAD added *in vitro* (Section 2.7.3). An activation coefficient >1.7 indicates deficiency. Normal values of the activation coefficient are seen in subjects whose habitual intake of riboflavin is between 1.2 and 1.5 mg/d.

11.8 Niacin

Niacin is not strictly a vitamin, since it can be synthesised in the body from the essential amino acid tryptophan. Indeed, it is only when tryptophan metabolism is deranged that dietary preformed niacin becomes important. Nevertheless, niacin was discovered as a nutrient during studies of the deficiency disease pellagra, associated with diets based largely on maize, which was a major public health problem in the southern United States throughout the first half of the 20th century and continued to be a problem in parts of India and sub-Saharan Africa until the 1990s.

Two compounds, nicotinic acid and nicotinamide, have the biological activity of niacin. When nicotinic acid was discovered to be a curative and preventive factor for pellagra, it was already known as a chemical compound, and was therefore never assigned a number amongst the B vitamins. The name niacin was coined in the United States when it was decided to enrich maize meal with the vitamin to prevent pellagra—it was considered that the name nicotinic acid was not desirable because of the similarity to nicotine. In the United States, the term *niacin* is commonly used to mean specifically nicotinic acid, and nicotinamide is known as niacinamide; elsewhere 'niacin' is used as a generic descriptor for both vitamers. Figure 2.20 shows the structures of nicotinic acid, nicotinamide, and the nicotinamide nucleotide coenzymes, NAD and NADP.

11.8.1   Metabolism of niacin

The nicotinamide ring of NAD can be synthesised in the body from the essential amino acid tryptophan (Figures 11.14 and 11.15). In adults, an amount of tryptophan equivalent to almost all of the dietary intake is metabolised by this pathway and hence is potentially available for NAD synthesis; only a relatively small amount of tryptophan is required for the synthesis of serotonin (Figure 11.15). A number of studies have investigated the

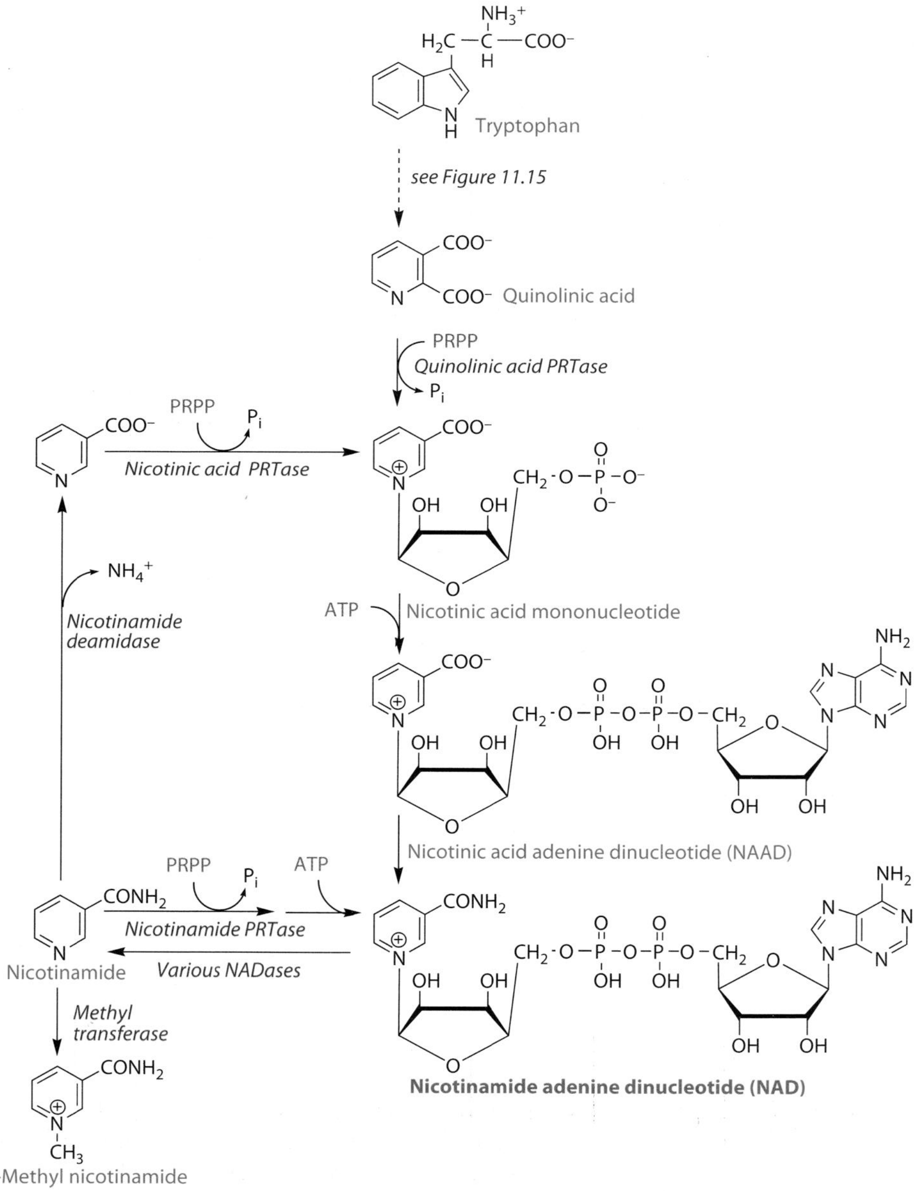

Figure 11.14 The metabolism of the nicotinamide nucleotide coenzymes.

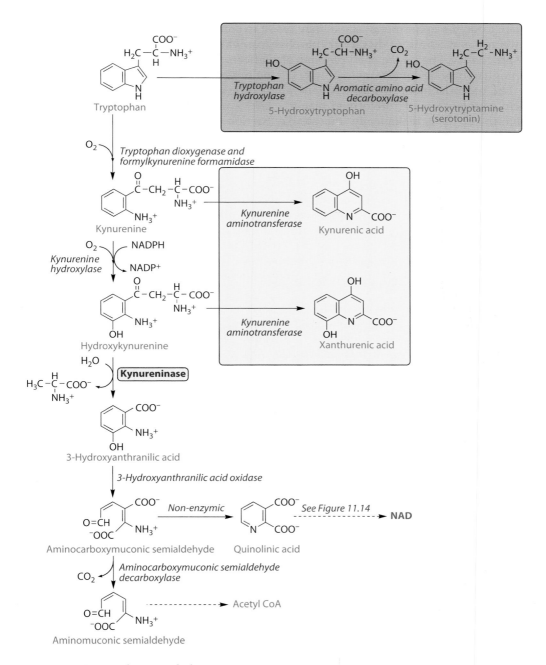

Figure 11.15 Tryptophan metabolism.

equivalence of dietary tryptophan and preformed niacin as precursors of the nicotinamide nucleotides, generally by determining the excretion of niacin metabolites in response to test doses of the precursors, in subjects maintained on deficient diets. There is a considerable variation between subjects in the response to tryptophan and niacin, and to allow for this, it is generally assumed that 60 mg of tryptophan is equivalent to 1 mg of preformed niacin. Changes in hormonal status may result in considerable changes in this ratio, with between 7 and 30 mg of dietary tryptophan equivalent to 1 mg of preformed niacin in late pregnancy. The intake of tryptophan also affects the ratio, and at low intakes, 1 mg of tryptophan may be equivalent to only 1/125 mg preformed niacin.

The niacin content of foods is generally expressed as mg niacin equivalents; 1 mg niacin equivalent = mg preformed niacin + 1/60 × mg tryptophan. Because most of the niacin in cereals is biologically unavailable (Section 11.8.1.1), it is conventional to ignore preformed niacin in cereal products.

11.8.1.1   *Unavailable niacin in cereals*

Chemical analysis reveals niacin in cereals (largely in the bran), but this is biologically unavailable because it is bound as niacytin–nicotinoyl esters to polysaccharides, polypeptides, and glycopeptides. Treatment of cereals with alkali (for example, soaking overnight in calcium hydroxide solution, the traditional method for the preparation of tortillas in Mexico) releases much of the nicotinic acid. This may explain why pellagra has always been rare in Mexico, despite the fact that maize is the dietary staple. Up to 10% of the niacin in niacytin may be biologically available as a result of hydrolysis by gastric acid.

11.8.1.2   *Absorption and metabolism of niacin*

Niacin is present in tissues, and therefore in foods, mainly as the nicotinamide nucleotide coenzymes. The *post mortem* hydrolysis of NAD(P) is extremely rapid in animal tissues, so much of the niacin in meat (a major dietary source of the vitamin) is free nicotinamide. Both nicotinic acid and nicotinamide are absorbed from the small intestine by a sodium-dependent saturable process.

11.8.1.3   *Metabolism of the nicotinamide nucleotide coenzymes*

The nicotinamide nucleotide coenzymes can be synthesised from either of the niacin vitamers and from quinolinic acid, an intermediate in the metabolism of tryptophan (Figure 11.14). In the liver, oxidation of tryptophan results in a considerably greater synthesis of NAD than is required, and this is catabolised to release nicotinic acid and nicotinamide, which are taken up and used by other tissues for synthesis of the coenzymes.

The catabolism of NAD^+ is catalysed by four enzymes:

1. NAD glycohydrolase, which releases nicotinamide and ADP-ribose.
2. NAD pyrophosphatase, which releases nicotinamide mononucleotide. This can either be hydrolysed by NAD glycohydrolase to release nicotinamide or can be a re-utilised to form NAD.
3. ADP-ribosyltransferases.
4. Poly(ADP-ribose) polymerase.

The activation of ADP-ribosyltransferase and poly(ADP-ribose) polymerase by toxins that cause DNA damage may result in considerable depletion of intracellular NAD(P), and may indeed provide a suicide mechanism to ensure that cells that have suffered very severe damage die, as a result of NAD(P) depletion and hence severely impaired ATP synthesis. The administration of DNA-breaking carcinogens to experimental animals results in the excretion of large amounts of nicotinamide metabolites, and depletion of tissue NAD(P). Chronic exposure to such carcinogens and mycotoxins may be a contributory factor in the aetiology of pellagra when dietary intakes of tryptophan and niacin are marginal.

Under normal conditions, there is little or no urinary excretion of either nicotinamide or nicotinic acid. This is because both vitamers are actively reabsorbed from the glomerular filtrate. It is only when the concentration is so high that the transporter is saturated that there is any significant excretion. The main urinary metabolites of niacin are N^1-methyl nicotinamide and its onward metabolic products, methyl pyridone-2-carboxamide and methyl pyridone-4-carboxamide.

11.8.2   The synthesis of nicotinamide nucleotides from tryptophan

Under normal conditions, almost all of the dietary intake of tryptophan, apart from the small amounts that are used for net new protein synthesis and synthesis of 5-hydroxytryptophan, is metabolised by the oxidative pathway (Figure 11.15) and hence is potentially available for NAD synthesis.

The synthesis of NAD from tryptophan involves the non-enzymic cyclisation of aminocarboxymuconic semialdehyde to quinolinic acid. The alternative metabolic fate of aminocarboxymuconic semialdehyde is decarboxylation, catalysed by aminocarboxymuconic semialdehyde decarboxylase, leading to acetyl CoA and total oxidation. There is thus competition between an enzyme-catalysed reaction, which has hyperbolic, saturable kinetics (Section 2.3.3), and a non-enzymic reaction with linear kinetics. At low rates of flux through the pathway, most metabolism will be by way of the enzyme-catalysed pathway, leading to oxidation. As the rate of formation of aminocarboxymuconic semialdehyde increases and picolinate carboxylase nears saturation, an increasing proportion will be available to undergo cyclisation to quinolinic acid, and onward metabolism to NAD. There is thus not a simple stoichiometric relationship between tryptophan and niacin, and the equivalence of the coenzyme precursors will depend on the amount of tryptophan to be metabolised and the rate of its metabolism.

The activities of three enzymes, tryptophan dioxygenase, kynurenine hydroxylase, and kynureninase, affect the rate of formation of aminocarboxymuconic semialdehyde, as may the rate of uptake of tryptophan into the liver.

Tryptophan dioxygenase is the enzyme that controls the entry of tryptophan into the oxidative pathway. It has a short half-life (of the order of 2 h) and is subject to regulation by three mechanisms:

1. Hormonal induction in response to glucocorticoid hormones and glucagon. As discussed in Section 9.1.2.3, induction of tryptophan dioxygenase leads to depletion of an essential amino acid, leaving surplus amino acids that can no longer be used for protein synthesis, that are now available for gluconeogenesis (Section 5.7).
2. Feedback inhibition and repression by NAD(P).
3. Stabilisation by its haem cofactor.

The activities of both kynurenine hydroxylase and kynureninase are only slightly higher than that of tryptophan dioxygenase, and increased tryptophan dioxygenase activity in response to glucocorticoid action is accompanied by increased accumulation and excretion of kynurenine, hydroxykynurenine and their transamination products, kynurenic and xanthurenic acids. Impairment of the activity of either enzyme may impair the onward metabolism of kynurenine, and so reduce the accumulation of aminocarboxymuconic semialdehyde, and hence the synthesis of NAD.

Kynurenine hydroxylase is FAD dependent, and the activity of kynurenine hydroxylase in the liver of riboflavin deficient rats is only 30%–50% of that in control animals.

Riboflavin deficiency (Section 11.7.3) may thus be a contributory factor in the aetiology of pellagra when intakes of tryptophan and niacin are marginal.

Kynureninase is a pyridoxal phosphate (vitamin B_6)-dependent enzyme, and its activity is extremely sensitive to vitamin B_6 depletion. Indeed, the ability to metabolise a test dose of tryptophan has been used to assess vitamin B_6 nutritional status (Section 11.9.5.1). Deficiency of vitamin B_6 will lead to severe impairment of NAD synthesis from tryptophan. Kynureninase is also inhibited by oestrogen metabolites.

11.8.3   *Metabolic functions of niacin*

The best defined role of niacin is in oxidation and reduction reactions, as the functional nicotinamide part of the coenzymes NAD and NADP (Section 2.2.4.1.3). In general, NAD^+ is involved as an electron acceptor in energy-yielding metabolism, being oxidised by the mitochondrial electron transport chain (Section 3.3.1.2), whilst the major coenzyme for reductive synthetic reactions is NADPH. An exception to this general rule is the pentose phosphate pathway of glucose metabolism (Section 5.4.2), which results in the reduction of $NADP^+$ to NADPH, and is the source of half the NADPH required for fatty acid synthesis (Section 5.6.1).

11.8.3.1   *The role of NAD in ADP-ribosylation*

In addition to its coenzyme role, NAD^+ is the source of ADP-ribose for:

- ADP-ribosyltransferases, which modify the activities of enzymes by catalysing reversible ADP-ribosylation.
- Poly(ADP-ribose) polymerase, which is activated by binding to breakage points in DNA, and activates the DNA repair mechanism.

11.8.4   *Pellagra—a disease of tryptophan and niacin deficiency*

Pellagra became common in Europe when maize was introduced from the New World as a convenient high-yielding dietary staple, and by the late 19th century, it was widespread throughout southern Europe, north and south Africa, and the southern United States. The proteins of maize are particularly lacking in tryptophan, and as with other cereals, little or none of the preformed niacin is biologically available (Section 11.8.1.1).

Pellagra is characterised by a photosensitive dermatitis, like severe sunburn, affecting all parts of the skin that are exposed to sunlight. Similar skin lesions may also occur in areas not exposed to sunlight, but subject to pressure, such as the knees, elbows, wrists, and ankles. Advanced pellagra is also accompanied by dementia (more correctly a depressive psychosis), and there may be diarrhoea. Untreated pellagra is fatal. The depressive psychosis is due to reduced synthesis of the neurotransmitter serotonin (Figure 5.15) as a result of lack of the essential amino acid tryptophan, and not to a deficiency of niacin *per se*.

Although the nutritional aetiology of pellagra is well established, and either tryptophan or niacin will prevent or cure the disease, additional factors, including deficiency of riboflavin (and hence impaired activity of kynurenine hydroxylase) or vitamin B_6 (and hence impaired activity of kynureninase), may be important when intakes of tryptophan and niacin are only marginally adequate.

Of the 87,000 deaths caused by pellagra in the United States during the first half of the 20th century, twice as many women as men died. Reports of individual outbreaks of pellagra, both in the United States, and more recently elsewhere, show a similar sex ratio. This may well be the result of inhibition of kynureninase, and impairment of the activity of kynurenine hydroxylase by oestrogen metabolites, and hence reduced synthesis of NAD from tryptophan.

11.8.5   Niacin Requirements

Although the nicotinamide nucleotide coenzymes function in a large number of oxidation and reduction reactions, this cannot be exploited as a means of assessing niacin status because the coenzymes are not tightly bound to their apo-enzymes, but act as cosubstrates of the reactions, binding to and leaving the enzyme as the reaction proceeds. No specific metabolic lesions associated with NAD(P) depletion have been identified.

The two methods of assessing niacin nutritional status are measurement of the ratio of NAD/NADP in red blood cells and the urinary excretion of niacin metabolites, neither of which is wholly satisfactory.

On the basis of depletion/repletion studies in which the urinary excretion of niacin metabolites was measured after feeding tryptophan or preformed niacin, the average requirement for niacin is 1.3 mg niacin equivalents/MJ energy expenditure, and reference intakes are based on 1.6 mg/MJ. Average intakes of tryptophan in Western diets will more than meet requirements without the need for a dietary source of preformed niacin.

11.8.5.1   Niacin toxicity

Nicotinic acid has been used to lower blood triacylglycerol and cholesterol in patients with hyperlipidaemia. However, relatively large amounts are required (of the order of 1–3 g/day, compared with reference intakes of 18–20 mg/day). At this level of intake, nicotinic acid causes dilatation of blood vessels and flushing, with skin irritation, itching, and a burning sensation. This effect wears off after a few days.

High intakes of both nicotinic acid and nicotinamide, in excess of 1 g/day, also cause liver damage, and prolonged use can result in liver failure. This is especially a problem with sustained release preparations of niacin, which permits a high blood level to be maintained for a relatively long time.

11.9   Vitamin B_6

Apart from a single outbreak in the 1950s, due to overheated infant milk formula, vitamin B_6 deficiency is unknown except under experimental conditions. Nevertheless, there is a considerable body of evidence that marginal status, and biochemical deficiency, may be relatively widespread.

The generic descriptor vitamin B_6 includes six vitamers (Figure 11.16): the alcohol pyridoxine, the aldehyde pyridoxal, the amine pyridoxamine, and their 5′-phosphates. The vitamers are metabolically interconvertible and have equal biological activity; they are all converted in the body to the metabolically active form, pyridoxal phosphate. 4-Pyridoxic acid is a biologically inactive end product of vitamin B_6 metabolism.

When foods are heated, pyridoxal and pyridoxal phosphate can react with the ε-amino groups of lysine to form a Schiff base (aldimine). This renders both the vitamin B_6 and the lysine biologically unavailable (Section 9.1.3.2); more importantly, the pyridoxyl lysine released during digestion is absorbed and has antivitamin B_6 antimetabolite activity.

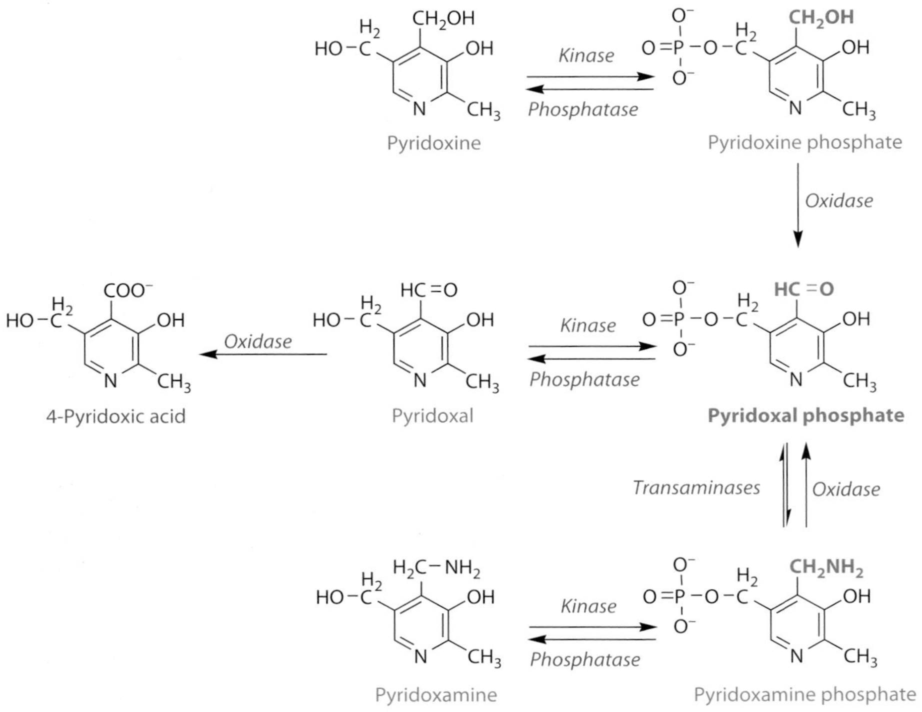

Figure 11.16 Interconversion of the vitamin B$_6$ vitamers.

11.9.1 Absorption and metabolism of vitamin B$_6$

The phosphorylated vitamers are hydrolysed by alkaline phosphatase in the intestinal mucosa; the dephosphorylated vitamers absorbed rapidly by diffusion, then phosphorylated, and pyridoxine and pyridoxamine phosphates are oxidised to pyridoxal phosphate. Much of the ingested vitamin is released into the portal circulation as pyridoxal, after dephosphorylation at the serosal surface of the mucosal cells.

Most of the absorbed vitamin enters the liver by diffusion, followed by metabolic trapping (Section 3.2.2.2) as the phosphate. Pyridoxal phosphate and some pyridoxal are exported from the liver bound to albumin. Free pyridoxal remaining in the liver is rapidly oxidised to 4-pyridoxic acid and excreted.

Extrahepatic tissues take up both pyridoxal and pyridoxal phosphate from the plasma. The phosphate is hydrolysed to pyridoxal, which can cross cell membranes, by extracellular alkaline phosphatase, then trapped intracellularly by phosphorylation.

Some 80% of the body's total vitamin B$_6$ is pyridoxal phosphate in muscle, mostly associated with glycogen phosphorylase (Section 5.6.3.1). This does not function as a reserve of the vitamin and is not released from muscle in times of deficiency; it is released into the circulation (as pyridoxal) in starvation, when glycogen reserves are exhausted and there is less requirement for phosphorylase activity. Under these conditions, it is available for redistribution to other tissues, and especially liver and kidney, to meet the increased requirement for transamination of amino acids (Section 9.3.1.2) for gluconeogenesis (Section 5.7).

11.9.2 Metabolic functions of vitamin B₆

Pyridoxal phosphate is a coenzyme in three main areas of metabolism:

1. Various reactions of amino acids, especially transamination, in which it functions as the intermediate carrier of the amino group (Section 9.3.1.2), and decarboxylation to form amines.
2. As the cofactor of glycogen phosphorylase (Section 56.3.1) in muscle and liver, where it is the phosphate group that is catalytically important.
3. In the regulation of the action of steroid hormones. Pyridoxal phosphate acts to remove the hormone-receptor complex from DNA binding, and so terminate the action of the hormones (Section 10.4).

11.9.3 Vitamin B₆ deficiency

Deficiency of vitamin B₆ severe enough to lead to clinical signs is extremely rare, and clear deficiency has only been reported in one outbreak, during the 1950s, when babies were fed on a milk preparation that had been severely overheated during manufacture. Many of the affected infants suffered convulsions, which ceased rapidly following the administration of vitamin B₆.

Moderate vitamin B₆ deficiency results in a number of abnormalities of amino acid metabolism and especially of tryptophan (Section 11.8.2) and methionine (Section 11.9.5.2). In experimental animals, it also leads to increased sensitivity of target tissues to steroid hormone action. This may be important in the development of hormone dependent cancer of the breast, uterus, and prostate, and vitamin B₆ status may therefore affect the prognosis.

11.9.4 Vitamin B₆ requirements

Most studies of vitamin B₆ requirements have followed the development of abnormalities of tryptophan (Section 11.8.2) and methionine (Section 11.9.5.2) metabolism during depletion, and normalisation during repletion with graded intakes of the vitamin. Adults maintained on vitamin B₆ deficient diets develop abnormalities of tryptophan and methionine metabolism faster, and their blood vitamin B₆ falls more rapidly, when their protein intake is relatively high (80–160 g/d in various studies) than on low protein intakes (30–50 g/d). Similarly, during repletion of deficient subjects, tryptophan and methionine metabolism and blood vitamin B₆ are normalised faster at low than at high levels of protein intake. From such studies, the average requirement for vitamin B₆ is estimated to be 13 μg/g dietary protein, and reference intakes are based on 15–16 μg/g dietary protein.

11.9.5 Assessment of vitamin B₆ status

Fasting plasma total vitamin B₆, or more specifically pyridoxal phosphate, is widely used as an index of vitamin B₆ nutritional status. Urinary excretion of 4-pyridoxic acid is also used, but it reflects recent intake of the vitamin rather than underlying nutritional status.

The most widely used method of assessing vitamin B₆ status is by the activation of erythrocyte transaminases by pyridoxal phosphate added *in vitro* (Section 2.7.3). The ability to metabolise test doses of tryptophan (Section 11.9.5.1) or methionine (Section 11.9.5.2) have also been used.

11.9.5.1   The tryptophan load test

The tryptophan load test for vitamin B$_6$ nutritional status (the ability to metabolise a test dose of tryptophan) is one of the oldest metabolic tests for functional vitamin nutritional status. It was developed as a result of observation of the excretion of an abnormal coloured compound, later identified as the tryptophan metabolite xanthurenic acid, in the urine of deficient animals.

Kynureninase (Figure 11.15) is a pyridoxal phosphate-dependent enzyme, and its activity falls markedly in vitamin B$_6$ deficiency, at least partly because it undergoes a slow mechanism-dependent inactivation that leaves catalytically inactive pyridoxamine phosphate at the active site. The enzyme can only be reactivated if there is an adequate supply of pyridoxal phosphate. This means that in vitamin B$_6$ deficiency, there is a considerable accumulation of both hydroxykynurenine and kynurenine, sufficient to permit greater metabolic flux than usual through kynurenine transaminase, resulting in increased formation of kynurenic and xanthurenic acids.

Xanthurenic and kynurenic acids, and kynurenine and hydroxykynurenine, are easy to measure in urine; thus, the tryptophan load test (the ability to metabolise a test dose of 2–5 g of tryptophan) has been widely adopted as a convenient and sensitive index of vitamin B$_6$ nutritional status. However, because glucocorticoid hormones increase tryptophan dioxygenase activity, abnormal results of the tryptophan load test must be regarded with caution and cannot necessarily be interpreted as indicating vitamin B$_6$ deficiency. Increased entry of tryptophan into the pathway will overwhelm the capacity of kynureninase, leading to increased formation of xanthurenic and kynurenic acids. Similarly, oestrogen metabolites inhibit kynureninase and reduce the activity of kynurenine hydroxylase, leading to results that have been misinterpreted as vitamin B$_6$ deficiency.

11.9.5.2   The methionine load test

The metabolism of methionine (Figure 6.22) includes two pyridoxal phosphate dependent steps: cystathionine synthetase and cystathionase. Cystathionase activity falls markedly in vitamin B$_6$ deficiency, and as a result, there is an increase in the urinary excretion of homocysteine and cystathionine, especially after a loading dose of methionine. However, homocysteine metabolism is more affected by folate status than vitamin B$_6$ status (Section 11.11.4), and like the tryptophan load test, the methionine load test is probably not a reliable index of vitamin B$_6$ status in field studies.

11.9.6   Non-nutritional uses of vitamin B$_6$

A number of studies have suggested that oral contraceptives cause vitamin B$_6$ deficiency. As a result of this, supplements of vitamin B$_6$ of between 50 and 100 mg/day, and sometimes higher, have been used to overcome the side-effects of oral contraceptives. Similar supplements have also been recommended for the treatment of the premenstrual syndrome, although there is little evidence of efficacy from placebo-controlled trials.

All of the studies that suggested that oral contraceptives cause vitamin B$_6$ deficiency used the tryptophan load test (Section 11.9.5.1). When other biochemical markers of status were also assessed, they were not affected by oral contraceptive use. Furthermore, most of these studies were performed using the now obsolete high-dose contraceptive pills. Oral contraceptives do not cause vitamin B_6 deficiency. The problem is that oestrogen metabolites inhibit kynureninase and reduce the activity of kynurenine hydroxylase. This results in the excretion of abnormal amounts of tryptophan metabolites, similar to what is seen in vitamin B_6 deficiency, but for a quite different reason.

Doses of 50–200 mg of vitamin B_6/day have an anti-emetic effect, and the vitamin has been widely used, alone or in conjunction with other anti-emetics, to minimise the nausea associated with radiotherapy and to treat pregnancy sickness. There is no evidence that vitamin B_6 has any beneficial effect in pregnancy sickness, nor that women who suffer from morning sickness have lower vitamin B_6 nutritional status than other pregnant women.

11.9.6.1   *Vitamin B_6 toxicity*

In experimental animals, doses of vitamin B_6 of 50 mg/kg body weight cause histological damage to dorsal nerve roots, and doses of 200 mg/kg body weight lead to the development of signs of peripheral neuropathy, with ataxia, muscle weakness, and loss of balance. Sensory neuropathy has been reported in seven patients taking 2–7 g of pyridoxine/day. Although there was some residual damage, withdrawal of these extremely high doses resulted in a considerable recovery of sensory nerve function. There is some evidence that intakes as low as 25–50 mg/day may also cause nerve damage.

11.10   *Vitamin B_{12}*

Dietary deficiency of vitamin B_{12} occurs only in strict vegans; the vitamin is found almost exclusively in animal foods. However, functional deficiency (pernicious anaemia, with spinal cord degeneration), as a result of impaired absorption, is relatively common, especially in elderly people with atrophic gastritis. The absorption of vitamin B_{12} is discussed in Section 4.5.2.1.

The structure of vitamin B_{12} is shown in Figure 11.17. The term *corrinoid* is used as a generic descriptor for cobalt-containing compounds of this general structure, which, depending on the substituents in the pyrrole rings, may or may not have vitamin activity. Some of the corrinoids that are growth factors for microorganisms not only have no vitamin B_{12} activity, but may be antimetabolites of the vitamin.

Vitamin B_{12} is found only in foods of animal origin. There are no plant sources of this vitamin, although it is also formed by some bacteria. This means that strict vegetarians (vegans), who eat no foods of animal origin, are at risk of dietary vitamin B_{12} deficiency. Preparations of vitamin B_{12} made by bacterial fermentation that are ethically acceptable to vegans are readily available.

There are claims that some plants (especially algae) contain vitamin B_{12}. This seems to be incorrect. The problem is that the officially recognised, and legally required, method of determining vitamin B_{12} in food analysis depends on the growth of *Lactobacillus* spp. for which vitamin B_{12} is an essential growth factor. However, these organisms can also use some corrinoids that have no vitamin activity. Therefore, analysis reveals the presence of something that appears to be vitamin B_{12} but in fact is not the active vitamin and is useless in human nutrition. Where biologically active vitamin B_{12} has been identified in algae, it is almost certainly the result of bacterial contamination of the lakes from which the algae were harvested.

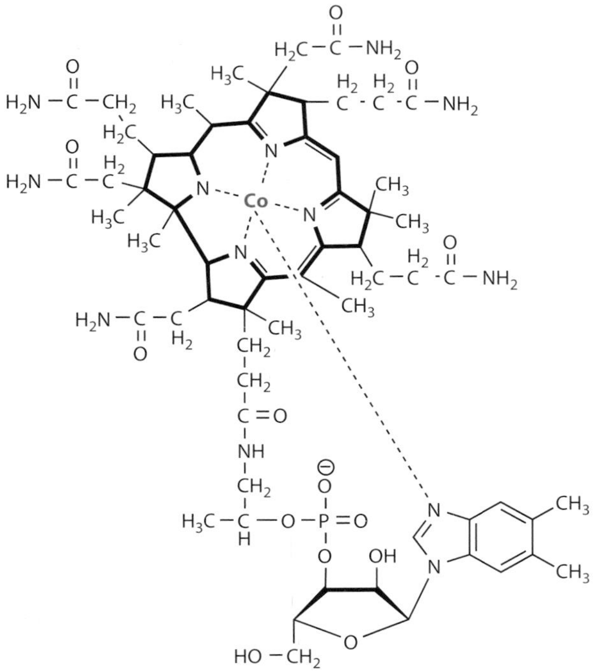

Figure 11.17 Vitamin B$_{12}$. Four coordination sites on the central cobalt atom are chelated by the nitrogen atoms of the corrin ring, and one by the nitrogen of the dimethylbenzimidazole nucleotide. The sixth coordination site may be occupied by: CN (cyanocobalamin), OH (hydroxocobalamin), H$_2$O (aquocobalamin, –CH$_3$ (methyl cobalamin), or 5'-deoxyadenosine (adenosylcobalamin).

11.10.1   Metabolic functions of vitamin B$_{12}$

There are two vitamin B$_{12}$-dependent enzymes in human tissues: methylmalonyl CoA mutase, and methionine synthetase. Methionine synthetase is discussed in Sections 6.6 and 11.11.3.2.

Methylmalonyl CoA is formed as an intermediate in the catabolism of valine and by the carboxylation of propionyl CoA arising in the catabolism of isoleucine, cholesterol, and (rare) fatty acids with an odd number of carbon atoms. It undergoes vitamin B$_{12}$-dependent rearrangement to succinyl CoA, catalysed by methylmalonyl CoA mutase (Figure 11.18). The activity of this enzyme is greatly reduced in vitamin B$_{12}$ deficiency, leading to an accumulation of methylmalonyl CoA, most of which is hydrolysed to yield methylmalonic acid, which is excreted in the urine; urinary excretion of methylmalonic acid provides a means of assessing vitamin B$_{12}$ nutritional status and monitoring therapy in patients with pernicious anaemia (Section 11.10.2).

11.10.2   Vitamin B$_{12}$ deficiency: pernicious anaemia

Vitamin B$_{12}$ deficiency causes pernicious anaemia; the release into the bloodstream of immature precursors of red blood cells (megaloblastic anaemia) because deficiency impairs the metabolism of folate and causes functional folate deficiency (Sections 11.11.3.2

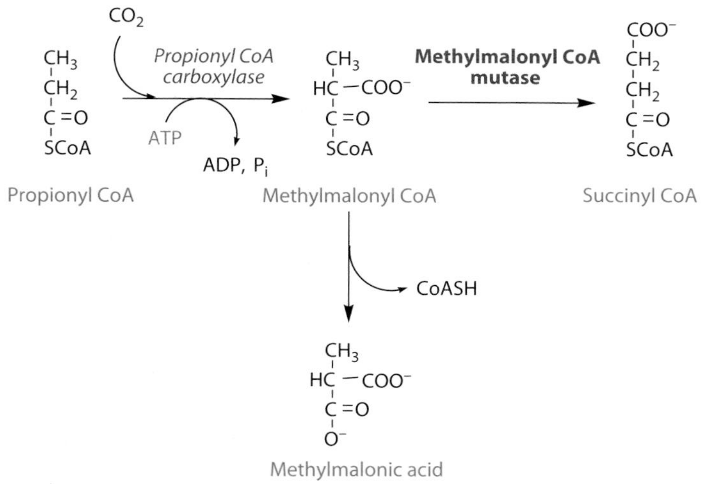

Figure 11.18 The reaction of methylmalonyl CoA mutase and formation of methylmalonic acid in vitamin B_{12} deficiency.

and 11.11.4). This disrupts the normal proliferation of red blood cells, causing immature precursors to be released into the circulation.

The other clinical feature of vitamin B_{12} deficiency, which is only rarely seen in folate deficiency, is degeneration of the spinal cord—hence the name 'pernicious' for the anaemia of vitamin B_{12} deficiency. The spinal cord degeneration is due to a failure of the methylation of one arginine residue in myelin basic protein, and occurs in about one third of people with megaloblastic anaemia due to vitamin B_{12} deficiency, and in about one third of deficient people who do not show signs of anaemia. The failure of arginine methylation in the central nervous system is due to a lack of methionine (Figure 6.22). Other tissues are protected in vitamin B_{12} deficiency because there is an alternative enzyme for the methylation of homo-cysteine to methionine that is not vitamin B_{12}-dependent and uses betaine as the methyl donor rather than methyl-tetrahydrofolate. This enzyme is absent from the nervous system.

The usual cause of pernicious anaemia is failure of the absorption of vitamin B_{12} (Section 4.5.2.1) rather than dietary deficiency. Failure of intrinsic factor secretion is commonly due to autoimmune disease; 90% of patients with pernicious anaemia have antibodies to the gastric parietal cells. Similar autoantibodies are found in 30% of the relatives of pernicious anaemia patients, suggesting that there is a genetic basis for the condition.

About 70% of patients also have anti-intrinsic factor antibodies in plasma, saliva, and gastric juice. Although the oral administration of partially purified preparations of intrinsic factor will restore the absorption of vitamin B_{12} in many patients with pernicious anaemia, this can result eventually in the production of anti-intrinsic factor antibodies; parenteral administration of vitamin B_{12} is the preferred means of treatment. For patients who secrete anti-intrinsic factor antibodies in the saliva or gastric juice, oral intrinsic factor will be useless.

11.10.3 Vitamin B_{12} requirements

The total body pool of vitamin B_{12} is of the order of 2.5 mg, with a minimum desirable body pool of about 1 mg. The daily loss is about 0.1% of the body pool in subjects with normal enterohepatic circulation of the vitamin (Section 4.5.2.1); on this basis, requirements are about 1–2.5 μg/day, and reference intakes for adults range between 1.4 and 2.0 μg.

11.10.4   *Assessment of vitamin B_{12} status*

A number of radioligand binding assays have been developed for measurement of plasma concentrations of vitamin B_{12}. They may give falsely high values if the binding protein is cobalophilin, which binds a number of metabolically inactive corrinoids; more precise determination of true vitamin B_{12} comes from assays in which the binding protein is purified intrinsic factor.

A serum concentration of vitamin B_{12} below 110 pmol/L is associated with megaloblastic bone marrow, incipient anaemia, and myelin damage. Below 150 pmol/L, there are early bone marrow changes, abnormalities of the dUMP suppression test (Section 11.11.6.2), and methylmalonic aciduria after a valine load (Section 11.10.1).

11.10.4.1   *The Schilling test for vitamin B_{12} absorption*

The absorption of vitamin B_{12} can be determined by the Schilling test. An oral dose of [^{57}Co] or [^{58}Co]vitamin B_{12} is given together with a parenteral flushing dose of 1 mg of non-radioactive vitamin to saturate body reserves and the urinary excretion of radioactivity is followed as an index of absorption of the oral material. Normal subjects excrete 16%–45% of the radioactivity over 24 h, whilst patients lacking intrinsic factor excrete less than 5%.

The test can be repeated, giving intrinsic factor orally together with the radioactive vitamin B_{12}; if the impaired absorption was due to a simple lack of intrinsic factor and not to anti-intrinsic factor antibodies in saliva or gastric juice, then a normal amount of the radioactive material should be absorbed and excreted.

11.11   *Folic acid*

Folate functions in the transfer of one-carbon fragments in a wide variety of biosynthetic and catabolic reactions; it is therefore metabolically related to vitamin B_{12}. Deficiency of either vitamin has similar clinical effects, and the haematological effects of vitamin B_{12} deficiency are exerted by effects on folate metabolism.

Although folate is widely distributed in foods, dietary deficiency is not uncommon, and a number of commonly used drugs can cause folate depletion. More importantly, there is good evidence that intakes of folate considerably higher than normal dietary levels reduce the risk of neural tube defects, and pregnant women are recommended to take supplements. There is also evidence that high intakes of folate may also be effective in reducing plasma homocysteine in subjects genetically at risk of hyperhomocystinaemia (some 10%–20% of the population), and hence reducing the risk of ischaemic heart disease and stroke (Section 6.6). High intakes of folate are also associated with a lower incidence of colorectal cancer, but may speed the development of cancerous lesions from benign colorectal polyps.

11.11.1   *Folate vitamers and dietary equivalence*

The structure of folic acid (pteroyl glutamate) is shown in Figure 11.19. The folate co-enzymes may have up to 7 additional glutamate residues linked by γ-peptide bonds, forming pteroyldiglutamate (PteGlu$_2$), pteroyltriglutamate (PteGlu$_3$), etc., collectively known as folate or pteroyl polyglutamate conjugates (PteGlu$_n$).

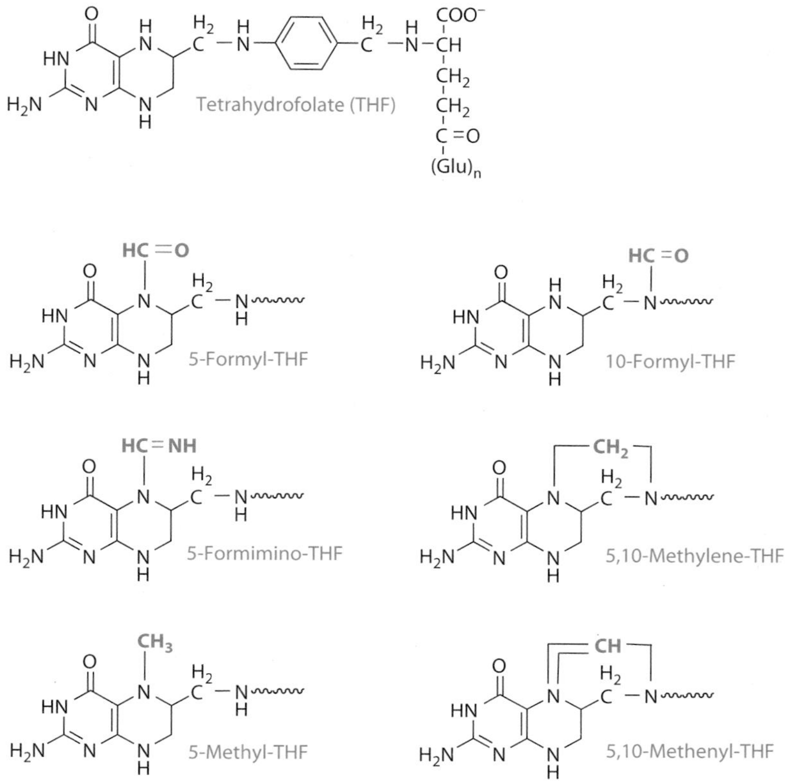

Figure 11.19 Folic acid and the various one-carbon substituted folates.

Folate is the preferred trivial name for pteroylglutamate, although both folate and folic acid may also be used as a generic descriptor to include various polyglutamates. PteGlu$_2$ is sometimes referred to as folic acid diglutamate, PteGlu$_3$ as folic acid triglutamate, etc.

Tetrahydrofolate can carry one-carbon fragments attached to N-5 (formyl, formimino, or methyl groups), N-10 (formyl), or bridging N-5–N-10 (methylene or methenyl groups). 5-Formyl-tetrahydrofolate is more stable to atmospheric oxidation than folate itself and is usually used in pharmaceutical preparations; it is also known as folinic acid, and the synthetic (racemic) compound as leucovorin.

The extent to which the different forms of folate can be absorbed varies; to permit calculation of folate intakes, the dietary folate equivalent has been defined as 1 μg mixed food folates or 0.6 μg free folic acid. On this basis, total dietary folate equivalents = μg food folate + 1.7 × synthetic (free) folic acid.

11.11.2   Absorption and metabolism of folate

About 80% of food folate consists of polyglutamates; a variable amount may be substituted with various one-carbon units or be present as dihydrofolate derivatives. Folate conjugates are hydrolysed in the small intestine by conjugase (pteroylpolyglutamate hydrolase), a zinc-dependent enzyme of the pancreatic juice, bile, and mucosal brush border; zinc deficiency (Section 11.15.2.6) can impair folate absorption. Free folate, released by conjugase action, is absorbed by active transport in the jejunum.

The folate in milk is mainly bound to a specific binding protein; the complex is absorbed intact, mainly in the ileum, by a mechanism that is distinct from the active transport system for the absorption of free folate. The biological availability of folate from milk or of folate from diets to which milk has been added is greater than that of unbound folate.

Much of the dietary folate undergoes methylation and reduction within the intestinal mucosa; thus, what enters the portal bloodstream is largely 5-methyl-tetrahydrofolate (Figure 11.19). Other substituted and unsubstituted folate monoglutamates and dihydrofolate are also absorbed; they are reduced and methylated in the liver, then secreted in the bile. The liver also takes up various folates released by tissues; again these are reduced, methylated, and secreted in the bile.

The total daily enterohepatic circulation of folate is equivalent to about one third of the dietary intake. Despite this, there is very little faecal loss of folate; jejunal absorption of methyl-tetrahydrofolate is a very efficient process, and the faecal excretion of some 200 µg (450 nmol) of folates per day represents synthesis by intestinal flora and does not reflect intake to any significant extent.

Methyl-tetrahydrofolate circulates bound to albumin, and is available for uptake by extra-hepatic tissues. Small amounts of other one-carbon substituted folates also circulate and will also enter cells by the same carrier-mediated process, where they are trapped by formation of polyglutamates, which do not cross cell membranes.

The main circulating folate is methyl-tetrahydrofolate, which is a poor substrate for polyglutamylation; demethylation by the action of methionine synthetase (Figure 6.22) is required for effective metabolic trapping of folate. In vitamin B_{12} deficiency, when methionine synthetase activity is impaired, there is therefore impaired retention of folate in tissues (Section 11.11.3.2).

The catabolism of folate is largely by cleavage of the C-9–N-10 bond, catalysed by carboxypeptidase G. The *p*-aminobenzoic acid moiety is amidated and excreted in the urine as conjugates; pterin is excreted either unchanged or as biologically inactive metabolites.

11.11.3   Metabolic functions of folate

The metabolic role of folate is as a carrier of one-carbon units, both in catabolism and in biosynthetic reactions. These may be carried as formyl, formimino, methyl, methylene, or methylene residues (Figure 11.19). The major sources of these one-carbon units and their major uses as well as the interconversions of the substituted folates are shown in Figure 11.20.

The major point of entry for one-carbon fragments into substituted folates is methylene-tetrahydrofolate, which is formed in the catabolism of glycine, serine, and choline.

Serine hydroxymethyltransferase is a pyridoxal phosphate dependent enzyme that catalyses the cleavage of serine to glycine and methylene-tetrahydrofolate. Whilst folate is required for the catabolism of number of compounds, serine is the most important source of substituted folates for biosynthetic reactions, and the activity of serine hydroxymethyltransferase is regulated by the availability of folate. The reaction is freely reversible, and under appropriate conditions in liver it functions to form serine from glycine, as a substrate for gluconeogenesis (Section 5.7).

The catabolism of histidine leads to the formation of formiminoglutamate (Section 11.11.6.1). The formimino group is transferred onto tetrahydrofolate to form formimino-tetrahydrofolate, which is subsequently deaminated to form methenyl-tetrahydrofolate.

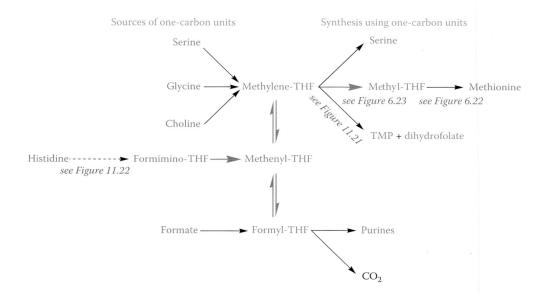

Figure 11.20 Sources and utilisation of folate derivatives carrying one-carbon fragments and inter-conversion of the one-carbon-substituted folates.

Methylene-, methenyl-, and 10-formyl-tetrahydrofolates are freely interconvertible. This means that when one-carbon folates are not required for synthetic reactions, the oxidation of the formyl group of formyl-tetrahydrofolate to carbon dioxide provides a means of maintaining an adequate tissue pool of free folate.

By contrast, the reduction of methylene-tetrahydrofolate to methyl-tetrahydrofolate is irreversible, and the only way in which free folate can be formed from methyl-tetrahydrofolate is by the reaction of methionine synthetase (Figure 6.22 and Section 11.11.3.2).

10-Formyl- and methylene-tetrahydrofolate are donors of one-carbon fragments in a number of biosynthetic reactions, including especially the synthesis of purines, pyrimidines, and porphyrins. In most cases, the reaction is a simple transfer of the one-carbon group from substituted folate onto the acceptor substrate. Two reactions are of especial interest: thymidylate synthetase and methionine synthetase.

11.11.3.1   *Thymidylate synthetase and dihydrofolate reductase*

The methylation of deoxyuridine monophosphate (dUMP) to thymidine monophosphate (TMP), catalysed by thymidylate synthetase (Figure 11.21), is essential for the synthesis of DNA, although preformed TMP can be reutilised by salvage from the catabolism of DNA.

The methyl donor is methylene-tetrahydrofolate; the reaction involves reduction of the one-carbon fragment to a methyl group at the expense of the folate, which is oxidised to dihydrofolate. Dihydrofolate is then reduced to tetrahydrofolate by dihydrofolate reductase.

Thymidylate synthase and dihydrofolate reductase are especially active in tissues with a high rate of cell division, and hence a high rate of DNA replication and a high requirement for thymidylate. Because of this, inhibitors of dihydrofolate reductase have been exploited as anti-cancer drugs. One of the earliest of these is methotrexate, an analogue of 10-methyl-tetrahydrofolate. Chemotherapy consists of alternating periods of

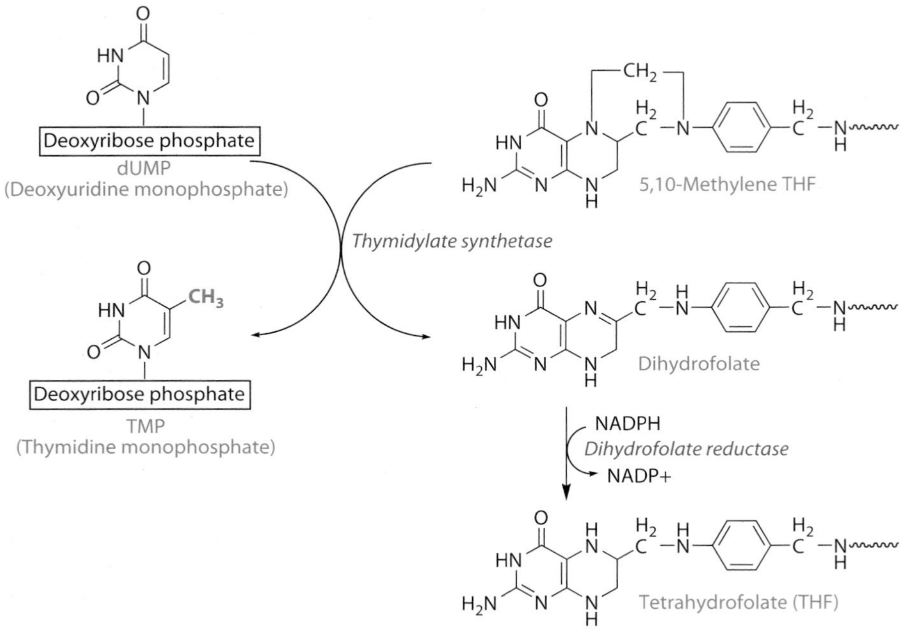

Figure 11.21 The reaction of thymidylate synthetase and dihydrofolate reductase.

administration of methotrexate and folate (normally as 5-formyl-tetrahydrofolate, leucovorin) to replete the normal tissues and avoid folate deficiency—so-called leucovorin rescue.

The dihydrofolate reductase of some bacteria and parasites differs significantly from the human enzyme, and inhibitors of the enzyme can be used as antibacterial drugs (e.g. trimethoprim) and antimalarial drugs (e.g. pyrimethamine).

11.11.3.2   *Methionine synthetase and the methyl-folate trap*

In addition to its role in the synthesis of proteins, methionine, as the *S*-adenosyl derivative, acts as a methyl donor in a wide variety of biosynthetic reactions; the resultant homocysteine may either be metabolised to yield cysteine or be remethylated to yield methionine (Figure 6.22).

Two enzymes catalyse the methylation of homocysteine to methionine:

1. Methionine synthetase is a vitamin B_{12}-dependent enzyme, for which the methyl donor is methyl-tetrahydrofolate.
2. Homocysteine methyltransferase utilises betaine (an intermediate in the catabolism of choline) as the methyl donor and is not vitamin B_{12} dependent.

Both enzymes are found in most tissues, but only the vitamin B_{12}-dependent methionine synthetase occurs in the central nervous system.

The reduction of methylene-tetrahydrofolate to methyl-tetrahydrofolate is irreversible and the major source of folate for tissues is methyl-tetrahydrofolate. The only metabolic role of methyl-tetrahydrofolate is the methylation of homocysteine to methionine, and this is the only way in which methyl-tetrahydrofolate can be demethylated to yield free folate in tissues. Methionine synthetase thus provides the link between the physiological functions of folate and vitamin B_{12}. Impairment of methionine synthetase activity in vitamin

B_{12} deficiency will result in the accumulation of methyl-tetrahydrofolate that can neither be utilised for any other one-carbon transfer reactions nor be demethylated to provide free folate. Therefore, there is functional deficiency of folate, secondary to the deficiency of vitamin B_{12}.

11.11.4 Folate deficiency: megaloblastic anaemia

Dietary deficiency of folate is not uncommon, and as noted above, deficiency of vitamin B_{12} also leads to functional folate deficiency. In either case, it is cells that are dividing rapidly, and therefore have a large requirement for thymidine for DNA synthesis, that are most severely affected. These are the cells of the bone marrow that form red blood cells, the cells of the intestinal mucosa, and the hair follicles. Clinically, folate deficiency leads to megaloblastic anaemia, the release into the circulation of immature precursors of red blood cells.

11.11.5 Folate requirements

Depletion/repletion studies to determine folate requirements using folic acid monoglutamate suggest a requirement of the order of 80–100 μg (170–220 nmol)/day. The total body pool of folate in adults is some 17 μmol (7.5 mg), with a biological half-life of 101 days. This suggests a minimum requirement for replacement of 85 nmol (37 μg) per day. Studies of the urinary excretion of folate metabolites in subjects maintained on folate free diets suggest that there is catabolism of some 80 μg of folate/day.

Because of the problems of determining the biological availability of the various folate polyglutamate conjugates found in foods, reference intakes allow a wide margin of safety, and are based on an allowance of 3 μg (6.8 nmol)/kg body weight.

11.11.5.1 Folate in pregnancy

During the 1980s, a considerable body of evidence accumulated that spina bifida and other neural tube defects (which occur in about 0.75%–1% of pregnancies) were associated with low intakes of folate and that increased intake during pregnancy might be protective. It is now established that supplements of folate begun periconceptually result in a significant reduction in the incidence of neural tube defects, and it is recommended that intakes be increased by 400 μg/day before conception. The studies were conducted using folate monoglutamate, and it is unlikely that an equivalent increase in intake could be achieved from unfortified foods; supplements are recommended where flour is not fortified with folic acid by law. Closure of the neural tube occurs by day 28 of pregnancy, which is before the woman knows she is pregnant. The advice therefore is that all women who are, or may be about to become, pregnant, should take folate supplements.

11.11.5.2 Higher levels of folate intake

Marginal folate status leads to reduced methylation of key regulatory areas of DNA involved in regulating gene expression (Section 6.4.1) and higher intakes of folate are associated with lower incidence of colorectal (and possibly other) cancer. There is some evidence that supplements of folate may be protective against some cancers, although high intakes may increase the rate of conversion of benign intestinal polyps to cancer.

Folate supplements of 400 μg/day reduce the incidence of spina bifida and neural tube defect; about 1% of pregnant women are at risk (Section 11.11.5.1). Similar supplements lower plasma homocysteine in people with the unstable variant of methylene tetrahydrofolate reductase (Section 6.6.1.2).

Folate supplements in excess of 350 µg/day may impair zinc absorption. More importantly, there are two potential problems that have to be considered when advocating either widespread use of folate supplements or widespread enrichment of foods with folate:

1. High levels of folate intake mask the megaloblastic anaemia of vitamin B_{12} deficiency (Section 11.10.2), so that the presenting sign is irreversible nerve damage. This is especially a problem for the elderly, who may have impaired absorption of vitamin B_{12} as a result of gastric atrophy (Section 4.5.2.1). It has been suggested that the addition of crystalline vitamin B_{12} to foods as well as folate would permit absorption of adequate amounts of vitamin B_{12} to prevent deficiency developing.
2. Antagonism between folate and the anticonvulsants used in the treatment of epilepsy is part of their mechanism of action; about 2% of the population have (drug-controlled) epilepsy. Relatively large supplements of folic acid (in excess of 1000 µg/day) may antagonise the anticonvulsants and lead to an increase in the frequency of epileptic attacks.

11.11.6   Assessment of folate status

The serum or red blood cell concentration of folate can be measured by radioligand binding assays, but there are a number of problems, and in some centres microbiological determination is preferred. In addition, there are two tests for functional folate status, the FIGLU test and the dUMP suppression test.

11.11.6.1   Histidine metabolism—the FIGLU test

The ability to metabolise a test dose of histidine provides a sensitive functional test of folate nutritional status; formiminoglutamate (FIGLU) is an intermediate in histidine catabolism (Figure 11.22) and is metabolised by a folate-dependent enzyme. In

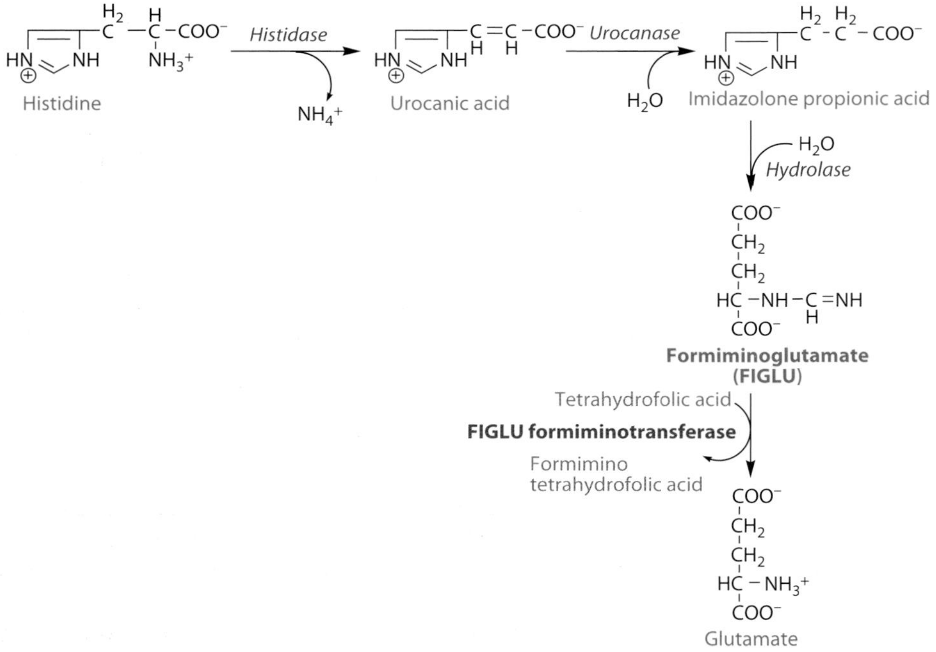

Figure 11.22 The metabolism of histidine—the FIGLU test for folate status.

deficiency, the activity of this enzyme is impaired, and formiminoglutamate accumulates and is excreted in the urine, especially after a test dose of histidine—the so-called FIGLU test.

Although the FIGLU test depends on folate nutritional status, the metabolism of histidine will also be impaired, and hence, a positive result obtained, in vitamin B_{12} deficiency because of the secondary deficiency of free folate. About 60% of vitamin B_{12}-deficient subjects show increased FIGLU excretion after a histidine load.

11.11.6.2 The dUMP suppression test

Rapidly dividing cells can either use preformed TMP for DNA synthesis or can synthesise it *de novo* from dUMP (Section 11.11.3.1). Isolated bone marrow cells or stimulated lymphocytes incubated with [^{3}H]TMP will incorporate label into DNA. In the presence of adequate amounts of methylene-tetrahydrofolate, the addition of dUMP as a substrate for thymidylate synthetase reduces the incorporation of [^{3}H]TMP as a result of dilution of the pool of labelled material by newly synthesised TMP and inhibition of thymidylate kinase by thymidine triphosphate.

This suppression of the incorporation of [^{3}H]thymidine into DNA in rapidly dividing cells by added deoxyuridine provides an index of folate status. In normal cells, the incorporation of [^{3}H]thymidine into DNA after preincubation with dUMP is less than 2% of that without preincubation. By contrast, cells that are deficient in folate form little or no thymidine from dUMP and hence incorporate nearly as much of the [^{3}H]thymidine after incubation with dUMP as they do without preincubation.

Either a primary deficiency of folate or functional deficiency secondary to vitamin B_{12} deficiency will have the same effect. In folate deficiency, addition of any biologically active form of folate, but not vitamin B_{12}, will normalise the dUMP suppression of [^{3}H]thymidine incorporation. In vitamin B_{12} deficiency, addition of vitamin B_{12} or methylene-tetrahydrofolate, but not methyl-tetrahydrofolate, will normalise dUMP suppression.

11.12   Biotin

Biotin was originally discovered as part of the complex called *bios*, which promoted the growth of yeast, and separately, as vitamin H, the protective or curative factor in 'egg white injury'—the disease caused experimentally by feeding diets containing large amounts of uncooked egg white.

Biotin is widely distributed in many foods. It is synthesised by intestinal flora, and in balance studies the total output of biotin in urine plus faeces is threefold to sixfold greater than the intake, reflecting bacterial synthesis. It is not known to what extent this bacterially synthesised biotin is available to the host.

11.12.1   Absorption and metabolism of biotin

Most biotin in foods is present as biocytin (ε-amino-biotinyl lysine, Figure 11.23), which is released on proteolysis, then hydrolysed by biotinidase in the pancreatic juice and intestinal mucosal secretions, to yield free biotin. The extent to which bound biotin in foods is biologically available is not known.

Free biotin is absorbed from the small intestine by active transport and circulates in the bloodstream both free and bound to a serum glycoprotein that has biotinidase activity, catalysing the hydrolysis of biocytin.

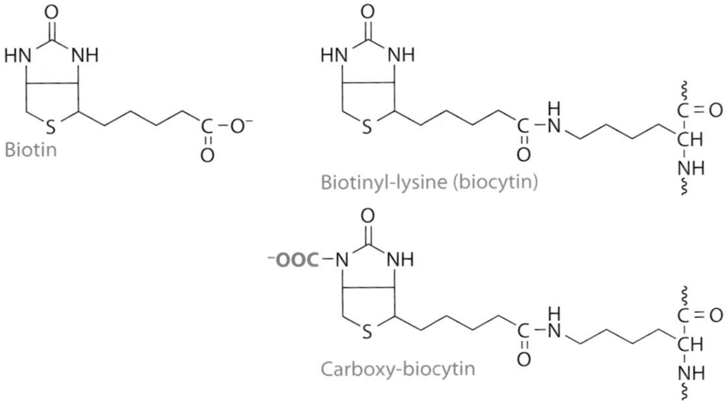

Figure 11.23 Biotin, biocytin (ε-amino biotinyllysine) and carboxy-biocytin.

Biotin enters tissues by a saturable facilitated transport system, and is then incorporated into biotin dependent enzymes as the ε-amino-lysine peptide, biocytin. Unlike other B vitamins, where concentrative uptake into tissues can be achieved by facilitated diffusion followed by metabolic trapping, the incorporation of biotin into enzymes is relatively slow and cannot be considered part of the uptake process. On catabolism of the enzymes, biocytin is hydrolysed by biotinidase, permitting reutilisation.

11.12.2   *Metabolic functions of biotin*

Biotin functions to transfer carbon dioxide in a small number of carboxylation reactions. The reactive intermediate is 1-*N*-carboxy-biocytin (Figure 11.23), formed from bicarbonate in an ATP-dependent reaction. A single holocarboxylase synthetase acts on the apo-enzymes of acetyl CoA carboxylase (a key enzyme in fatty acid synthesis, Section 5.5.6.1), pyruvate carboxylase (a key enzyme in gluconeogenesis Section 5.7), propionyl CoA carboxylase (Figure 11.18), and methylcrotonyl CoA carboxylase, to form the active holo-enzymes from (inactive) apo-enzymes and free biotin.

11.12.3   *Biotin deficiency and requirements*

Biotin is widely distributed in foods, and deficiency is unknown, except amongst people maintained for many months on total parenteral nutrition and a very small number of people who eat very large amounts of uncooked egg. Avidin, a protein in egg white, binds biotin extremely tightly and renders it unavailable for absorption. It is denatured by cooking and loses its ability to bind biotin. The amount of avidin in uncooked egg white is relatively small, and problems of biotin deficiency have only occurred in people eating abnormally large amounts—a dozen or more raw eggs a day, for some years.

The few early reports of human biotin deficiency all concerned people who consumed large amounts of uncooked eggs. They developed a fine scaly dermatitis and hair loss (alopecia). Histology of the skin showed an absence of sebaceous glands and atrophy of the hair follicles. Provision of biotin supplements of between 200 and 1000 µg/day resulted in cure of the skin lesions and regrowth of hair, despite continuing their abnormal diet. There have been no studies of provision of smaller doses of biotin to such people. More recently, similar signs of biotin deficiency have been observed in patients receiving total parenteral nutrition for prolonged periods, after major resection of the gut. The signs resolve following the provision of biotin, but again there have been no studies of the amounts of biotin required; intakes have ranged between 60 and 200 µg/day.

There is no evidence on which to estimate requirements for biotin. Average intakes are between 10 and 200 µg/day. Since dietary deficiency does not occur, such intakes are obviously more than adequate to meet requirements.

11.13 Pantothenic acid

Pantothenic acid (sometimes known as vitamin B_5) has a central role in energy-yielding metabolism as the functional moiety of coenzyme A (Figure 5.23) and in the biosynthesis of fatty acids as the prosthetic group of acyl carrier protein (Section 5.6.1).

Pantothenic acid is widely distributed in all foodstuffs; the name derives from the Greek for 'from everywhere', as opposed to other vitamins, which were originally isolated from individual rich sources. As a result, deficiency has not been unequivocally reported in human beings except in specific depletion studies, which have generally used the antagonist ω-methyl pantothenic acid.

11.13.1 Absorption, metabolism, and metabolic functions of pantothenic acid

About 85% of dietary pantothenic acid is as coenzyme A or phosphopantetheine, which is hydrolyzed to pantothenic acid. The intestinal absorption of pantothenic acid is by facilitated diffusion, and occurs at a constant rate throughout the length of the small intestine; intestinal bacterial synthesis may contribute to pantothenic acid nutrition.

The first step in pantothenic acid utilisation is phosphorylation. Pantothenate kinase is rate limiting; thus, unlike vitamins that are accumulated by metabolic trapping, there can be significant accumulation of free pantothenic acid in tissues.

11.13.1.1 Coenzyme A and acyl carrier protein

All tissues are capable of forming coenzyme A from pantothenic acid. CoA functions as the carrier of fatty acids, as thio-esters, in mitochondrial β-oxidation (Section 5.5.2). The resultant two-carbon fragments, as acetyl CoA, then undergo oxidation in the citric acid cycle (Section 5.4.4). CoA also functions as a carrier in the transfer of acetyl (and other fatty acyl) moieties in a variety of biosynthetic and catabolic reactions, including

- Synthesis of cholesterol and steroid hormones.
- Synthesis of long-chain fatty acid from palmitate and elongation of polyunsaturated fatty acids, in mitochondria (Section 5.6.1.1).
- Acylation of serine, threonine, and cysteine residues on proteolipids and acetylation of neuraminic acid.

Fatty acid synthesis (Section 5.6.1) is catalysed by a cytosolic multi-enzyme complex in which the growing fatty acyl chain is bound by thio-ester linkage to an enzyme-bound 4'-phospho-pantetheine residue, rather than to free CoA, as in β-oxidation. This component of the fatty acid synthetase complex is the acyl carrier protein.

11.13.2   Pantothenic acid deficiency: safe and adequate levels of intake

Prisoners of war in the Far East in the 1940s who were severely malnourished showed, amongst other signs and symptoms of vitamin deficiency diseases, a new condition of paraesthesia and severe pain in the feet and toes, which was called the 'burning foot syndrome', or nutritional melalgia. Although it was tentatively attributed to pantothenic acid deficiency, no specific trials of pantothenic acid were carried out; rather the subjects were given yeast extract and other rich sources of all vitamins as part of an urgent programme of nutritional rehabilitation.

Experimental pantothenic acid depletion, commonly together with the administration of ω-methyl pantothenic acid, results in the following signs and symptoms after 2–3 weeks:

- Neuromotor disorders, including paraesthesia of the hands and feet, hyperactive deep tendon reflexes and muscle weakness. These can be explained by the role of acetyl CoA in the synthesis of the neurotransmitter acetylcholine, and impaired formation of threonine acyl esters in myelin. Dysmyelination may explain the persistence and recurrence of neurological problems many years after nutritional rehabilitation in people who had suffered from burning foot syndrome.
- Mental depression, which again may be related to either acetylcholine deficit or impaired myelin synthesis.
- Gastrointestinal complaints, including severe vomiting and pain, with depressed gastric acid secretion in response to gastrin.
- Decreased serum cholesterol and decreased urinary excretion of 17-ketosteroids, reflecting the impairment of steroidogenesis.
- Decreased acetylation of *p*-aminobenzoic acid, sulphonamides, and other drugs, reflecting reduced availability of acetyl CoA for these reactions.

There is no evidence on which to estimate pantothenic acid requirements. Average intakes are between 3 and 7 mg/day, and since deficiency does not occur, such intakes are obviously more than adequate to meet requirements.

11.14   Vitamin C (ascorbic acid)

Vitamin C is a vitamin for only a limited number of vertebrate species: human beings and other primates, the guinea pig, bats, the passeriform birds, and most fishes. Ascorbate is synthesised as an intermediate in the gulonolactone pathway of glucose metabolism; in those vertebrate species for which it is a vitamin, one enzyme of the pathway, gulonolactone oxidase, is absent.

The vitamin C deficiency disease, scurvy, has been known for many centuries, and was described in the Ebers papyrus of 1500 BC and by Hippocrates. The Crusaders are said to have lost more men through scurvy than were killed in battle, whilst in some of the long voyages of exploration of the 14th and 15th centuries up to 90% of the crew died from scurvy. Cartier's expedition to Quebec in 1535 was struck by scurvy; local native Americans taught him to use an infusion of swamp spruce leaves to prevent or cure the condition.

Recognition that scurvy was due to a dietary deficiency came relatively early. James Lind demonstrated in 1757 that orange and lemon juice were protective, and Cook maintained his crew in good health during his circumnavigation of the globe (1772–1775) by stopping frequently to take on fresh fruit and vegetables. In 1804, the British Navy decreed

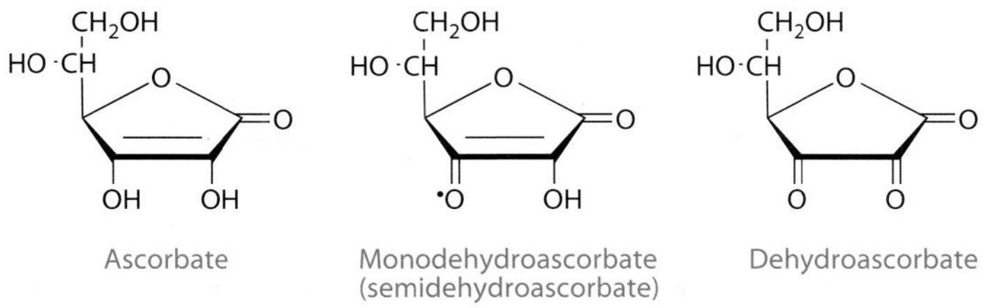

Figure 11.24 Vitamin C.

a daily ration of lemon or lime juice for all ratings, a requirement that was extended to the Merchant Navy in 1865.

Both ascorbic acid and dehydroascorbic acid have vitamin C activity (Figure 11.24).

Vitamin C is found in fruits and vegetables. Very significant losses of vitamin C occur as vegetables wilt, or when they are cut, as a result of release of ascorbate oxidase from the plant tissue. Significant losses of the vitamin also occur in cooking, both through leaching into the cooking water and atmospheric oxidation, which continues when foods are left to stand before serving.

11.14.1   Absorption and metabolism of vitamin C

At intakes up to about 100 mg/day, between 80% and 95% of dietary ascorbate is absorbed by active transport (Section 3.2.2.3) at the intestinal mucosal brush border membrane. As the transporter becomes saturated, a lower proportion of high intakes is absorbed.

About 70% of blood ascorbate is in plasma and erythrocytes (which do not concentrate the vitamin from plasma). The remainder is in white cells, which have a marked ability to concentrate it (Section 11.14.5). There is no specific storage organ for ascorbate; apart from leukocytes (which account for only 10% of total blood ascorbate), the only tissues showing a significant concentration of the vitamin are the adrenal and pituitary glands.

Ascorbic acid is excreted in the urine, either unchanged or as dehydroascorbate and diketogulonate. Both ascorbate and dehydroascorbate are filtered at the glomerulus, then reabsorbed. When glomerular filtration of ascorbate and dehydroascorbate exceeds the capacity of the transport systems, at a plasma concentration of ascorbate between 70 and 85 µmol/L, the vitamin is excreted in the urine in amounts proportional to intake.

11.14.2   Metabolic functions of vitamin C

Ascorbic acid has specific roles in two groups of enzymes: the copper-containing hydroxylases (Section 11.14.2.1) and the α-ketoglutarate-linked iron-containing hydroxylases (Section 11.14.2.2). It also increases the activity of a number of other enzymes *in vitro*, although this is a non-specific reducing action rather than reflecting any metabolic function of the vitamin. In addition, it has a number of non-enzymic effects due to its action as a reducing agent and oxygen radical quencher (Section 6.5.3.4).

11.14.2.1   Copper-containing hydroxylases

Dopamine β-hydroxylase is a copper-containing enzyme involved in the synthesis of the catecholamines noradrenaline and adrenaline from tyrosine in the adrenal medulla and central nervous system. The enzyme contains Cu^+, which is oxidised to Cu^{2+} during the hydroxylation of the substrate; reduction back to Cu$^+$ specifically requires ascorbate, which is oxidised to monodehydroascorbate.

A number of peptide hormones have a carboxy terminal amide that is essential for biological activity. The amide group is derived from a glycine residue that is on the carboxyl side of the amino acid that will become the amidated terminal of the mature peptide. This glycine is hydroxylated on the α-carbon by a copper-containing enzyme, peptidylglycine hydroxylase. The α-hydroxyglycine residue then decomposes non-enzymically to yield the amidated peptide and glyoxylate. The copper prosthetic group is oxidised in the reaction, and as in dopamine β-hydroxylase, ascorbate is specifically required for reduction back to Cu$^+$.

11.14.2.2   α-Ketoglutarate-linked iron-containing hydroxylases

A number of iron-containing hydroxylases share a common reaction mechanism, in which hydroxylation of the substrate is linked to decarboxylation of α-ketoglutarate. Many of these enzymes are involved in the modification of precursor proteins to yield the final, mature, protein. This is a process of postsynthetic modification—modification of an amino acid residue after it has been incorporated into the protein during synthesis on the ribosome (Section 9.2.3.4).

- Proline and lysine hydroxylases are required for the postsynthetic modification of procollagen in the formation of mature, insoluble, collagen, and proline hydroxylase is also required for the postsynthetic modification of the precursor proteins of osteocalcin and the C1q component of complement.
- Aspartate β-hydroxylase is required for the postsynthetic modification of the precursor of protein C, the vitamin K-dependent protease that hydrolyses activated Factor V in the blood clotting cascade (Figure 11.12).
- Trimethyllysine and γ-butyrobetaine hydroxylases are required for the synthesis of carnitine (Section 5.5.1).

Ascorbate is oxidised during the reaction of these enzymes, but not stoichiometrically with the decarboxylation of α-ketoglutarate and hydroxylation of the substrate. The purified enzyme is active in the absence of ascorbate, but after some 5–10 s (about 15–30 cycles of enzyme action), the rate of reaction begins to fall. At this stage, the iron in the catalytic site has been oxidised to Fe^{3+}, which is catalytically inactive; activity is restored only by ascorbate, which reduces it back to Fe^{2+}. The oxidation of Fe^{2+} is the consequence of accidental oxidation by the bound oxygen rather than the main reaction of the enzyme, which explains why the enzyme can remain active for several seconds in the absence of ascorbate, and why the consumption of ascorbate is not stoichiometric.

11.14.3   Vitamin C deficiency: scurvy

The vitamin C deficiency disease, scurvy, was formerly a common problem at the end of winter, when there had been no fresh fruits and vegetables for many months.

Although there is no specific organ for storage of vitamin C in the body, signs of deficiency do not develop in previously adequately nourished subjects until they have been deprived of the vitamin for 4–6 months, by which time plasma and tissue concentrations have fallen considerably. The earliest signs in volunteers maintained on a vitamin C free diet are skin changes, beginning with plugging of hair follicles by horny material, followed by enlargement of the hyperkeratotic follicles and petechial haemorrhage as a result of increased fragility of blood capillaries.

At a later stage, there is also haemorrhage of the gums. This is frequently accompanied by secondary bacterial infection and considerable withdrawal of the gum from the necks of the teeth. As the condition progresses, there is loss of dental cement, and the teeth become loose in the alveolar bone and may be lost.

Wounds show only superficial healing in scurvy, with little or no formation of (collagen-rich) scar tissue; healing is delayed and wounds can readily be reopened. Scorbutic scar tissue has only about half the tensile strength of that normally formed.

Advanced scurvy is accompanied by intense pain in the bones, which can be attributed to changes in bone mineralisation as a result of abnormal collagen synthesis. Bone formation ceases and the existing bone becomes rarefied, and the bones fracture with minimal trauma.

The name *scurvy* is derived from the Italian *scorbutico,* meaning an irritable, neurotic, discontented, whining, and cranky person. The disease is associated with listlessness and general malaise, and sometimes changes in personality and psychomotor performance and a lowering of the general level of arousal. These behavioural effects can be attributed to impaired synthesis of the catecholamine neurotransmitters (noradrenaline and adrenaline), as a result of low activity of dopamine β-hydroxylase.

Most of the other clinical signs of scurvy can be accounted for by the effects of ascorbate deficiency on collagen synthesis, as a result of impaired proline and lysine hydroxylase activity. Depletion of muscle carnitine (Section 5.5.1), as a result of impaired activity of trimethyllysine and γ-butyrobetaine hydroxylases, may account for the lassitude and fatigue that precede clinical signs of scurvy.

11.14.3.1   Anaemia in scurvy

Anaemia is frequently associated with scurvy and may be either macrocytic, indicative of folate deficiency (Section 11.11.4) or hypochromic, indicative of iron deficiency (Sections 11.15.2.3 and 11.16).

Folate deficiency may be epiphenomenal, since the major dietary sources of folate are the same as those of ascorbate. However, some patients with clear megaloblastic anaemia respond to the administration of vitamin C alone, suggesting that there may be a role of ascorbate in the maintenance of normal pools of reduced folates, although there is no evidence that any of the reactions of folate is ascorbate dependent.

Iron deficiency in scurvy may well be secondary to reduced absorption of inorganic iron (Section 4.5.3.1) and impaired mobilisation of tissue iron reserves (Section 11.11.4). At the same time, the haemorrhages of advanced scurvy will cause a significant loss of blood.

There is also evidence that erythrocytes have a shorter half-life than normal in scurvy, possibly as a result of oxidative damage to membrane lipids due to impairment of the reduction of tocopheroxyl radical by ascorbate (Section 6.5.3.4).

11.14.4   Vitamin C requirements

Vitamin C illustrates extremely well how different criteria of adequacy, and different interpretations of experimental evidence (Section 11.1), can lead to different estimates of requirements, and to reference intakes ranging between 30 and 90 mg/day for adults.

The requirement for vitamin C to prevent clinical scurvy is less than 10 mg/day. However, at this level of intake, wounds do not heal properly and an intake of 20 mg/day is required for optimum wound healing. Allowing for individual variation in requirements, this gives a reference intake for adults of 30 mg/day, which was the UK reference intake until 1991.

The 1991 UK Reference Nutrient Intake for vitamin C is based on the level of intake at which the plasma concentration increases sharply, showing that requirements have now been met, tissues are saturated, and there is spare vitamin being transported between tissues, available for excretion. This criterion of adequacy gives an RNI of 40 mg/day for adults.

The alternative approach to determining requirements is to estimate the total body content of vitamin C, then measure the rate at which it is metabolised, by giving a test dose of isotopically labelled vitamin. This was the basis of both the 1989 U.S. RDA of 60 mg/day for adults and the Netherlands RDA of 80 mg/day. Indeed, it also provides an alternative basis for the RNI of 40 mg/day adopted in Britain in 1991.

The problem lies in deciding what is an appropriate body content of vitamin C. The American studies were performed on subjects whose total body vitamin C was estimated to be 1500 mg at the beginning of a depletion study. However, there is no evidence that this is a necessary, or even a desirable, body content of the vitamin. It is simply the body content of the vitamin amongst a small group of young people eating a self-selected diet rich in fruit and vegetables. There is good evidence that a body pool of 900 mg is more than adequate. It is three times larger than that at which the first signs of deficiency are observed and will protect against the development of any signs of deficiency for several months on a completely vitamin C-free diet.

There is a further problem in interpreting the results of this kind of study. The rate at which vitamin C is catabolised varies with the intake and body pool. This means that as the experimental subjects become depleted, the rate at which they catabolise the vitamin decreases. Thus calculation of the amount required to maintain the body content depends on the way in which results obtained during depletion studies are extrapolated to the rate in subjects consuming a normal diet—and on the amount of vitamin C in that diet.

An intake of 40 mg/day is more than adequate to maintain a total body content of 900 mg of vitamin C—the same as the UK RNI. At a higher level of habitual intake, 60 mg/day is adequate to maintain a total body content of 1500 mg (the 1989 U.S. RDA). Making allowances for changes in the rate of metabolism with different levels of intake and allowing for incomplete absorption of the vitamin gives the Netherlands RDA of 80 mg/day.

The 2000 U.S. RDA for vitamin C, shown in Table 11.3, is based achieving near complete saturation of neutrophils with the vitamin, with minimal urinary loss, giving an RDA of 90 mg/day for men and an extrapolated RDA of 75 mg/day for women.

11.14.4.1   *Possible benefits of high intakes of vitamin C*

At intakes above about 100 mg/day, the body's capacity to metabolise vitamin C is saturated, and any further intake is excreted in the urine unchanged. Therefore, it would not seem justifiable to recommend higher levels of intake. However, vitamin C enhances the intestinal absorption of inorganic iron (Section 4.5.3.1), both by maintaining it in the Fe^{2+} state and also by chelating it. A dose of 25 mg of vitamin C taken together with a meal increases the absorption of iron some 65%, whilst a 1 g dose gives a ninefold increase. This occurs only when ascorbic acid is present together with the test meal; neither intravenous administration of vitamin C nor intake several hours before the test meal has any effect on iron absorption. Optimum iron absorption may therefore require significantly more than 100 mg of vitamin C/day.

The safety of nitrates and nitrites used in curing meat, a traditional method of preservation, has been questioned because of the formation of nitrosamines by reaction between nitrite and amines naturally present in foods under the acid conditions in the stomach (Section 6.7.4). In experimental animals, nitrosamines are potent carcinogens, and some authorities have limited the amounts of these salts that are permitted, although there is little evidence of any hazard to human beings from endogenous nitrosamine formation. Ascorbate can prevent the formation of nitrosamines by reacting non-enzymatically with nitrite and other nitrosating reagents, forming NO, NO_2, and N_2. Again, this is an effect of ascorbate present in the stomach at the same time as the dietary nitrites and amines, rather than an effect of vitamin C nutritional status.

11.14.4.2   Pharmacological uses of vitamin C

A number of studies have reported low ascorbate status in patients with advanced cancer—perhaps an unsurprising finding in seriously ill patients. With very little experimental evidence, it has been suggested that very high intakes of vitamin C (of the order of 10 g/day or more) may be beneficial in enhancing host resistance to cancer and preventing the development of AIDS in people who are HIV positive. Controlled studies with patients matched for age, sex, site, and stage of primary tumours and metastases, and for previous chemotherapy, have not shown any beneficial effect of high dose ascorbic acid in the treatment of advanced cancer.

High doses of vitamin C have been recommended for the prevention and treatment of the common cold, with some evidence from some studies that the vitamin reduces the duration and severity of symptoms, although other studies show no beneficial effects.

11.14.4.3   Toxicity of vitamin C

Regardless of whether or not high intakes of ascorbate have any beneficial effects, large numbers of people habitually take between 1 and 5 g/day of vitamin C supplements (compared with reference intakes of 40–90 mg/day), and some take considerably more. There is little evidence of any significant toxicity. Once the plasma concentration of ascorbate reaches the renal threshold, it is excreted more or less quantitatively with increasing intake, and there is no evidence that higher intakes increase the body pool above about 1500 mg/kg body weight. Unabsorbed ascorbate in the intestinal lumen is a substrate for bacterial fermentation, and may cause diarrhoea and intestinal discomfort.

High concentrations of vitamin C can react with proteins non-enzymatically, glycating them in the same way as high concentrations of glucose glycate proteins in poorly controlled diabetes mellitus (Section 10.7.1). There is some evidence that a high intake of vitamin C from supplements is associated with a higher risk of cardiovascular disease in post-menopausal women with type II diabetes.

Up to 5% of the population are at risk from the development of renal oxalate stones. The risk is from both ingested oxalate and that formed endogenously, mainly from the metabolism of glycine. A number of reports have suggested that people consuming high intakes of vitamin C excrete more oxalate in the urine, but no pathway for the formation of oxalate from ascorbate is known. High intakes of vitamin C acidify the urine, and this reduces the solubility of oxalate and uric acid salts as well as xanthine and cysteine, resulting in an increased risk of renal stone formation. By contrast, the more acidic urine increases the solubility of phosphates and reduces the formation of calcium and magnesium phosphate stones.

11.14.5   Assessment of vitamin C status

It is relatively easy to assess the state of body reserves of vitamin C by measuring the excretion after a test dose. A subject whose tissue reserves are saturated will excrete more or less the whole of a test dose of 500 mg of ascorbate over 6 h.

The plasma concentration of vitamin C falls relatively rapidly during experimental depletion studies, to undetectably low levels within 4 weeks of initiating a vitamin C free diet, although clinical signs of scurvy may not develop for a further 3–4 months, and tissue concentrations of the vitamin may be as high as 50% of saturation.

The concentration of ascorbate in leukocytes is correlated with the concentrations in other tissues, and falls more slowly than the plasma concentration in depletion studies. The reference range of leukocyte ascorbate is 1.1–2.8 mol/10^6 cells; a significant loss of leukocyte ascorbate coincides with the development of clinical signs of scurvy.

Without a differential white cell count, leukocyte ascorbate concentration does not give a meaningful index of vitamin C status. The different types of leukocyte have different capacities to accumulate ascorbate. This means that a change in the proportion of granulocytes, platelets, and mononuclear leukocytes will result in a change in the total concentration of ascorbate/10^6 cells, although there may well be no change in vitamin nutritional status. Stress, myocardial infarction, infection, burns, and surgical trauma all result in changes in leukocyte distribution, with an increase in the proportion of granulocytes (which are saturated at a lower concentration of ascorbate than other leukocytes), and hence, an apparent change in leukocyte ascorbate. This has been widely misinterpreted to indicate an increased requirement for vitamin C in these conditions.

11.15   Minerals

Those inorganic minerals that have a function in the body must obviously be provided in the diet, since elements cannot be interconverted. Many of the essential minerals are of little practical nutritional importance, since they are widely distributed in foods, and most people eating a normal mixed diet are likely to receive adequate intakes.

In general, mineral deficiencies are a problem when people live largely on foods grown in one region, where the soil may be deficient in some minerals. Iodine deficiency is a major problem in many areas of the world (Section 11.15.3.3). For people whose diet consists of foods grown in a variety of different regions, mineral deficiencies are unlikely. Iron deficiency is a problem in most parts of the world because if iron losses from the body are relatively high (e.g. from heavy menstrual blood loss), it is difficult to achieve an adequate intake to replace the losses (Section 11.15.2.3).

Mineral deficiency is unlikely amongst people eating an adequate mixed diet. More importantly, many of the minerals, including those that are dietary essentials, are toxic in even fairly modest excess. This is unlikely to be a problem with high mineral content of foods, although crops grown in regions where the soil content of selenium is especially high may provide dangerously high levels of intake of this mineral (Section 11.15.2.5). Toxicity arises when people take inappropriate supplements of minerals or are exposed to contamination of food and water supplies.

11.15.1   Calcium

The most obvious requirement for calcium in the body is in the mineral of bones and teeth—a complex mixture of calcium carbonates and phosphates (hydroxyapatite), together with magnesium salts and fluorides. An adult has about 25 mol (1 kg) of calcium in the body, 99% of which is in the skeleton and teeth. This means that calcium requirements are especially high in times of rapid growth—during infancy and adolescence and in pregnancy and lactation.

Although the major part of the body's calcium is in bones, the most important functions of calcium are in the maintenance of muscle contractility and responses to hormones and neurotransmitters. To maintain these essential regulatory functions, bone calcium is mobilised in deficiency to ensure that the plasma concentration is kept within the range of 2.2–2.6 mmol/L.

Just under half of the serum calcium is present as free ionised calcium; most of the remainder is bound to serum albumin, with 9% complexed by citrate. Hyperventilation leads to alkalosis as carbon dioxide is exhaled. This leads to release of protons from serum albumin to maintain plasma pH, and as a result, free ionised calcium falls as it binds to negatively charged albumin, leading to tetany, as neuromuscular regulation is disturbed by the loss of free ionised calcium.

$$H^+ + HCO_3^- \rightleftharpoons H_2CO_3 \rightleftharpoons \uparrow CO_2 + H_2O$$
$$\text{Albumin-H} \rightleftharpoons H^+ + \text{albumin}^-$$
$$\text{Albumin}^- + Ca^{2+} \rightleftharpoons \text{albumin-Ca}$$

Inositol trisphosphate released as a second messenger in response to hormone action (Section 10.3.3) leads to release of calcium from the endoplasmic reticulum into the cytosol, and the intracellular concentration of calcium increases rapidly from 0.1 to 1.0 µmol/L. This increase in cytosolic calcium activates protein kinase C and calmodulin (Section 10.3.3) as well as enzymes that are directly responsive to calcium. Responses to increased intracellular calcium include

- Secretion of digestive enzymes from the acinar cells of the pancreas, and of amylase from the parotid salivary gland, in response to acetylcholine released by nerves.
- Contraction of vascular and gastric smooth muscle, again in response to cholinergic innervation.
- Glycogenolysis in liver (Section 5.6.3.1), in response to vasopressin.
- Aggregation, shape change, and hormone secretion by blood platelets in response to thrombin.
- Histamine secretion by mast cells in response to antigens.
- DNA synthesis and cell division in fibroblasts in response to peptide growth factors.

The main sources of calcium are milk and cheese; dietary calcium is absorbed by an active process in the mucosal cells of the small intestine (Section 3.2.2.3) and is dependent on vitamin D (Section 11.3.3). Calcitriol, the active metabolite of vitamin D, induces the synthesis of a calcium binding protein, which permits the mucosal cells to accumulate calcium from the intestinal lumen, and in vitamin D deficiency, the absorption of calcium is seriously impaired.

Although the effect of vitamin D deficiency is impairment of the absorption and utilisation of calcium, rickets (Section 11.3.4) is not simply the result of calcium deficiency. Calcium-deficient children with adequate vitamin D nutritional status do not develop rickets but have a much reduced rate of growth. Nevertheless, calcium deficiency may be a contributory factor in the development of rickets when vitamin D status is marginal.

11.15.1.1   *Calcium homeostasis*

The average daily intake of calcium is 25 mmol, of which 10–14 mmol is normally absorbed. This is countered by secretion of 7 mmol of calcium into the intestinal lumen, and faecal excretion is 18–22 mmol/day (Figure 11.25). About 240 mmol of calcium is filtered in the

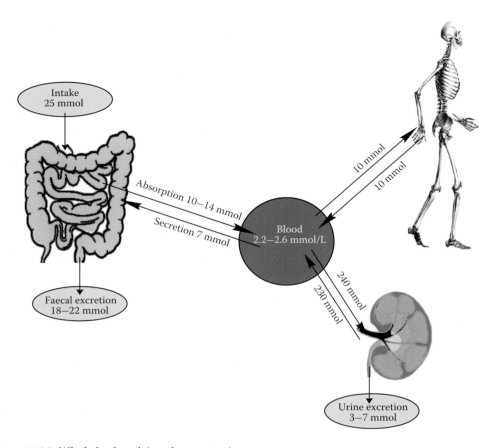

Figure 11.25 Whole body calcium homeostasis.

kidneys, almost all of which is reabsorbed; urinary excretion is 3–7 mmol/day. There is also continual turnover of bone, with release and replacement of 10 mmol of calcium/day. This means that the plasma concentration of calcium can be maintained in three ways: by regulating intestinal absorption, by regulating renal reabsorption, or by regulating bone turnover. The regulation of intestinal absorption of calcium by calcitriol is discussed in Section 11.3.3.

Three hormones are responsible for regulating calcium homeostasis:

1. Calcitriol, the active metabolite of vitamin D, which has hypercalcaemic actions. As discussed in Section 11.3.2.2, the synthesis of active calcitriol or inactive 24-hydroxy-calcidiol is regulated by reciprocal changes in the activities of calcidiol 1-hydroxylase and 24-hydroxylase in response to calcium availability and parathyroid hormone.
2. Parathyroid hormone, secreted by the parathyroid glands, which also has hypercalcaemic actions. Although, as shown in Figure 11.1, there are normally four parathyroid glands embedded in the thyroid, the number and their position are variable, and abnormalities occur in about 1 in 10 glands. Although parathyroid hormone is an 84-amino acid peptide, only the 34 amino acids at the amino terminal are required for activity, and synthetic parathyroid hormone is this 34-amino acid peptide. Like other peptide hormones, parathyroid hormone acts via cell surface G-protein-coupled

receptors, linked to the formation of cAMP (Section 10.3.2). cAMP is released from the kidney in response to parathyroid hormone action and can be measured in plasma or urine as a marker of parathyroid hormone action. The main regulator of parathyroid hormone secretion is serum calcium; parathyroid cells have a cell surface calcium receptor that activates phospholipase C, leading to production of inositol trisphosphate and diacylglycerol (Section 10.3.3). Hypercalcaemia inhibits parathyroid hormone secretion, and hypocalcaemia increases it. As well as increasing the renal reabsorption of calcium, parathyroid hormone also increases renal excretion of phosphate.

3. Calcitonin, secreted by the parafollicular or C cells of the thyroid, which acts to lower serum calcium. These cells are embryologically distinct from the remainder of the thyroid gland and are derived from the neural crest. Calcitonin is a 32-amino acid peptide, but the gene codes for 136 amino acids. The same gene is transcribed and translated in the brain to yield the calcitonin gene-related peptide (CGRP), as a result of differential splicing of the primary transcript. CGRP mRNA shares three introns with calcitonin mRNA, but not the fourth; instead, it has two introns that are absent from calcitonin mRNA (Section 9.2.2.1).

Almost all of the calcium that is filtered in the glomerulus is reabsorbed. There is paracellular reabsorption in the proximal renal tubule and thick ascending limb; this is unregulated. In both the thick ascending limb and distal tubule, there is transcellular transport, which is regulated by hormones. Parathyroid hormone increases calcium uptake in both the thick ascending limb and distal tubule; calcitriol increases it in the distal tubule. In both regions, calcitonin reduces calcium transport.

All three hormones are also involved in the regulation of bone turnover (Figure 11.26). Osteoblasts, the cells that secrete new bone matrix, are stimulated by calcitriol and parathyroid hormone to secrete factors that both increase differentiation of osteoclasts and also activates them. Activated osteoclasts secrete enzymes that hydrolyse bone matrix, releasing calcium into the circulation. If calcium is available, then after this erosion by osteoblasts, bone is replaced by osteoblast action. The osteoblasts become surrounded by the new bone matrix they secrete and differentiate into osteocytes. Calcitonin, secreted in response to a rising concentration of calcium, inactivates osteoclasts.

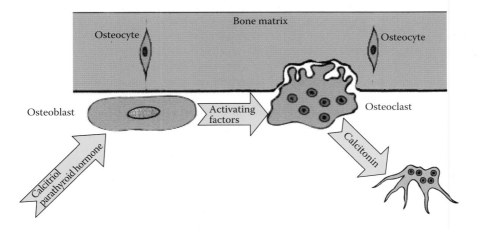

Figure 11.26 Bone mineral mobilisation in response to calcitriol and parathyroid hormone.

Hyperparathyroidism, as a result of either a benign tumour of one of the parathyroid glands or as an adaptive response to longstanding hypocalcaemia, results in excessive resorption of bone, leading to cyst formation and bone pain as well as possibly renal calcium phosphate stones because of the hypercalcaemia caused by excessive parathyroid hormone.

Hypoparathyroidism may be iatrogenic, the result of accidental removal of parathyroid glands during thyroid surgery or may be idiopathic—failure of parathyroid hormone secretion although the cause is unknown. In either case, there is a low circulating concentration of parathyroid hormone, with hypocalcaemia and hyperphosphatemia. Pseudohypoparathyroidism is the result of defects of the parathyroid hormone receptors in bone and kidney, resulting in impaired responsiveness to the hormone. In this case there is a high circulating concentration of parathyroid hormone, but again hypocalcaemia and hyperphosphataemia are seen. The hypercalcaemia causes paraesthesia, tetany, and sometimes epilepsy as a result of increased excitability of nerves. Treatment of hypoparathyroidism or pseudohypoparathyroidism is by providing supplements of calcium and calcitriol.

11.15.1.2   Osteoporosis

Osteoporosis is a progressive loss of bone with increasing age, after the peak bone mass has been achieved at the age of about 30 years old. The cause is the normal process of bone turnover with reduced replacement of the tissue that has been broken down. Both mineral and the organic matrix of bone are lost in osteoporosis, unlike osteomalacia (Section 11.3.4), where there is loss of bone mineral, but the organic matrix is unaffected.

Osteoporosis can occur in relatively young people, as a result of prolonged bed rest (or weightlessness in space flight)—bone continues to be degraded, but without physical activity, there is less stimulus for replacement of the lost tissue. More importantly, it occurs as an apparently unavoidable part of the ageing process. Here the main problem is the reduced secretion of oestrogens (in women) and androgens (in men) with increasing age; amongst other actions, the sex steroids are required for the differentiation of osteoblasts for new bone formation. The problem is especially serious in women, since there is a much more abrupt fall in oestrogen secretion at the menopause than the more gradual (and less severe) fall in androgen secretion in men with increasing age. As a result, many more elderly women than men suffer from osteoporosis. Post-menopausal hormone replacement therapy with oestrogens has a protective effect.

People with higher peak bone mass are less at risk from osteoporosis, since they can tolerate more loss of bone before there are serious effects. Therefore, adequate calcium and vitamin D nutrition through adolescence and young adulthood is likely to provide protection against osteoporosis in old age. High intakes of calcium have less effect once peak bone mass has been achieved. However, there are no adverse effects either because of the close regulation of calcium homeostasis; problems of hypercalcaemia and calcinosis (the calcification of soft tissues) occur as a result of vitamin D intoxication (Section 11.3.5.1) or other disturbances of calcium homeostasis, not as a result of high intakes of calcium.

11.15.2   Minerals that function as prosthetic groups in enzymes

11.15.2.1   Cobalt

In addition to its role in vitamin B_{12} (Figure 11.17), cobalt provides the prosthetic group of a small number of enzymes. It is therefore a dietary essential, despite the fact that vitamin B_{12} cannot be synthesised in the body. However, no clinical signs of cobalt deficiency are known, except in ruminant animals, whose intestinal bacteria synthesise vitamin B_{12}. Inorganic cobalt salts are toxic, and even a moderately excessive intake can lead to damage to heart muscle.

11.15.2.2   Copper
Copper provides the essential functional part of a number of enzymes involved in oxidation and reduction reactions, including dopamine β-hydroxylase in the synthesis of noradrenaline and adrenaline (Section 11.14.2.1), cytochrome oxidase in the electron transport chain (Section 3.3.1.2), and superoxide dismutase, one of the enzymes involved in protection against oxygen radicals (Section 6.5.3.1). Copper is also important in the oxidation of lysine to form the cross links in collagen and elastin. In copper deficiency, the bones are abnormally fragile because the abnormal collagen does not permit the normal flexibility of the bone matrix. More importantly, elastin is less elastic than normal, and copper deficiency can lead to death following rupture of the aorta.

11.15.2.3   Iron
The most obvious function of iron is in the haem of haemoglobin, the oxygen-carrying protein in red blood cells and myoglobin in muscles. Haem is also important as the co-enzyme for oxidation and reduction reactions in a variety of enzymes, including the cytochromes (Section 3.3.1.2). A number of enzymes, including the iron–sulphur proteins of the electron transport chain (Figure 3.20) also contain non-haem iron (i.e., iron bound to the enzyme other than in haem), which is essential to their function.

Deficiency of iron leads to reduced synthesis of haemoglobin, and hence a lower than normal amount of haemoglobin in red blood cells. Iron-deficiency anaemia is a major problem worldwide, especially amongst women. The problem is due to a loss of blood greater than can be replaced by absorption of dietary iron. In developing countries, intestinal parasites (especially hookworm), which cause large losses of blood in the faeces, are a common cause of anaemia in both men and women. In developed countries, it is mainly women who are at risk of iron deficiency as a result of heavy menstrual losses of blood. Probably 10%–15% of women have menstrual losses of iron greater than can be met from a normal dietary intake, and are therefore at risk of developing anaemia unless they take iron supplements

Iron in foods occurs in two forms: haem in meat and meat products and inorganic iron salts in plant foods. The absorption of haem iron is better than that of inorganic iron salts; as discussed in Section 4.5.3.1, only about 10% of the inorganic iron of the diet is absorbed, although this is increased by vitamin C (Section 11.14.4.1).

11.15.2.4   Molybdenum
Molybdenum functions as the prosthetic group of a small number of enzymes, including xanthine oxidase, which is involved in the metabolism of purines to uric acid for excretion, and pyridoxal oxidase, which metabolises vitamin B_6 to the inactive excretory product pyridoxic acid (Section 11.9.1). It occurs in an organic complex, molybdopterin, which is chemically similar to folate (Section 11.11) but can be synthesised in the body as long as adequate amounts of molybdenum are available.

Molybdenum deficiency has been associated with increased incidence of cancer of the oesophagus, but this seems to be an indirect association. The problem occurs amongst people living largely on maize grown on soil that is poor in molybdenum. Molybdenum-deficient maize plants are more susceptible to attack by fungi that produce carcinogenic toxins. Thus, while the people living on this diet are at risk of molybdenum deficiency, the main problem is not one of molybdenum deficiency in the people, but rather of fungal spoilage of their food.

11.15.2.5 *Selenium*

Selenium functions in a number of enzymes, including glutathione peroxidase (Section 6.5.3.2) and thyroxine deiodinase, which forms the active thyroid hormone, tri-iodothyronine, from thyroxine secreted by the thyroid gland (Figure 11.28). It is present as the selenium analogue of the amino acid cysteine, selenocysteine. The STOP codon UGA codes for selenocysteine in a context-sensitive manner (Section 2.1.2). Free selenocysteine is not incorporated into proteins. There is a specific tRNA for selenocysteine, and it is esterified to serine by amino acyl tRNA synthase. The seryl tRNA is then phosphorylated, and the phosphoseryl tRNA reacts with selenophosphate to form selenocysteinyl tRNA (Figure 11.27).

Selenium deficiency is widespread in parts of China, and in some parts of the United States and Finland. The soil is so poor in selenium that it is added to fertilisers to increase the selenium intake of the population, and so prevent deficiency. In New Zealand, despite the low selenium content of the soil, it was decided not to use selenium-rich fertilisers because of the hazards of selenium toxicity. By contrast, in some parts of the world, the soil is so rich in selenium that locally grown crops would provide more than the recommended upper limit of selenium intake if they were the main source of food, and it is not possible to graze cattle safely on the pastures in these regions.

The average requirement for selenium is 45 µg/day, with a reference intake of 55 µg. There is cause for concern in the UK (and elsewhere) that the average intake of selenium is only about 40 µg/day. Intakes have fallen since the latter part of the 20th century as a result of increasing use of wheat grown in Europe, where soils are relatively selenium depleted, replacing wheat from North America and Australia, where soil selenium levels are higher.

Selenium is extremely toxic in even modest excess; signs of poisoning can be seen at intakes above 400 µg/day, which has been set as the upper tolerable intake by the U.S. Institute of Medicine; the World Health Organization recommends that selenium intakes should not exceed 200 µg/day. Signs of selenium poisoning (selenosis) include brittleness, then loss of hair and nails, as well as a strong and unpleasant odour from volatile selenium compounds exhaled in the breath and excreted in sweat. There is no benefit from intakes of selenium greater than about 55–100 µg/day; once requirements have been met, the activity of glutathione peroxidase (Section 6.5.3.2) and other selenoproteins does not increase any further.

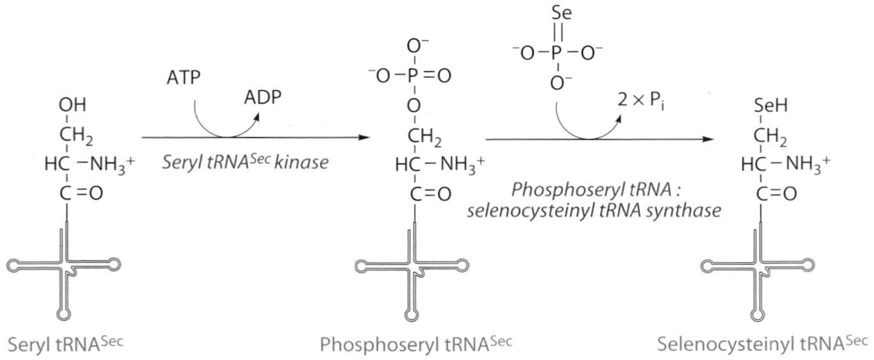

Figure 11.27 Formation of selenocysteinyl tRNA.

11.15.2.6   Zinc

Zinc provides the prosthetic group of more than a hundred enzymes, with a wide variety of functions. It is also involved in the receptor proteins for steroid and thyroid hormones, calcitriol, and vitamin A. In these proteins, zinc forms an integral part of the region of the protein (the zinc finger) that interacts with the promoter site on DNA to initiate gene transcription in response to hormone action (Section 10.4).

Overt zinc deficiency occurs only amongst people living in tropical or subtropical areas whose diet is very largely based on unleavened whole-meal bread. The problem is seen mainly as delayed puberty; thus, young men of 18–20 years are still prepubertal. This is a result of reduced sensitivity of target tissues to androgens because of the role of zinc in steroid hormone receptors. Two separate factors contribute to the deficiency:

1. Wheat flour provides very little zinc, and in unleavened wholemeal bread, much of the zinc that is present is not available for absorption because it is bound to phytate and dietary fibre.
2. Sweat contains a relatively high concentration of zinc, and in tropical conditions, there can be a considerable loss of zinc in sweat.

Marginal zinc deficiency is associated with poor wound healing, increased susceptibility to infection, and impairment of the senses of taste and smell.

11.15.3   Minerals that have a regulatory role (in neurotransmission, as enzyme activators or in hormones)

11.15.3.1   Calcium

In addition to its role in bone mineral, calcium has a major function in metabolic regulation (Section 10.3.3), nerve conduction, and muscle contraction. Calcium nutrition and homeostasis are discussed in Section 11.14.1.

11.15.3.2   Chromium

Chromium is involved, as an organic complex, the glucose tolerance factor, in the interaction between insulin and its cell surface receptor (Section 10.3.4), and deficiency is associated with impaired glucose tolerance (Section 10.7). There is no evidence that increased intakes of chromium have any beneficial effect in diabetes, and whilst there is no evidence of harm from organic chromium complexes, inorganic chromium salts are highly toxic.

11.15.3.3   Iodine

Iodine is required for the synthesis of the thyroid hormones, thyroxine, and tri-iodothyronine. Deficiency leads to goitre, a visible enlargement of the thyroid gland, as a result of hypertrophy to attempt to synthesise enough thyroxine. It is widespread in inland upland areas over limestone soil. This is because the soil over limestone is thin, and minerals, including iodine, readily leach out; thus, locally grown plants are deficient in iodine. Near the coast, sea spray contains enough iodine to replace these losses. Worldwide, many millions of people are at risk of deficiency, and in parts of central Brazil, the Himalayas, and central Africa, goitre may affect more than 90% of the population.

Thyroid hormones regulate metabolic activity, and people with thyroid deficiency have a low basal metabolic rate (Section 5.1.3.1), and hence gain weight readily. They tend to be lethargic and have a dull mental apathy. Children born to iodine-deficient mothers are especially at risk, and more so if they are then weaned onto an iodine-deficient diet. They may suffer from very severe mental retardation (goitrous cretinism) and congenital deafness. There is evidence that even mild iodine deficiency or inadequacy in pregnancy can lead to intellectual impairment in children. Although hypothyroidism as a result of iodine deficiency leads to a low metabolic rate and weight gain, once iodine requirements have been met, additional intake does not have any further effect and does not help weight loss in overweight people.

By contrast, overactivity of the thyroid gland, and hence overproduction of thyroid hormones, leads to a greatly increased metabolic rate, possibly leading to very considerable weight loss, despite an apparently adequate intake of food. Hyperthyroid people are lean and have a tense nervous energy.

Iodide is accumulated in the thyroid gland, where specific tyrosine residues in the protein thyroglobulin are iodinated to yield di-iodotyrosine, catalysed by a peroxidase (Figure 11.28). The next stage is the transfer of the di-iodophenol residue of one di-iodotyrosine onto another, the coupling reaction, yielding protein-bound thyroxine, which is stored in the colloid of the thyroid gland. In response to stimulation by thyrotropin, thyroglobulin is hydrolysed, releasing thyroxine into the circulation. The active hormone is tri-iodothyronine, which is formed from thyroxine by a selenium-dependent deiodinase (Section 11.15.2.5), both in the thyroid gland and, more importantly, in target tissues. Because of this role of selenium in the metabolism of the thyroid hormones, the effects of iodine deficiency will be exacerbated by selenium deficiency.

In developed countries where there is a risk of iodine deficiency, supplementation of foods is common. Iodised salt may be available or bread may be baked using iodised salt.

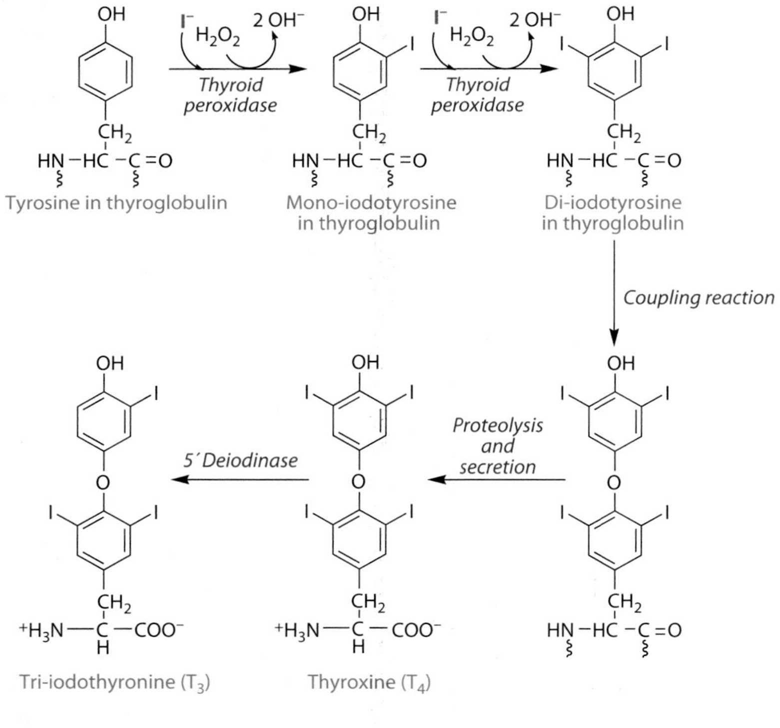

Figure 11.28 Synthesis of the thyroid hormones.

In remote regions of developing countries, this is rarely possible, and the treatment and prevention of iodine deficiency depends on periodic visits by medical teams who give relatively large doses of iodised oil by intramuscular injection.

The problem of widespread iodisation of foods in areas of deficiency is that adults whose thyroid glands have enlarged, in an attempt to secrete an adequate amount of thyroid hormone despite iodine deficiency, now become hyperthyroid. This is considered an acceptable risk to prevent the much more serious problems of goitrous cretinism amongst the young.

11.15.3.4 Magnesium
Magnesium is a cofactor for enzymes that utilises ATP and also several of the enzymes involved in DNA replication and transcription (Sections 9.2.1.1 and 9.2.2.1). It is not clear whether or not magnesium deficiency is an important nutritional problem, since there are no clear signs of deficiency. However, it has been established that intravenous administration of magnesium salts is beneficial immediately after a heart attack.

11.15.3.5 Manganese
Manganese functions as the prosthetic group of a variety of enzymes, including superoxide dismutase, a part of the body's antioxidant defence system (Section 6.5.3.1), pyruvate carboxylase in gluconeogenesis (Section 5.7), and arginase in urea synthesis (Section 9.3.1.4). Deficiency has only been observed in deliberate depletion studies.

11.15.3.6 Sodium and potassium
The maintenance of the normal composition of intracellular and extracellular fluids, and osmotic homeostasis depends largely on the maintenance of relatively high concentrations of potassium inside cells and sodium outside. The gradient of sodium and potassium across cell membranes is maintained by active (ATP-dependent) pumping (Section 3.2.2.6). Nerve conduction depends on the rapid reversal of this transmembrane gradient to create and propagate the electrical impulse, followed by a more gradual restoration of the normal ion gradient.

There is little or no problem in meeting sodium requirements; indeed, the main problem with sodium is an excessive intake, rather than deficiency (Section 6.3.4).

11.15.4 Minerals known to be essential, but whose function is not known

11.15.4.1 Silicon
Silicon is known to be essential for the development of connective tissue and the bones, although its function in these processes is not known. The silicon content of blood vessel walls decreases with age and with the development of atherosclerosis. It has been suggested, although the evidence is not convincing, that silicon deficiency may be a factor in the development of atherosclerosis.

11.15.4.2 Vanadium
Experimental animals maintained under very strictly controlled conditions show a requirement for vanadium for normal growth. There is some evidence that vanadium has a role in regulation of the activity of sodium/potassium pumps (Section 3.2.2.6), although this has not been proven. A number of studies have shown that vanadium salts potentiate or mimic insulin action and may reduce insulin requirements in patients with diabetes mellitus. Some athletes and weight trainers take vanadium supplements, but there is no evidence of any beneficial effect.

11.15.4.3 *Nickel and tin*

There is some evidence from experimental animals maintained under strictly controlled conditions and fed a highly purified diet that a dietary intake of nickel and tin is required for optimum growth and development. No metabolic function has been established for either mineral.

11.15.5 *Minerals that have effects in the body but whose essentiality is not established*

11.15.5.1 *Fluoride*

Fluoride has clear beneficial effects in modifying the structure of bone mineral and dental enamel, strengthening the bones, and protecting teeth against decay. The use of fluoride toothpaste, and the addition of fluoride to drinking water in many regions, has resulted in a very dramatic decrease in the incidence of dental decay despite high consumption of sucrose and other extrinsic sugars (Section 6.3.3.1). These benefits are seen at levels of fluoride of the order of 1 part/million (ppm) in drinking water. Such concentrations occur naturally in many parts of the world, and this is the concentration at which fluoride is added to water in many areas.

Excessive intake of fluoride leads to brown discoloration of the teeth (dental fluorosis). A concentration above about 12 ppm in drinking water, as occurs naturally in some parts of the world, is associated with excessive deposition of fluoride in the bones, leading to increased fragility (skeletal fluorosis).

Although fluoride has beneficial effects, there is no evidence that it is a dietary essential. Fluoride prevents dental decay, but it is not correct to call dental decay a fluoride deficiency disease.

11.15.5.2 *Lithium*

Lithium salts are used in the treatment of bipolar manic-depressive disease; they act by altering the responsiveness of some neurons to stimulation. However, this seems to be a purely pharmacological effect, and there is no evidence that lithium has any essential function in the body nor that it provides any benefits for healthy people.

11.15.5.3 *Other minerals*

In addition to minerals that are known to be dietary essentials, there are a number that may be consumed in relatively large amounts, but which have, as far as is known, no function in the body. Indeed, excessive accumulation of these minerals may be dangerous, and a number of them are well-known as poisons. Such elements include aluminum, arsenic, antimony, boron, cadmium, cesium, germanium, lead, mercury, silver, and strontium.

11.16 *Nutritional anaemias*

A variety of micronutrient deficiencies may lead to the development of anaemia. Three types of anaemia can be distinguished by microscopic examination of a blood film:

1. Microcytic, hypochromic anaemia, with small red blood cells that are underpigmented due to lack of haemoglobin.
2. Macrocytic, normochromic anaemia, with large red blood cells that contain a normal amount of haemoglobin. This is a problem of vitamin B_{12} (Section 11.10.2) and folate

(Section 11.11.4) deficiency. The absorption of vitamin B_{12} declines with the development of atrophic gastritis in the elderly, and infection with the fish tape worm can lead to impairment of vitamin B_{12} absorption (Section 4.5.2.1) and hence to megaloblastic anaemia.

3. Haemolytic anaemia, with excessive haemolysis of red blood cells, haemoglobin visible in the plasma, and empty red cell ghosts. This is a problem of vitamin E deficiency (Section 11.4.4), and potentially a problem for people with the genetic disease favism (lack of glucose 6-phosphate dehydrogenase, Section 5.4.2.1).

The commonest cause of hypochromic anaemia is iron deficiency. As discussed in Section 4.5.3.1, the absorption of iron is tightly regulated, and absorption especially of inorganic iron is limited. Whilst this protects against the problems of iron overload, it also means that blood losses can outstrip the ability to replace the lost iron, leading to iron deficiency anaemia. Even in developed countries, many women of child-bearing age have extremely low iron reserves, or are clearly iron deficient and anaemic because of relatively high menstrual blood losses. In addition to menstrual blood losses, a variety of intestinal parasites can lead to considerable blood loss, as can deficiency of vitamin K, leading to clotting disorders (Section 11.5.3). The bleeding associated with scurvy (vitamin C deficiency, Sections 11.14.3 and 11.14.3.1) can also result in iron deficiency anaemia if losses exceed absorption of iron from the diet.

A number of compounds in foods can inhibit the absorption of iron, including calcium, dietary fibre, oxalates, phosphates, phytates, polyphenols, soya, and egg protein. Equally, some compounds enhance iron absorption, including alcohol, organic acids and amino acids, and meat protein, as well as vitamin C. A low intake of vitamin C can be a factor in the development of iron-deficiency anaemia, and it is well known that when iron supplements are given they should be taken together with vitamin C or fruit juice to provide enough vitamin C to maximise absorption of the iron.

Copper and riboflavin (vitamin B_2) are required for iron metabolism and, very rarely, deficiency of either of these may be a cause of iron deficiency anaemia. The first step in haem biosynthesis is the reaction of δ-aminolevulinic acid synthetase. This is a pyridoxal phosphate-dependent enzyme, and, rarely, vitamin B_6 deficiency is a cause of hypochromic anaemia.

Key points

- Vitamins are organic nutrients with essential metabolic functions, generally required in small amounts in the diet, which cannot be synthesised by the body. The lipid-soluble vitamins (A, D, E, and K) are hydrophobic molecules requiring normal fat absorption for their absorption and the avoidance of deficiency symptoms.
- Vitamin A (retinol), present in meat, and the provitamin (β-carotene), found in plants, form retinaldehyde, utilised in vision, and retinoic acid, which acts in the control of gene expression.
- Vitamin D is a prohormone yielding the active derivative, calcitriol, which regulates calcium and phosphate metabolism; deficiency leads to rickets and osteomalacia.
- Vitamin E (tocopherol) is an important antioxidant in the body, acting in the lipid phase of membranes to protect against the effects of free radicals.
- Vitamin K is the cofactor for a carboxylase that acts on glutamate residues of precursor proteins of blood clotting factors and bone proteins to enable them to chelate calcium.

- Thiamin is the cofactor in oxidative decarboxylation of α-keto acids and of transketolase in the pentose phosphate pathway.
- Riboflavin and niacin are cofactors in oxidation and reduction reactions.
- Pantothenic acid is present in coenzyme A and acyl carrier protein, which act as carriers for acyl groups in metabolic reactions.
- Vitamin B_6, as pyridoxal phosphate, is the coenzyme for enzymes of amino acid metabolism, and of glycogen phosphorylase; it also acts to terminate the actions of nuclear-acting hormones.
- Biotin is the coenzyme for carboxylation reactions.
- Vitamin B_{12} and folate are involved in metabolism of one-carbon units.
- Vitamin C is a water-soluble antioxidant that maintains vitamin E and many metal cofactors in the reduced state and is the cofactor for a number of hydroxylation reactions.
- Inorganic mineral elements that have a function in the body must be provided in the diet. When intake is insufficient, deficiency may develop, and excessive intakes may be toxic.
- The serum concentration of calcium is tightly regulated. Calcium homeostasis is regulated by three hormones: calcitriol (the active metabolite of vitamin D) and parathyroid hormone, which have a hypercalcaemia action, and calcitonin, which has a hypocalcaemia action.
- Whilst iron deficiency is the most important cause of anaemia worldwide, a variety of other micronutrient deficiencies can also lead to anaemia.

Index

Page numbers followed f and t indicate figures and tables, respectively.